MATERNITY CARE

MATERNITY CARE

Helen Farrer RN RM

SECOND EDITION

CHURCHILL LIVINGSTONE
MELBOURNE EDINBURGH LONDON AND NEW YORK 1990

CHURCHILL LIVINGSTONE
Medical Division of Longman Group UK Limited

Distributed in Australia by Longman Cheshire Pty Limited, Longman House, Kings Gardens, 95 Coventry Street, South Melbourne 3205, and by associated companies, branches and representatives throughout the world.

First edition 1983 (Pitman Publishing Ltd)
Second edition 1990

ISBN 0-443-04209-8

British Library Cataloguing in Publication Data
Farrer, Helen, *1946–*
Maternity care. — 2nd ed.
1. Obstetrics. Nursing
I. Title
610.73′678

Library of Congress Cataloging in Publication Data
Farrer, Helen.
Maternity care/Helen Farrer. — 2nd ed.
p. cm.
ISBN 0-443-04209-8
1. Obstetrical nursing. 2. Perinatology. I. Title.
[DNLM: 1. Obstetrical Nursing. 2. Perinatology— nurses' instruction. 3. Pregnancy — nurses' instruction.
WY 157.3 F242m]
RG951.F37 1990
610.73′678 — dc20
DNLM/DLC
for Library of Congress 89-25367

Produced by Longman Singapore Publishers (Pte) Ltd.
Printed in Singapore

PREFACE

Maternity Care is designed to assist those studying the maternity or obstetric component of Family Health Care nursing. Although primarily concerned with the normal aspects of childbirth, this book gives a basic coverage of the more common complications and interventions as well. The nursing student will thus, it is hoped, have a greater appreciation of what she might encounter during her period of clinical placement and so understand more fully the need for preventive care.

This second edition of *Maternity Care* has been written to take account of the many developments which have occurred in the last few years—developments not only in the speciality itself but also in the education of nurses. As well, it reflects the growing involvement of childbearing families as participating receivers of our care, and the re-emergence of midwives as those families' advocates. There is less emphasis on the medical model.

The scope and depth of most of the book have been expanded, while the text has been tightened where appropriate. New areas covered include the complications of early pregnancy (miscarriage, ectopic pregnancy, hydatidiform mole) and family planning. Social, emotional and cultural aspects are discussed in greater detail, and the section on postnatal community care and support has been enlarged. Newborn baby care in general and breast feeding in particular have been revised in line with current teaching and practice.

H. F.

ACKNOWLEDGEMENTS

The revision of *Maternity Care* has given me the opportunity to respond to the helpful and constructive criticisms which have come from users of the first edition, particularly from nurse educators. I am grateful to them all for their comments. Thanks are also due to those who have helped directly in gathering and assessing new or revised material. Mrs Susan Braybrook, Miss Nan Cook, Dr Cliff Flower, Miss Rose Morrison, Mrs Pauline Walker and the late Miss Pamela Rose all gave their time and critical help. I would also like to thank Dr Howard Welch and Miss Maree Lunt for their help from the very start.

H. F.

Note

A decision had to be made on the gender of pronouns in this book. While acknowledging that there are both male and female midwives, nurses, doctors and babies, to avoid confusion or the clumsy repetition of he/she, midwives and nurses are referred to as 'she' and doctors and babies as 'he'. Similarly, the marital status of women having babies is not assumed: the word 'husband' should be taken to include 'partner'.

CONTENTS

CONTENTS

1

MATERNITY CARE TODAY

Chapter outline
Rights and responsibilities
The maternity caregivers
Choosing the type and place of confinement
Childbirth in a multicultural society
Maternity care and the nursing student

Maternity care has changed over the years, particularly over the last 10 years, and it continues to change still. The experience of pregnancy and childbirth is no longer that of a meekly submissive 'patient' who is occasionally allowed to suggest preferences in the type of care she receives, and whose husband and family are granted, somewhat grudgingly, limited involvement in even more limited areas of her care. Maternity care today considers the mother-to-be in the context of her family and the pregnancy and childbirth experience as a significant life event, about which the couple has the right to make choices.

Antenatal care and education have brought about these changes in attitude. The media and community special interest groups reinforce and promote it. And the maternity caregivers, most especially the doctors and midwives, have adapted their practices to help achieve the ideals of a good childbirth experience. Doctors and midwives are, on the whole, not just going along with change because of consumer demand, but in many cases are actively involved in creating improvements in care, teaching their own students and colleagues and lending their support to consumer groups.

RIGHTS AND RESPONSIBILITIES

Having a baby is a normal natural physiological event for which a woman's body is designed, although it has never been considered to be free of risk. In modern society we do not always allow nature her full reign. It is becoming more common for a woman to wait for several years after her body is physically mature and ready for childbirth before embarking upon a first pregnancy. She may then have relatively few pregnancies (compared with women 50 or 100 years ago) and will anticipate an outcome of the pregnancies that she does have of not just survival but good quality life for both mother and baby.

Good quality life for mother and baby is not an unreasonable expectation. Fetal maturity and wellbeing can now be monitored early and easily, and many babies born immaturely have a good chance of normal mental and physical development because of the incredible advance of neonatal intensive care in recent years. Infection, once a major cause of maternal and neonatal mortality and morbidity, is now prevented or easily treated by modern techniques and antibiotics. Severe conditions of pregnancy such as pre-eclampsia and eclampsia are now becoming rarer because of generally improved health and nutrition, early detection through antenatal care, and skilled management before the condition worsens.

There are high-risk pregnancies, and in such cases both the mother's and the baby's condition need to be assessed more frequently and more intensively. Labor may need to be managed actively, with induction, acceleration, continuous monitoring and assisted delivery in order to obtain the best outcome and quality of life for both mother and baby. Such active management and intervention can cause distress and resentment in a couple who had anticipated a normal birth experience and consequently feel deprived of their rights to that experience. Those who give information about childbirth are aware, therefore, of the importance of balancing discussion of parents' rights with their associated responsibilities. A fetus in the uterus is an innocent passenger who also has rights, particularly the right to adequate oxygenation and nutrition, and sometimes intervention must take place when these rights are threatened. Even where intervention is necessary, however, there is now a very much greater sensitivity on the part of maternity care providers and they do attempt to make the pregnancy and childbirth experience as positive for the couple as they can.

THE MATERNITY CAREGIVERS

Midwives

The word midwife means 'with woman'. It is an ancient title and there have been records of midwives from Old Testament times. Modern-day midwives must first be registered nurses before they undergo further study, experience and examination in the care of the pregnant, labouring and postnatal woman and her baby. They are then qualified to perform all normal pregnancy care (after a doctor has excluded possible or potential abnormalities), to supervise labour and conduct normal deliveries and to care for the postnatal woman and the normal newborn baby. In some birthing centres the entire care is given by midwives; in others, and in most hospitals, the care is given under the direction of a doctor. It is, however, the midwife who does stay 'with woman', especially during her labour.

Midwives are employed in hospitals, antenatal clinics, antenatal wards and labour wards, in nurseries, and in postnatal wards and clinics. They also work in the community as visiting midwives (particularly after a mother and baby are discharged early from hospital), in community health centres and family planning clinics. They are involved in antenatal education, labour preparation and parentcraft teaching. Midwives are also moving into specialist areas such as lactation consultancy, and some work in independent practice.

Obstetricians

Obstetricians are highly qualified medical practitioners who have undergone postgraduate experience and examination in the care of women during pregnancy, labour and the puerperium. They work in public or community hospitals as consultants where each clinic or unit is headed by a senior obstetrician who may be assisted by other obstetricians. The unit may also include doctors undergoing their postgraduate education aimed at qualification as obstetricians. Obstetricians also provide maternity care on a private or one-to-one basis and the woman attends for antenatal visits at the obstetrician's private consulting rooms. Most obstetricians have access to a limited number of private beds at public hospitals and at the larger private hospitals.

General practitioners

General practitioners are also involved in maternity care. They sometimes have the advantage of already knowing and caring for the family unit and so of understanding wider needs or problems which may affect the pregnancy. General practitioners usually have an arrangement with a number of obstetricians for consultation and referral if they feel that specialist care might be needed. Some general practitioners hold a Diploma of Osbstetrics and Gyanecology which qualifies them to perform certain obstetric interventions, such as uncomplicated forceps delivery and vacuum extraction.

Other health professionals in maternity care

The pregnant woman may be referred to, or may choose to attend, other health professionals for extra advice, education or treatment during pregnancy. Nutritional advisors may be consulted for dietary planning and nutrition education; physiotherapists for antenatal exercises, labour preparation and relaxation techniques; breast consultants for breast and nipple preparation and later for supervision and help in establishing breast feeding; parentcraft teachers for advice on planning beyond the birth in such matters as purchasing baby equipment, simple budgeting, safety aspects and basic babycare skills. Social workers, chaplains and pharmacists may also contribute to the care of the pregnant woman and her family.

CHOOSING THE TYPE AND PLACE FOR CONFINEMENT

Confinement is a rather old-fashioned word used to cover the childbearing time, but specifically used for the time of childbirth and the days following when the woman was confined, or restricted to her bed, as she used to be barely more than a generation ago.

A choice must be made early in pregnancy about where the woman is to spend this time of confinement. She and her family may be very keen to have a particular type of birth experience or a particular doctor or midwife. Because the most popular centres are booked up quickly, the couple may have to make their choice very early, perhaps even before they have met or had a chance to talk with the obstetrician who will supervise their care. An informed choice is not always possible if there is little time, and some matters (such as whether a particular hospital has plenty of car parking for visitors) which might seem important on first consideration, may seem far less significant later on. Then, because of their further knowledge gained from many sources, they may be concerned more by such matters as flexibility of practice in, for example, birthing positions or baby care and feeding.

Some points about which the couple should know, as different centres do have different practices, are:

- attitudes to the husband's participation
- other family members' or friends' participation
- the type of accommodation available
- procedures such as shaving and enemas
- what is meant by that centre's definition of 'natural childbirth'
- usual management of pain during labour
- activity, food and drink during labour
- common positions during delivery
- episiotomies
- students and observers
- immediate care of the baby at birth
- later care of the baby (whether routinely nursery-based)
- rooming-in
- demand feeding
- night feeding
- access to the baby, when and by whom
- provision and laundering of baby clothing
- cost of the confinement
- usual length of hospital stay
- possible costs involved.

Most hospitals and some doctors' rooms are able to provide booklets or leaflets which deal with these points. Anyone involved with maternity care has a responsibility to ensure that the couple receives as much information as necessary to make a well-informed choice, even at this very early stage. Otherwise there could be disappointment and misunderstanding when the time of confinement arrives.

Home confinement

When a pregnancy is normal and there appears to be no foreseeable complication, a home confinement could prove to be a special and delightful experience in the life of the woman and her family. In most Australian cities, a small number of doctors and midwives provide this option and are dedicated to its success. There are, however, problems with home confinements being accepted widely because our medical and emergency services and personnel are not specifically equipped to deal with complications of childbirth. Even in the UK, where an obstetric 'flying squad' service operates, home confinements are now less common. There, first-time mothers are now routinely advised to accept hospital care and certain conditions must be met for home confinements of subsequent babies.

Another problem related to home confinement is that if an emergency does arise, the couple may find themselves in the nearest specialist maternity unit, where the medical and midwifery practices may not match the couple's ideals, and they are not booked into a centre which does.

Birthing centres

Birthing centres were first designed to bridge the gap betwen home confinement and, what was at the time, usual hospital management. Hospital management has changed considerably since then and many hospital labour wards offer several of the features of birthing centres. They were set up to meet the needs of the growing number of families who were dissatisfied with hospital care or were attracted by the idea of home birth. Birthing centres allow the mother to experience childbirth in conditions as close as possible to home and as a totally natural event, while (in a hospital-based birthing centre) providing immediate access to emergency facilities she or her baby could need if complications arise. Figure 1.1 shows the Family Birthing Centre at the Royal Women's Hospital in Melbourne.

When a birthing centre is chosen as the place for confinement, the woman applies to be accepted into its program. The conditions for acceptance are not rigid, but must fall into the category of normal, based upon the woman's history and the doctor's examination from the first visit. Only about half of those who apply are suitable for birthing centre pregnancy care and confinement.

Most of the subsequent antenatal care and education, and the delivery, are conducted in the birthing centre by midwives. Any problems are referred to the woman's doctor or to a hospital unit doctor. Birthing centre midwives are skilled in all aspects of normal midwifery and need to be able to recognise immediately any departure from normal. A close relationship develops between the midwives and the families in their care, and as the midwives usually work on a rotating shift basis, their midwife during labour will be known to them from the antenatal visits.

Other features of birthing centre management include:

- minimal medical and nursing intervention—no shaving, enemas, induction or acceleration of labour, or stirrups
- statistically, there are fewer episiotomies performed in birthing centres
- the baby is fully examined within 12 hours of birth, and mother and baby can go home within 24 hours if all is normal
- visits from a domiciliary midwife continue for the 1st week after the birth and the family

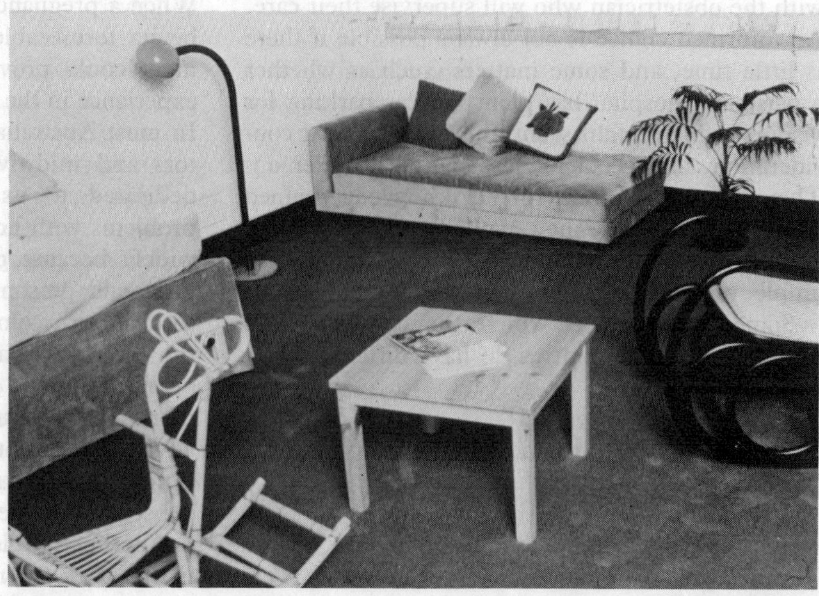

Figure 1.1 Part of the Family Birthing Centre at the Royal Women's Hospital, Melbourne

then return to the birth centre for further checking at 1 week and at 6 weeks postnatally.

Other conditions of acceptance into the birthing centre programme, apart from the probability of a normal pregnancy and labour can include:

- provision of adequate help for the mother at home for at least the first 3 postnatal days
- co-operation of a local doctor who can deal with any situation arising in the later weeks of pregnancy and in the postnatal period
- satisfactory attendance at the birthing centre, co-operation with its teachings and recommendations, and willingness to transfer, without fuss, to a more traditional medical setting if complications beyond the scope of birthing centre management should arise.

Hospital confinement

Hospital care is the most commonly chosen and available option for childbirth. In many places it is the only option, but even where home confinements and birthing centres are available, the majority of women are happy to receive hospital care. It is difficult to generalise, but far greater attention is now being given to the significance of the birth experience in the life of a family, and the staff of most hospitals, even though they may be big and busy institutions, have relaxed their approach to maternity care as a result. Much of the change has come about by consumer demand, but midwives and doctors have responded and, with few exceptions, aim to give the family the best possible experience. Hospitals have facilities for treatment of antenatal conditions and complications, for immediate intervention or emergency care, and for the resuscitation and care of sick babies.

CHILDBIRTH IN A MULTICULTURAL SOCIETY

Birth, like death and marriage, is a critical time in the life of a family, and cultural influences can play a significant part in the responses of those concerned; these can sometimes be more intense than the parents-to-be might have anticipated. Those who give maternity care have a responsibility to take into account the effects of cultural and religious practices and restrictions which may be observed during pregnancy and confinement and to accept them as being important for families, even if they are sometimes hard to understand or appear to interfere with what may be regarded as the normal or ideal maternity care.

With the wide range of cultures represented in Australian society it is impossible in a book such as this to cover the specific ways in which cultural or religious practices will be observed in the maternity setting. One point of great importance is, however, that people are never stereotyped because they come from a particular background, not only because presumptions should never be made about any groups of people, but also because some people remain more closely attached to their cultural origins, and are stricter in observing related customs, than others.

Language problems

Inability to communicate in a common language can make caring for the pregnant woman and her husband very much more difficult than when her caregivers can be sure that the couple has a clear understanding of the process of pregnancy and childbirth. Unless the couple have had access to childbirth education in their own language or the presence of interpreters has enabled basic communication, they could feel particularly isolated and afraid. The absence of an extended family or community support for new immigrants can also make this a difficult time. Much can be achieved by non-verbal communication, and the couple is likely to be especially alert for all gestures and expressions coming from the doctors and midwives. Caregivers must be particularly careful in their way of moving and use of voice tone to avoid transmitting further unease to the couple.

'Women's business'

In many cultures childbirth is very much 'women's business'. The labouring woman's mother, her sisters and other female relatives may see themselves as her rightful companions at this time. They may resent the husband being welcomed into the labour ward while they are excluded. They may sit outside in the waiting room, conducting a vigil until the baby has been born, because they simply cannot contemplate going home in case they are, after all, needed. The husband is caught in the middle: his presence is approved by the staff, and usually by his wife, but he is aware of the feelings of deprivation being experienced by his wife's family. Labour ward midwives are sensitive to this partly cultural and partly 'generation-gap' situation, knowing that it often upsets the woman in their care if the matter is not resolved; it could in, fact, have an effect upon family relationships for a long time into the future.

In some cultures the woman and her husband are comfortable to be together while she labours, but physical contact between them is restricted or prohibited from the first sign of a 'show' of blood. This means that the husband is unable to contribute in any physical way to his wife's comfort, yet he remains in her presence which, to observers, could be seen as uncaring if they do not understand the reasons behind his behaviour. From the time of any issue of blood, until a set time (usually 40 days) after the birth, the woman is regarded as 'unclean' and her husband may not touch her until she has been ritually purified.

Sometimes the husband would prefer to be on the outside and, if so, he is not pressured to remain with his wife. Or it may be his wife's preference that he does not stay with her during labour and he is happy to agree. The reactions of staff to this departure from what they now regard as 'normal' should not be disapproving, even if it did take them many years of campaigning for the rights of husbands to remain with their wives during labour and delivery and the early minutes of bonding with the baby.

Modesty

Cultural and religious influences may make the matter of modesty particularly important to a woman. In some cultures no part of a woman apart from her face (and even that may be partially covered) and her hands may normally be seen by anyone other than her husband. She may be allowed to be attended by female doctors and midwives only, and even then may be reluctant to expose any part of her body for palpation, fetal heart recording or examination. Her modesty is respected and adaptations to usual practices made where possible.

Response to pain

In some cultures the expression of all emotions including that of being hurt by pain is encouraged, while in others it is discouraged and repressed. Either situation can cause confusion for those who attend a woman during pregnancy and labour, and their response to her apparent distress or stoicism may lead to inappropriate administration or withholding of pain-relief measures. After wide experience, and by trusting their clinical assessment skills, this becomes less of a problem, but their decisions about appropriate pain relief and its timing may not be understood by those with less knowledge, such as student observers or members of the woman's family.

Response to midwives and nurses

The professions of midwifery and nursing require a high standard of schooling before entry into an exacting programme of theory and practice before qualification and registration, and are held in high esteem by most members of the community. In some of the countries from which immigrants have come, however, midwifery and nursing are low-status jobs, requiring minimal education and attracting only low class or low caste women. In these cases, there is little reason for people to accept them as having sound knowledge or to take recommendation or direction from them. This affects midwives and nurses in two ways: firstly, they may find themselves being treated very much as menials, 'slushies', fetchers and carriers or the like, and when this happens they can find it difficult to create a satisfactory relationship with those under their care; and secondly, because their skills and knowledge are not acknowledged, they may find that they are not trusted and the woman and (particularly) her husband may be anxious that the doctor is not present throughout the entire labour. They may continually ask for the doctor to be contacted or summoned, and it is not unknown for a husband to go outside and telephone the doctor himself: even then, some are unconvinced that they are in safe hands and that all is proceeding normally. Once again, a trusting relationship between the midwife and the labouring woman is hard to achieve and sustain, and the labour is rarely helped by the prevalence of such anxiety. Good antenatal education dispels inaccurate conceptions of the role and functions of the midwife, but the opportunity to attend these classes may not be taken by those who do not understand the benefits gained.

Unfamiliar dietary laws, fasting during or before holy days, the special customs observed during religious festivals and refusal of certain forms of treatment as a religious principle may all be met by those involved in maternity care. Most hospitals which cater frequently or regularly for women from particular cultures are geared to their special needs, and are ready to adapt their patterns of care to provide the best experience possible for families from differing cultures.

MATERNITY CARE AND THE NURSING STUDENT

The nursing student will find maternity care different from almost all other areas of health care she has experienced; in some cases time is needed for the student to adjust to the different focus and attitudes. The maternity 'patient' is not sick: she is going through what ought to be a natural life experience. She and her family may appear to have worries and concerns which, compared with those of other patients the nursing student has encountered, may seem to be minimal. The pace of maternity care is non-urgent, except during a busy day in the labour ward. Even there, inside individual rooms, all may be quiet. When a baby is born, great drama and excitement may accompany the birth, or the process may be achieved in a very low-key way.

Few nursing students are unaffected by the experience of witnessing the birth of a baby. Most will regard it as a great privilege. To see how a new baby first adapts to life outside the uterus, to watch the first feed being given and to witness on subsequent days the establishment of lactation and the progress of the mother as she learns to care for her baby: all of these features of normal human experience will enhance the student's understanding of family relationships and her appreciation of behavioural adaptations when the family's welfare is threatened by illness or other stress.

If the student is able to respond to what she encounters and bases her observation upon a sound theoretical basis, she will gain much from this opportunity of involvement in maternity care.

2

GLOSSARY

Over the years, midwifery has developed a language of its own. As well as finding many new terms exclusive to the specialty, the student will discover that other words, more familiar to her, have quite different meanings when applied to midwifery.

Some of the terms and definitions given in this chapter do not come under the heading 'normal midwifery' but are included to make the reading of charts and discussion in the clinical area of more value to the student.

abortion: the termination of a pregnancy before the fetus is viable; may be spontaneous or induced; the term miscarriage is often substituted when referring to spontaneous abortion

abruptio placentae: the premature detachment of a normally situated placenta

accoucheur: the person delivering a baby

accreta: a placenta which is attached very closely to the uterine wall because of a deficiency in the basal decidua

afterbirth: the placenta

after-pains: painful uterine cramps occurring in the week following delivery; after-pains are often felt more by multiparae, and especially while breast feeding

amenorrhoea: absence of menstruation

amniocentesis: aspiration of a sample of amniotic fluid through a needle inserted into the uterine cavity via the mother's abdomen

amnion: the inner membrane enclosing the fetus and liquor

amnioscopy: visualisation of the amniotic fluid through the intact membranes with a hollow metal tube inserted into the cervical canal to inspect the colour and amount of liquor

amniotic fluid: the fluid surrounding the fetus in the uterus, also known as liquor

ante: a prefix meaning before, e.g. antenatal or antepartum, before birth

Apgar score: a scoring system, used at 1, 3 and 5 minutes after birth, to evaluate the condition of the baby

APH: antepartum haemorrhage–bleeding from the genital tract after the 20th week of pregnancy

apnoea: cessation of respiration

areola: the brown pigmented area surrounding the nipple

ARM: artificial rupture of the membranes–one method of inducing or accelerating labour

atelectasis: imperfect expansion of the lungs

attitude of the fetus: the posture of the fetus, i.e. the relationship of the fetal head and limbs to the fetal spine

auscultation: listening, e.g. to the fetal heart

bimanual: using two hands, e.g. in vaginal examination or compression of the uterus

binovular: developing from two ova

blastocyst: the fertilised ovum after 1 week's development and at the time of implantation–separation into inner and outer cell masses has occurred

Brandt-Andrews method: one method of delivery of the placenta, using controlled cord traction while elevating the fundus of the uterus

Braxton-Hicks contractions: painless contractions of the uterus occurring throughout pregnancy, but not usually felt by the woman until the last 2 months

breech: referring to the buttocks; a breech presentation is one in which the buttocks of the fetus lie lowest in the pelvis

bregma: name given to the anterior (large) fontanelle in the fetal skull

caesarean section: operative delivery of the viable fetus through an abdominal incision

caput succedaneum: an oedematous swelling below the baby's scalp but above the skull bone, formed during labour because of pressure on the presenting part by the cervix, after the membranes have ruptured

cardiotocograph: a tracing from a fetal monitoring machine, which shows both the fetal heart rate and the uterine contraction patterns

carneous: fleshy; carneous mole is a blood clot surrounding a dead embryo in the uterus

cephalhaematoma: bleeding below the periosteum of one or more bones of the baby's skull

cephalic: pertaining to the head

chloasma: brown pigmentation of the face during pregnancy–the 'mask of pregnancy'

choriocarcinoma: a malignant growth which sometimes complicates hydatidiform mole pregnancy

chorion: the outer membrane of the pregnancy sac, continuous with the placenta and adherent to the uterine lining

chorion villus sampling: removal of some of the villi (finger-like projections) arising from the chorion, to test for fetal abnormalities

chromosomes: small rod-shaped bodies present in the nucleus of each cell. They contain the genes or hereditary factors

circumcision: excision of a circular portion of the prepuce (foreskin) of the penis

colostrum: the yellowish fluid formed in the breasts during pregnancy and secreted until lactation is established (usually on the 3rd to 4th day following delivery)

complementary feeding: a feeding given to an unsettled baby after a breast feeding

conception: the union of the nucleus of the spermatozoon with the nucleus of the ovum, also called fertilisation

congenital: existing at birth

contraction: temporary shortening of a muscle

cotyledon: lobe (as in the placenta)

crowning: the moment during birth when the largest diameter of the fetal head has just passed under the symphysis pubis

curettage: scraping out (of the uterine cavity)

decidua: that which is shed; the name given to the lining of the uterus during pregnancy

demand feeding: a system of baby feeding where the baby is fed when he appears to be hungry, rather than at set intervals

disproportion: in midwifery this refers to the relationship between the size of the fetal head and the size of the maternal pelvis; either the head is too large or the pelvis too small

Dextrostix: a commonly-used method and simple way of estimating blood glucose levels

dyspareunia: pain or difficulty during intercourse

dystocia: difficult labour

eclampsia: a clinical state, peculiar to pregnancy, characterised by epileptic-type convulsions, and usually preceded by the pre-eclamptic syndrome

ectopic: out of place; an ectopic pregnancy is one in which implantation of the fertilised ovum occurs outside the body of the uterus

ECV: external cephalic version–turning a fetus by abdominal manipulation so that the fetal head is presenting

effacement: the 'taking up' or thinning and stretching (but not dilating) of the cervix as it merges into the lower segment of the uterus during labour

embryo: the name given to the unborn baby from the 3rd to the 8th week of development; after this, the term fetus is used

engagement: the setting of the widest presenting diameter of the fetal head into the pelvis, i.e., below the pelvic brim

engorgement: distension or congestion; engorgement of the breasts, making them full, hard and sore, is due to the increased blood supply before true lactation is established

epidural: outside the dura; epidural analgesia is one form of pain relief offered during labour

episiotomy: an incision into the perineum, to enlarge the vulval orifice during the delivery of an infant

exomphalos: a severe form of umbilical hernia, in which some of the intestines can protrude

external cephalic version: 'turning' the fetus by a doctor using abdominal manipulation, so that the head is the presenting part

fertilisation: the union of the nucleus of a spermatozoon with the nucleus of a mature ovum

fibroids: fibromyomata; benign growths of fibrous and muscular tissue, usually within the wall of the uterus

flaccid: limp, with poor muscle tone

fetus: the unborn baby from the end of the 8th week of development onwards

fontanelle: 'little fountain'; soft spot, or space, at the junction of three or more bones on a baby's skull, covered by membrane and skin

forewaters: amniotic fluid trapped between the presenting part and the cervix when the membranes are still intact

fourchette: the posterior junction of the labia minora

fundal: referring to the fundus (see below)

fundus: the top of the uterus

gamete: a reproductive cell capable of fertilising or being fertilised to produce a new individual; a mature spermatozoon or ovum

gavage: a method of feeding sick or small babies via a nasal or oral tube into the stomach

gestation: the period for which a pregnancy has existed

gravid: pregnant, gravida–a pregnant woman *or* the number of pregnancies a woman has had (including a current pregnancy)

Guthrie test: neonatal screening test for PKU (phenylketonuria), done on about the 5th day after birth, using blood samples collected from a heel prick

hind-milk: milk lying in the hind part of the breast, and obtained by the baby only when that breast is properly emptied; its composition differs from the milk obtained at the beginning of a feed (fore-milk), by having a higher proportion of fat and vitamins and lower fluid content

hyaline: cartilage-like

hydatidiform: resembling small drops or sacs

hydrocephalus: literally 'water on the brain'; a condition in which there is an excessive amount of cerebrospinal fluid in the ventricles of the brain

hyperemesis gravidarum: excessive vomiting during pregnancy

hysterotomy: opening into the uterus; an abdominal hysterotomy may be performed to terminate a pregnancy after the 12th week when other methods are unsuitable or dangerous

implantation: the embedding of the early pregnancy (at the blastocyst stage) into the lining of the uterus. Also called nidation

induction: the leading-in or 'bringing-on' of labour

inertia: weak or infrequent uterine contractions

introitus: entrance; the opening of the vagina

involution: the return to the non-pregnant size and state (especially of the uterus)

kernicterus: bile staining and necrosis of the brain cells, a complication of severe jaundice

labour: the process by which the fetus and placenta are expelled from the birth canal by the contraction of the uterine muscles

lactation: secretion of milk by the breasts

lanugo: the fine downy fetal hair which is often found on the face, shoulders, back and arms in premature babies

let-down reflex: contraction of the myoepithelial cells surrounding the alveoli in the breast, in response to a neurogenic stimulus, causing the milk to flow

lie: the relationship of the fetal spine to the maternal spine, normally longitudinal

lightening: the reduction of the fundal height when the fetal head sinks down into the pelvis (engages)

linea nigra: literally 'black line'; a pigmented line in the abdominal mid-line which becomes noticeably dark during pregnancy

liquor: the amniotic fluid surrounding the fetus in the uterus

lithotomy position: a position in which the woman lies on her back with her buttocks close to the edge of the bed and her feet elevated in supports or stirrups

'living ligatures': a term commonly used to describe the action of the criss-cross fibres of the middle layer of uterine muscle, which contract to restrict the blood flow to the placental site following delivery

LNMP: last normal menstrual period

lochia: the name given to the drainage from the uterus after delivery

lower uterine segment: the lower third of the uterine body coupled with the upper half of the cervix–this area thins and stretches during the later months of pregnancy

maceration: softening of the fetal tissues after fetal death in utero. The skin peels and lifts, and the bones soften and collapse

mastitis: inflammation of the breasts

mechanism: a series of passive movements by which the fetus passes through the birth canal

meconium: the dark green tarry substance that is formed in the bowel of the fetus and passed as the first bowel action after birth

mentum: chin

milia: small white spots which are common on the baby's face and chin; sebaceous glands which are, as yet, unfunctioning

miscarriage: a term often used for spontaneous abortion

missed abortion: the retention of the products of conception of an early pregnancy in which the embryo has died

mongolian spots: areas of dark skin pigmentation usually on the lower back, buttocks and genitals; more common in southern European, Asian and dark-skinned peoples

Montgomery's tubercles: prominent sebaceous follicles appearing on the areolae of the breasts during pregnancy

moulding: elongation of the baby's head as a result of the ability of the bones of the skull to slide over each other to lessen the largest presenting diameter

morula: the name give to the fertilised ovum when simple cell division is taking place

multigravida: a woman pregnant for the second or subsequent time

multipara: a woman who has given birth to her second or subsequent viable baby

natal: referring to birth

neonatal: newly born; covers the first 28 days after birth

normal labour: labour which is of spontaneous onset, vertex presentation, at term, completed within 4–24 hours and involves no artificial aids or complications

nullipara: a woman who has not had a pregnancy which has lasted to the stage of viability

omphalocele: umbilical hernia

operculum: the plug of mucus formed in the cervix during pregnancy and passed as the 'show' when the external cervical os dilates

oxytocic: an agent which acts to contract the uterus

palpation: assessment by feeling with the hands

Papanicolaou smear: a smear taken from the surface of the cervix to examine exfoliated cells for abnormal or suspicious changes

paracervical: beside the cervix

parity: the childbearing status of a woman

partogram: a graphical method of recording the events of the progress of labour

parturition: childbirth

pelvimetry: measurement of the pelvic capacity either clinically or by using X-rays

phenylketonuria: a disorder of protein metabolism; screening for phenylketonuria in the newborn is routine and is done using the Guthrie test after the baby has consumed milk for a certain number of days (usually performed on the 5th day after birth)

phototherapy: treatment by light–exposure of a jaundiced baby to light in order to reduce the amount of unconjugated bilirubin by converting it to a water-soluble form for excretion

placenta: the temporary organ which supplies the needs of the embryo/fetus until birth; often called the 'afterbirth' because it is expelled shortly after the baby is born

placenta praevia: low implantation of the placenta, sometimes giving rise to antepartum haemorrhage as the lower uterine segment begins to stretch

polyhydramnios: excessive amniotic fluid

postmaturity: strictly, a baby born after 40 weeks gestation; in practice, intervention to terminate the pregnancy is usually not made for postmaturity until 7–10 days following term

postpartum: following delivery

PPH: postpartum haemorrhage (defined as a blood loss of 600 ml or more following delivery

precipitate: extremely fast (precipitate labour is one completed within four hours)

pre-eclampsia: a syndrome of elevated blood pressure, proteinuria and oedema (or two of these three signs), which can often precede eclampsia

pre-term: born before 37 weeks gestation

primigravida: pregnant for the first time

primipara: a woman who has given birth to her first viable baby

prostaglandins: a group of substances, found in semen and in menstrual blood. They have an oxytocic effect and are used for the induction of abortion and to ripen the cervix and induce labour.

pruritus: itching

pseudocyesis: 'phantom' or false pregnancy, in which several of the symptoms of pregnancy may be apparent without a pregnancy existing

psychoprophylaxis: mental preparation to overcome the discomforts or pain of labour

pudendal: pertaining to the external genital organs. Pudendal block–local analgesia injected around the pudendal nerve

puerperal: pertaining to the puerperium or the period of up to 6 weeks following the birth of a child

quickening: the first fetal movements felt by the mother

retraction: the ability of uterine muscle fibres to retain some of their shortening after a contraction, rather than fully relaxing

retrolental: behind the lens of the eye

Rhesus factor: an antigenic factor found in the blood of 85% of people who are termed Rhesus (Rh) positive

Shirodkar suture: a removable purse-string type suture inserted into the external cervix to prevent premature dilatation

'show': the mucoid discharge from the cervix as a result of dilatation of the external cervical os

speculum: an instrument which, by displacing adjacent tissues, allows visualisation of an internal organ or structure

station: the level of the presenting part of the fetus in relation to the ischial spines in the pelvis

stillborn: a baby who is born after the 20th week of gestation and who is born dead, with no heart-beat and no respiratory efforts

stress incontinence: the escape of urine from the bladder when stress in the form of increased intra-abdominal pressure occurs. Due to weakness of the pelvic floor or the urethral sphincters

striae gravidarum: stretch marks of pregnancy

supplementary feeding: a feeding given to a breast-fed baby as a substitute for a breast feed

surfactant: a detergent-like substance of lecithin which lines the lung alveolar walls to prevent them from adhering and collapsing after expiration. Present in sufficient quantities after 34 weeks gestation

suture: the line of union of adjacent bones of the fetal skull

Syntocinon: a synthetic oxytocic drug, commonly used for induction of labour

talipes: turning of the feet; *talipes equino varus* involves downwards and inwards turning, *talipes calcaneo-valgus* involves upwards and outwards turning

transition: the period during labour at the end of first stage, when the cervix is almost, but not quite, fully dilated.

transverse lie: condition in which the longitudinal axis of the fetus is lying transversely, i.e. across, the mother's uterus

trimester: one-third of pregnancy (a 3-month period)

trophoblast: the outer cell mass of the fertilised ovum at the blastocyst stage which develops to form the placenta and outer membrane

ultrasonography: a non-invasive method of diagnosing the presence, position and size of a mass using high frequency sound waves; in early pregnancy it is necessary for the woman to have a full bladder to displace the uterus upwards out of the pelvis

uniovular: from one ovum

uterine isthmus: the junction of the cervix and the body of the uterus

vernix caseosa: the white, greasy protective substance which covers the fetal skin for most of the pregnancy; it can be found in the skin folds, e.g. axillae and groins, at term

version: turning

vertex: the top of the skull

viable: capable of independent existence after birth:

Wharton's jelly: the gelatinous substance contained in the umbilical cord which protects the umbilical blood vessels from pressure

zygote: an organism produced by two gametes; the fertilised ovum before cleavage

3

ANATOMY AND PHYSIOLOGY

The whole reproductive system is designed with one ultimate aim—reproduction. Each organ and structure has a specific contribution to make to the achievement of this aim, from the structures which aid in sexual arousal and vaginal lubrication, through to the muscular powers which expel the fetus at term. Some structures have a protective role, preventing infection from ascending and possibly causing blockage of the fallopian tubes. Other structures are designed to support the uterus in the best position for spermatozoa to enter, and to continue supporting it when it increases enormously in size and weight during pregnancy.

Each structure is described as it appears during the period of reproductive maturity, i.e., during those years between puberty and the climacteric.

EXTERNAL GENITALIA

VULVA

The vulva is the name given to the external genital structures (Fig. 3.1). The word means a cover or wrapper. The vulva extends from the mons pubis anteriorly to the perineum posteriorly, and it is bounded each side by the labia majora. Within these boundaries is included the labia minora, the clitoris, the vestibule and the fourchette. Opening into the vestibule are the urethral orifice and the vaginal orifice, and also the ducts of the para-urethral (Skene's) glands and Bartholin's glands.

Mons pubis
The mons pubis is the pad of fatty tissue lying above the symphysis pubis. It is covered by skin and pubic hair. The mons has a cushioning effect during sexual intercourse. The skin contains specialised sweat glands, the secretions of which have a characteristic odour. These secretions are believed to be of some sexual significance to the male.

Labia majora
The labia majora ('large lips') are two folds of skin with underlying fat which continue down as extensions of the mons pubis and merge into the perineum. The labia majora have hair and glands on their lateral aspects, but the inner surfaces are smooth.

Their function is protective—they close the

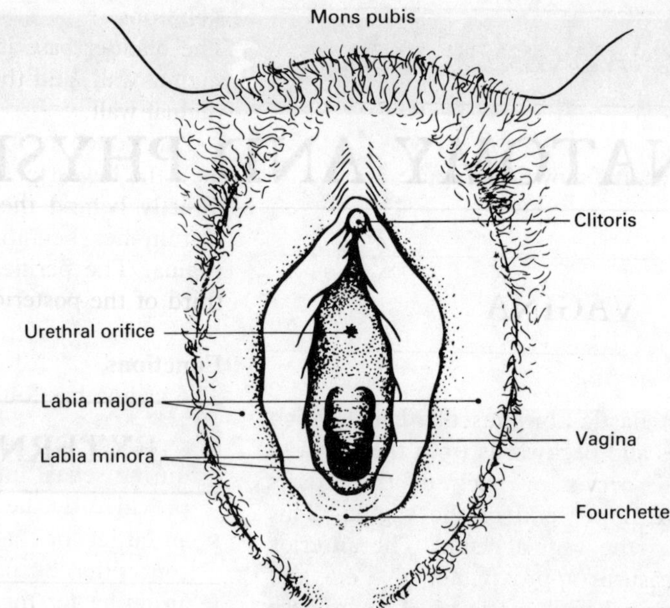

Figure 3.1 The vulva

entrance to the vagina and their fatty padding acts as a cushion.

Labia minora
The labia minora ('small lips') are two thin folds of skin lying inside the labia majora. They are joined at the front, and within that junction is the clitoris. Posteriorly they rejoin to form the fourchette. The labia minora have no subcutaneous fat. Their inner surfaces are normally in contact with each other and thus they add to the guarding of the entrance to the vagina.

Clitoris
The clitoris is a small projection of erectile tissue, situated within the anterior junction of the labia minora. It is richly supplied with blood and nerves, and is one of the major erotic zones of the female.

Vestibule
The vestibule is the name given to the space enclosed by the labia minora. The urethral orifice opens into the vestibule just below the clitoris. The ducts of the two para-urethral or Skene's glands also open into the vestibule, one on each side of the urethral orifice.

The vaginal orifice also opens into the vestibule. It is surrounded by a fold of thin membrane, the *hymen*, which does not completely close off the entrance to the vagina. After either the first act of intercourse, digital interference or the insertion of tampons, the hymen is usually torn. Following the vaginal delivery of a child the hymen disappears except for a few tags of skin known as *carunculae myrtiformes*. The function of the hymen is to guard the entrance to the vagina during the pre-pubertal years.

The ducts of the Bartholin's glands open outside the hymen, one on each side, just posterior to the vaginal orifice. The two Bartholin's glands secrete a mucoid lubricating substance, especially during sexual excitement.

Perineum
The perineum is made up of the perineal body—the central junction of the muscles of the pelvic floor—covered by the perineal skin. It extends from the fourchette (the posterior junction of the labia minora) to the anus.

INTERNAL GENITALIA

The pelvic organs are shown in Figure 3.2

VAGINA

The vagina is an elastic fibromuscular canal which extends upwards and backwards from the vulva to the uterus. The cervix or neck of the uterus projects into the upper end of the vagina. This area is known as the vaginal vault. The anterior vaginal wall measures approximately 7.5 cm and the posterior vaginal wall measures 9 cm. These walls are normally in close contact but can be separated easily. The lining of the vagina is arranged in folds (*rugae*). This allows the vagina to expand enormously, as it needs to, to accommodate the fetal head during delivery.

Structure

The vaginal wall has four layers:

- a lining of stratified squamous epithelium; there are no glands but some fluid seeps through the epithelium to provide moisture
- areolar connective tissue, well supplied with blood vessels
- smooth muscle tissue of longitudinal and circular fibres
- an outer layer of white fibrous connective tissue which blends with the surrounding pelvic fascia.

Fornices

Fornix comes from the Latin word for gutter. Where the cervix dips into the vaginal vault, a gutter is created surrounding the cervix. As the vaginal canal slopes backward and the uterus normally turns forward, there is a larger space at the posterior part of the gutter. The gutter is divided into four sections: a posterior, anterior and two lateral fornices.

Relations

The bladder base is related to the upper anterior vaginal wall, and the urethra to the lower anterior vaginal wall.

The pouch of Douglas (or uterorectal cul-de-sac), the lowest point of the peritoneal cavity, lies directly behind the posterior vaginal fornix—the rectum lies behind the upper two-thirds of the vagina. The perineal body lies behind the lower third of the posterior vaginal wall.

Functions

The vagina has four main functions:

- a passage for spermatozoa; they are deposited during sexual intercourse into the space provided by the posterior fornix
- an outlet for the fetus and other products of conception during labour
- an outlet for the menstrual flow
- by its acid secretions, it provides a barrier to ascending infection.

UTERUS

The uterus is a thick-walled, hollow muscular organ, lying between the bladder in front and the rectum behind (see Fig. 3.2). It consists of two parts, the corpus or body, and the cervix or neck. The cervix constitutes the lower third of the uterus, half of the cervix projecting into the vagina.

The uterus measures approximately 7.5 cm in length, 5.5 cm in width and 2.5 cm in depth. The walls are very thick, about 1.2 cm, thus the hollow cavity is extremely small.

Projecting laterally from the upper uterus are the fallopian tubes or oviducts. The points of insertion of these tubes are termed the *cornua* (or horns) of the uterus. That part of the uterus which is above the cornua is known as the *fundus*, while the junction of the cervix and the body of the uterus is called the *isthmus uteri* (Fig. 3.3).

The hollow part of the cervix is called the cer-

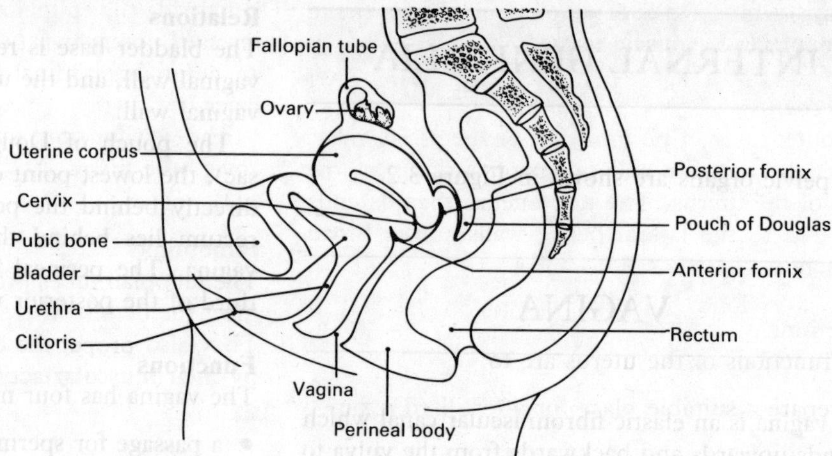

Figure 3.2 The pelvis — sagittal section

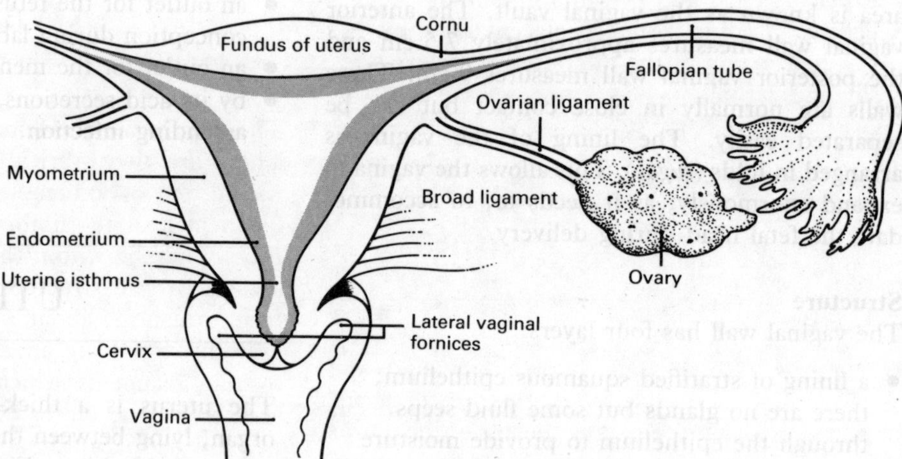

Figure 3.3 The internal reproductive organs — cross-section — viewed from behind

vical canal. The opening of the cervical canal into the vagina is called the external os and the opening of the canal at the level of the uterine isthmus is called the internal os.

Structure

Lining

The body of the uterus is lined by *endometrium*, which is epithelial tissue containing glands and stroma. The endometrium has a surface layer which is built up and then shed during each menstrual cycle, and a basal layer which remains constant.

The cervical canal is lined with columnar epithelium, and contains large glands secreting a clear mucus which forms a protective 'plug' at certain times, especially during pregnancy.

The vaginal projection of the cervix is lined with stratified squamous epithelium, continuous with the lining of the vagina.

Muscle layer

The middle layer of the uterine wall is muscular and is termed the *myometrium*. There is an outer longitudinal, middle oblique and inner circular arrangement of muscle fibres, interspersed with a small amount of fibrous tissue. The lower cervix contains a much greater amount of fibrous tissue in proportion to muscle tissue.

Outer coat
The outer layer of peritoneum, or the *perimetrium*, covers the anterior and posterior surfaces of the body of the uterus. The peritoneum then extends in a fold to the lateral pelvic walls as the broad ligament.

Functions
The functions of the uterus are to:

- prepare a suitable place for a fertilised ovum to embed
- provide protection and nourishment for the embryo/fetus until it is mature
- expel the fetus and placenta in labour
- control bleeding from the placental site by the contraction of the interlaced muscles—the 'living ligatures'.

FALLOPIAN TUBES

The fallopian tubes are also known as oviducts and sometimes as the uterine tubes. They extend, one on each side, from the cornua (horns) of the uterus towards the lateral pelvic walls. They are covered by the peritoneum forming the broad ligament. They are about 10 cm long, but do not stretch straight out; they bend and turn posteriorly. Their distal ends open out into the peritoneal cavity and can move freely. The ends are fimbriated, and these fimbriae embrace the ovary at ovulation thereby helping to attract the ovum into the tube. The lumen of the fallopian tube is very narrow, especially where the tube enters the uterus. At this point, the *interstitial* part of the tube, the lumen is less than 1 mm.

Structure
The tube is lined by ciliated epithelium arranged in many folds, which slow down the progress of the ovum to the uterus. Some of the cells secrete a serous fluid which may nourish the ovum.

Outside the epithelial lining, separated by a fine layer of connective tissue, are two muscle coats, an outer longitudinal layer and an inner circular layer.

The peritoneum forming the broad ligament covers the tubes.

Functions
The fallopian tubes provide a passage for sperm to meet the ovum, where fertilisation can take place. They also propel the ovum through to the uterus by their muscular action, aided by cilia and fluid.

OVARIES

The ovaries are the female gonads or sex glands. There are two ovaries, one on each side, lying within the abdominal cavity, behind the broad ligament near the fimbriated end of the fallopian tube. They lie within the peritoneal cavity. They are grey-white structures, with an irregular surface, measuring about 3 cm by 1.5 cm.

Both ovaries are attached to the uterus by the ovarian ligaments which run from the posterior surfaces of the uterus close to the cornua. There is extra support from the infundibulopelvic ligaments which extend to the side walls of the pelvis.

One surface of the ovary is in contact with the posterior surface of the broad ligament. This point of contact is the mesovarium. At the centre of the mesovarium is the hilum, and it is through this gateway that the ovarian blood vessels, lymphatics and nerves pass.

Structure
The ovary consists of a medulla and a cortex. The medulla is the inner portion, containing blood and lymphatic vessels supported by connective tissue. The cortex is the outer portion containing the ovarian follicles or egg cells, embedded in stroma.

The ovary is not covered by true peritoneum. It has instead a modified form of peritoneum, the germinal epithelium (Fig. 3.4).

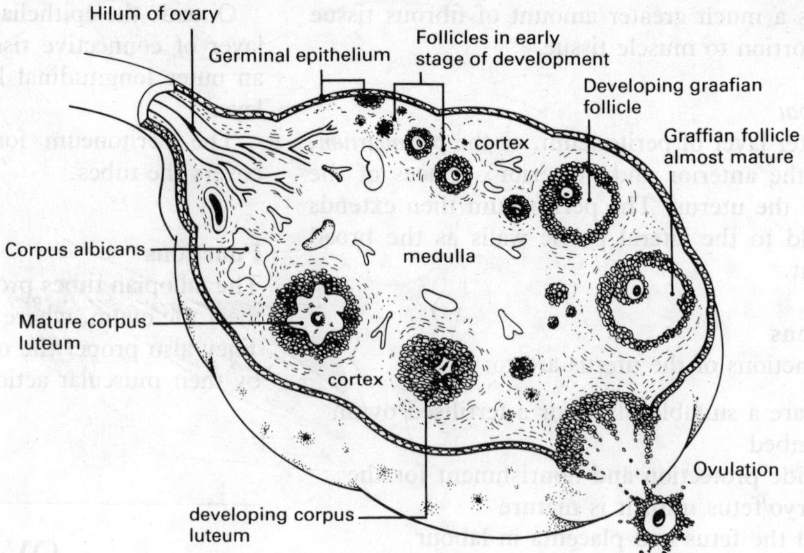

Figure 3.4 The ovary

Functions
The functions of the ovaries are:

- the production, storage and ripening of ovarian follicles and the release of ova
- the production of the ovarian hormones, oestrogen and progesterone.

PELVIC SUPPORTS

UTERINE LIGAMENTS

The pelvic connective tissue supporting the uterus consists of the broad ligament, the round ligaments, the uterosacral ligament and the pubocervical ligament.

Broad ligament
The broad ligament is a raised fold of peritoneum and fibromuscular tissue stretching from the uterus to the side wall of the pelvis.

The broad ligaments give very little support to the uterus, but at the base of these ligaments the fascia becomes dense, to form the *cardinal ligaments* (Fig. 3.5), from the cervix to the lateral pelvic walls.

Round ligaments
The round ligaments pass from the anterior cornua of the uterus forward and down through the inguinal canal to be inserted into the subcutaneous fat in the labia majora. They aid in holding the uterus anteverted or turned forward.

Uterosacral ligament
The uterosacral ligament (Fig. 3.6) extends backwards from the cervix and the cardinal ligaments to the sacrum. It divides to pass around the rectum, then reunites. By pulling the cervix back and up, it also helps to maintain anteversion of the uterus.

Pubocervical ligament
The pubocervical ligament runs from the front of the cervix forwards to the back of the pubic bone, dividing to pass around the urethra.

PELVIC FLOOR

The term 'pelvic floor' includes all of the tissues which fill the pelvic outlet and support the organs above.

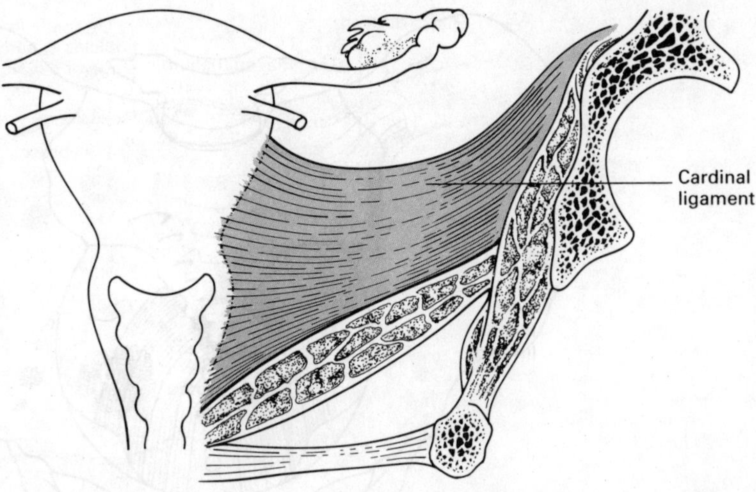

Figure 3.5 The cardinal ligament

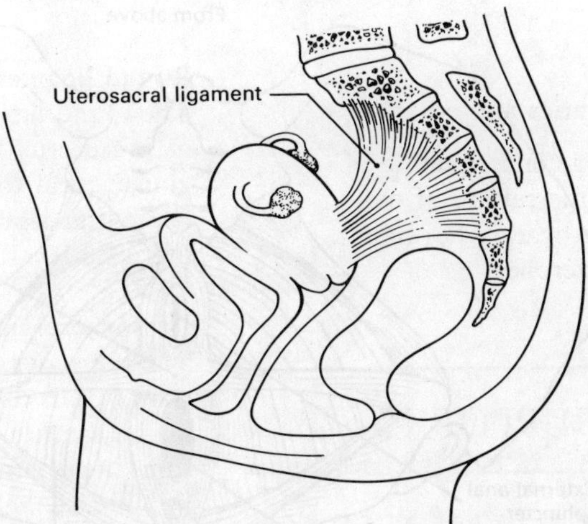

Figure 3.6 The uterosacral ligament

Levator ani muscles

The levator ani are the strongest supports of the pelvic floor (Fig. 3.7). These muscles form a broad sheet from the back of the pubis to the sacrum and coccyx, extending to the lateral pelvic walls. From the side walls, they sweep downwards and inwards to meet in the centre. The urethra, vagina and rectum pass through this muscular sheet. This weakens it to some extent, but it is normally an adequate support for the pelvic contents when a woman is standing erect (Fig. 3.8).

Superficial perineal muscles

The superficial perineal muscles lie below the levator ani sheet. They come in from the pubis, the sacrum and the lateral pelvic walls to unite between the vagina and the rectum (Fig. 3.7), thereby forming the superficial half of the perineal body.

Perineal body

The perineal body lies between the lower vagina and the lower rectum. It is a wedge-shaped body of muscle made up of the inferior surface of the junction of the levator ani muscles and the junction of the superficial perineal muscles. The perineal body must be displaced and flattened by the presenting part of the fetus just before delivery.

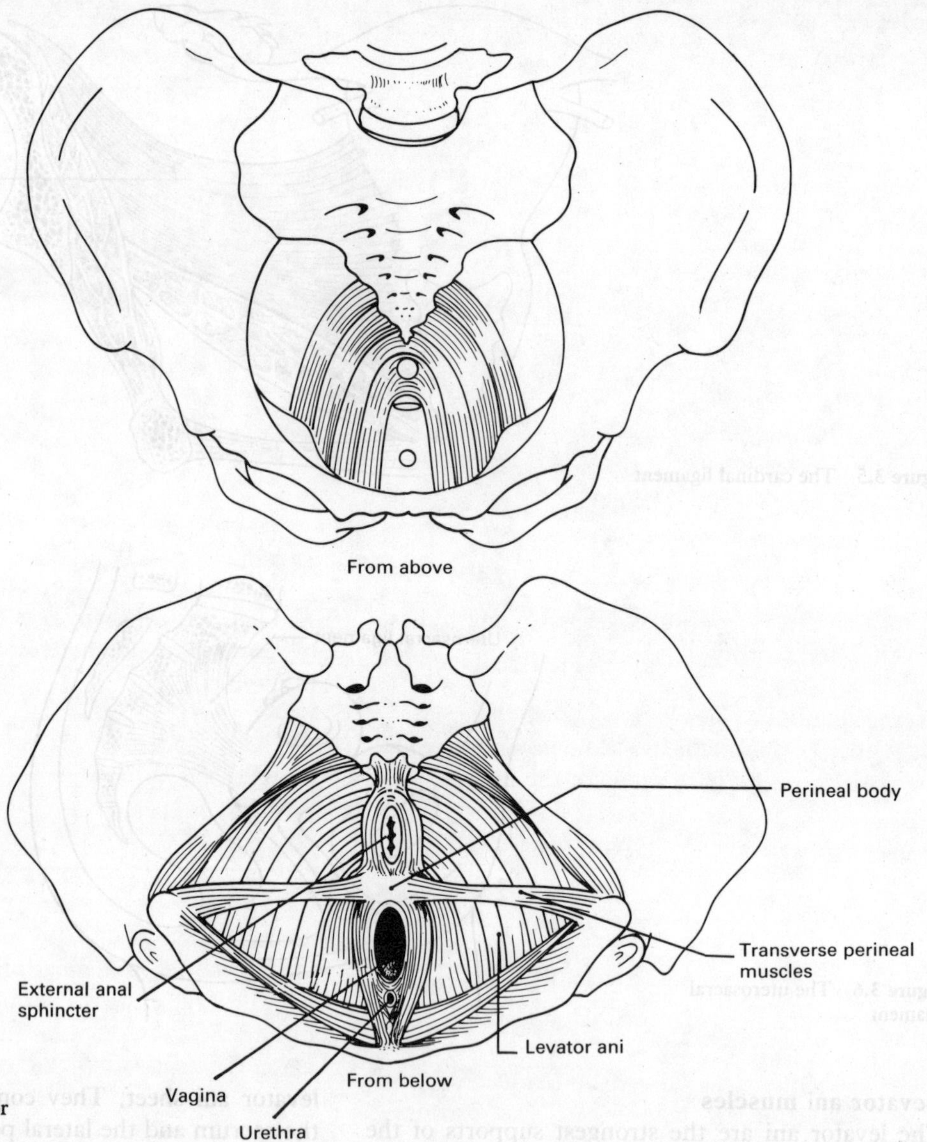

Figure 3.7 The pelvic floor muscles

BLOOD SUPPLY

ARTERIES

Internal genitalia

The uterus gets its blood supply from two large arteries on each side. It is essential that the uterus receives a large blood supply to cope with the great demands during pregnancy.

The *uterine artery* branches from the internal iliac artery. It runs through the base of the broad ligament to the internal os. It then divides and one branch goes upwards to the fundus with coiled branches, to allow for uterine expansion, going off to enter the uterus all along its length. A separate branch goes down to supply the cervix and vagina.

The *ovarian artery* is a branch of the abdominal aorta. A large branch enters the ovary and then

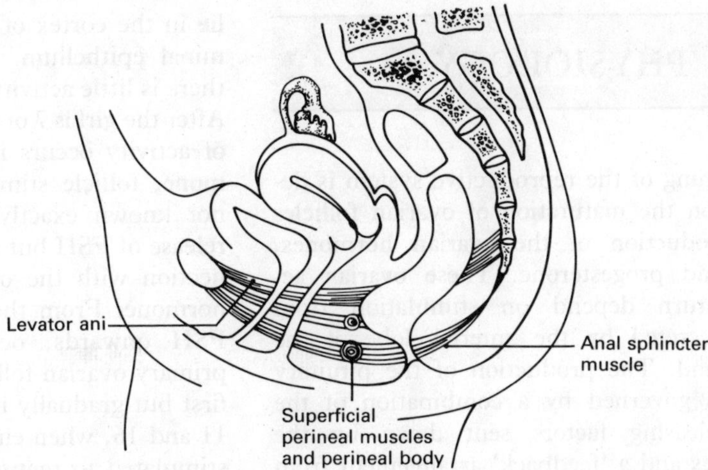

Figure 3.8 The muscles of the pelvic floor — sagittal section

the ovarian artery continues across to anastomose with the uterine artery.

External genitalia
The vulva is supplied by the *internal pudendal artery*, which is another branch of the internal iliac artery.

VEINS

The veins of the pelvic organs normally travel beside the arteries of these organs, an exception being the left ovarian vein which usually drains into the left renal vein.

LYMPHATICS

The pelvic lymph drainage follows the blood vessels. The lymph channels drain into groups of nodes near the major arteries of the pelvis. There is a cross-drainage from one side of the vulva to the other, which is why both inguinal lymph nodes are removed when there is a malignant lesion on only one side.

PELVIC NERVES

The vulva, perineum and lower vagina are innervated from the pudendal nerve. The skin of the vulva is very sensitive; perineal injuries (including episiotomies) can often be quite painful. The lower vagina is sensitive but the upper vagina is insensitive to ordinary stimuli.

The uterus is innervated by the autonomic nervous system. The cervix is able to be cut, pierced or diathermied without discomfort. It is, however, extremely sensitive to stretch; the dilatation of the cervix is responsible for a significant proportion of the discomfort of the first stage of labour.

The ovary is insensitive except to squeezing (as in bimanual examination). This explains why ovarian growths may not be noticed until they are quite large.

Unlike the ovaries and uterus, the fallopian tubes are sensitive to cutting, touching, crushing and stretching.

PHYSIOLOGY

The functioning of the reproductive system is dependent upon the maturation of ovarian follicles and the production of the ovarian hormones, oestrogen and progesterone. These ovarian activities in turn depend on stimulation from hormones secreted by the anterior lobe of the pituitary gland. The production of the pituitary secretions is governed by a combination of the hormone releasing factors sent down by the hypothalamus and a 'feedback' arrangement from the level of ovarian hormones circulating in the bloodstream. The levels of circulating ovarian hormones also send 'feedback' to, and so affect, the hypothalamus.

As well as this purely chemical system of hormonal control, there is a direct influence upon the hypothalamus from the cerebral cortex; therefore emotional factors can also affect the course of normal workings of any of the structures involved.

It is obvious then that an understanding of the 'menstrual cycle' and menstrual disorders involves far more than just knowing about the changes that occur in the uterine lining. It has to be thought of as the 'hypothalamic-pituitary-ovarian-endometrial' relationship. It is presented here as simply as possible in order not to confuse, but it is a complex topic and its finer points are still not fully understood.

The physiology of the reproductive system is discussed under the following headings:

- the ovulation
- the menstrual cycle
- actions of the ovarian hormones
- changes caused by aging and childbearing.

OVULATION

At birth, the ovaries of a baby girl contain something like 200 000 primary ovarian follicles. These lie in the cortex of the ovary, just below the germinal epithelium. During the very early years, there is little activity associated with these follicles. After the girl is 7 or 8 years old a gradual awakening of activity occurs in response to a pituitary hormone, follicle stimulating hormone (FSH). It is not known exactly what triggers off the initial release of FSH but it is believed to have some connection with the output of the pituitary growth hormone. From the time of the first releasing of FSH onwards, oestrogen is produced by the primary ovarian follicles, in very small amounts at first but gradually increasing. Between the ages of 11 and 16, when enough of the follicles have been stimulated to mature, the effects of oestrogen on its 'target' organs become evident, and for the first time an ovarian follicle ripens fully, to become a *graafian follicle* which will rupture to release its ovum, i.e. ovulation will occur.

Several hundreds of follicles probably start to ripen each month (once the cycle is established), each producing a certain amount of oestrogen. At some stage during this process, one follicle ripens more than the others and it produces a much greater output of oestrogen. This causes all those other ripening follicles to cease oestrogen production and to atrophy; they simply disappear into the substance of the ovary. The one follicle which has continued to grow and produce hormones is called, at this stage, a graafian follicle (see Fig. 3.4).

The mature graafian follicle consists of a layer of granulosa cells surrounding a space filled with follicular fluid. At one side of this space is the ovum. When the follicle is fully mature and is bulging out from the ovarian capsule, the outer cells of the follicle rupture and the ovum is discharged, along with most of the fluid, directly into the peritoneal cavity. From here it should be picked up by the fimbriae of the fallopian tubes which almost embrace the ovary at the time of ovulation.

Following the release of the ovum, the cells of the ruptured follicle join together to form a ring. They immediately start to grow and swell under the influence of another pituitary hormone, the luteinising hormone (LH) which has been released in response to the high levels of oestrogen, to form the *corpus luteum* (yellow body). The corpus luteum produces large quantities of progesterone and also continues oestrogen production. It has, however, a limited lifespan of about 10–12 days. It can be maintained by the hormone chorionic gonadotrophin which is normally produced only by the outer cell mass of a fertilized ovum. If there is no embedded fertilised ovum, the corpus luteum will degenerate and the levels of its hormone secretions will fall. The degenerated corpus luteum atrophies to remain as scar tissue on the surface of the ovary and is then known as a *corpus albicans* (white body).

MENSTRUAL CYCLE

Approximately every 28 days, the adult female body is prepared for pregnancy. It should be noted here that days is the *average* length of established menstrual cycles. There can be variations from between 21 days and 35 days which are considered normal for those who experience these intervals regularly. The cycle days are always counted from the first day of bleeding until the first day of bleeding of the next cycle.

Menstrual loss

The menstrual loss is usually about 50 to 100 ml in amount, spread over a period of 3–5 days. It is usually moderate on the first day and heavier on the second day, after which it gradually tapers off. The blood loss should *not* contain clots. It is believed that an enzyme, released from the endometrium, prevents this blood from clotting. If the flow is heavy and fast, the enzyme may be insufficient in amount or too slow in action to prevent clots from forming as the blood reaches the vagina.

HORMONAL CONTROL

This is shown diagrammatically in Figure 3.9. Follicle stimulating hormone is released when there is a low level of oestrogen in the bloodstream; it is inhibited by a high level of oestrogen.

Luteinising hormone is released in response to a high or rising level of oestrogen in the bloodstream. Its output falls when the progesterone level rises.

FSH stimulates the follicles to ripen and as they ripen they produce oestrogen. This oestrogen reaches a certain level to which the body responds by releasing LH and inhibiting FSH. After ovulation, if the corpus luteum is not maintained by pregnancy, the levels of both oestrogen and progesterone will fall. FSH is once again released in response to the lowered level of oestrogen and the cycle is continued.

CHANGES IN THE LINING OF THE UTERUS

The endometrium consists of a basal layer and a functional layer. It is the latter which changes in response to the production and withdrawal of oestrogen and progesterone.

Following menstruation, the functional layer starts to grow up from the basal layer as the oestrogen level starts to rise. This continues until ovulation occurs, and is known as the *proliferative phase*. The endometrium is repaired and rebuilt, and the tiny blood vessels swell and fill with blood. Once ovulation has occurred and the level of progesterone rises, the glands of the endometrium come into action and begin to secrete mucus, glycogen and other substances specifically to aid in the embedding and nourishment of the fertilised ovum. This is known as the *secretory phase*. Here it is important to understand that there is probably a 'threshold' for bleeding, dependent on the level of oestrogen in the bloodstream. If the amount of oestrogen is insufficient to cause the building up of the endometrium, no bleeding will occur. If the amount of oestrogen is kept above a certain level, it will maintain the endometrium and so no bleeding will occur. It is when the endometrium has been primed with sufficient oestrogen and then the level of oestrogen falls that bleeding occurs. When

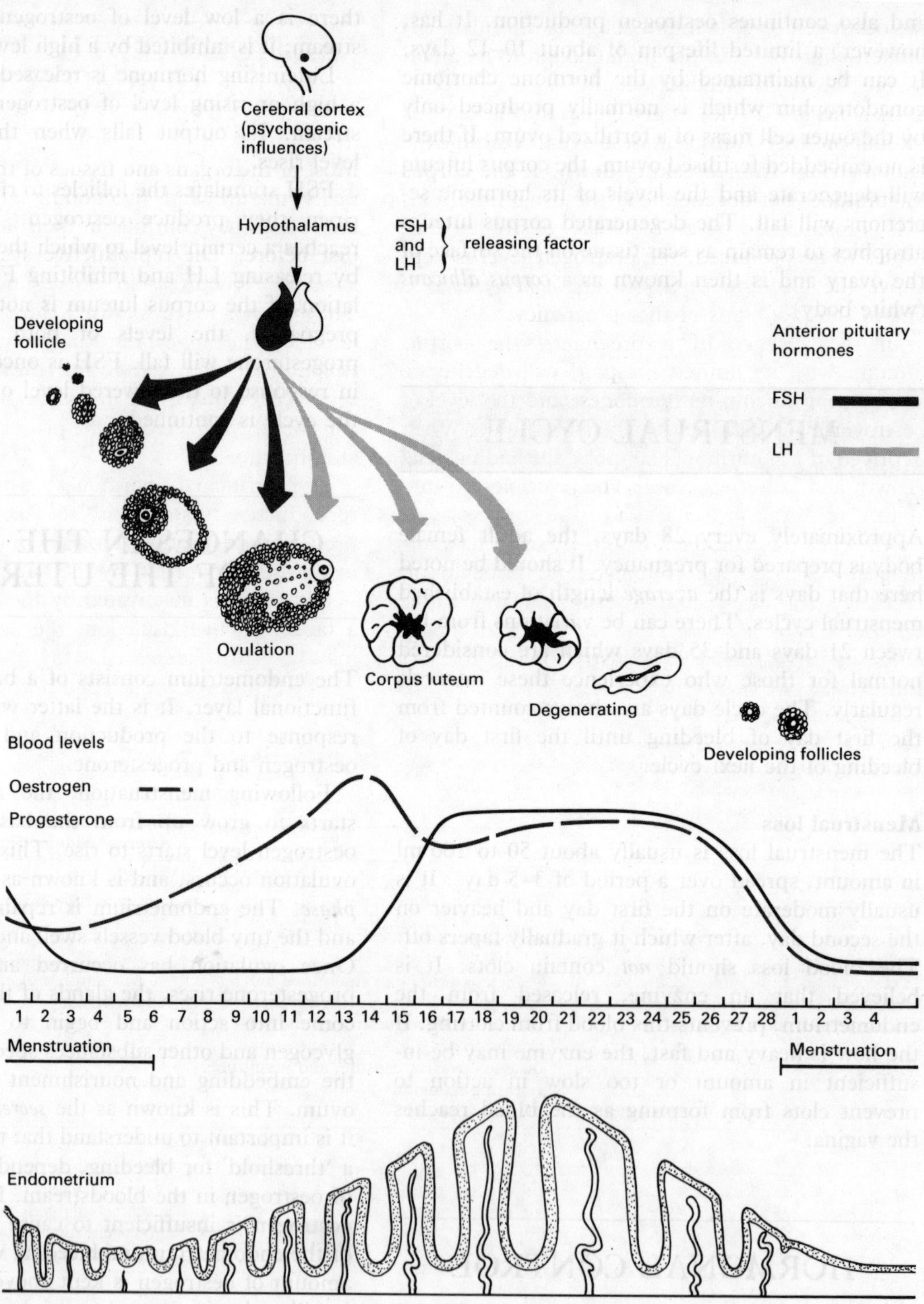

Figure 3.9 The menstrual cycle

the oestrogen level is high enough to stimulate endometrial growth but not high enough to maintain it, breakthrough bleeding occurs.

In a normal cycle, after ovulation, the corpus luteum produces sufficient oestrogen to inhibit the endometrium from breaking down. If the corpus luteum does not degenerate at the usual time, i.e., if it is maintained by a pregnancy, oestrogen continues to be produced, the oestrogen level is kept above the bleeding threshold and *amenorrhoea* is one of the first signs of that pregnancy.

In the absence of a pregnancy the corpus luteum, with its limited lifespan, will degenerate and stop producing its hormones, and the level of oestrogen will fall below the threshold. When deprived of the hormonal support, the endometrial growth and secretion cease. The arterioles go into spasm, resulting in ischaemia of the surface layer. As the cells die from lack of blood, small haemorrhages occur into the endometrium. It begins to break down, more bleeding results and the whole functional layer is shed. This, together with blood, is the menstrual flow, or menstruation. Table 3.1 summarises the menstrual cycle.

ACTIONS OF THE OVARIAN HORMONES

Most of the organs and tissues of the body are normally mature and functioning at birth or soon after, and they continue in their job until death or just before. The reproductive system and its associated structures do not follow this pattern. They do not reach maturity until they are stimulated by the appropriate hormones, they do not function if the source of these hormones is removed or disturbed in some way, and they are considerably affected by the processes of aging and childbearing.

The principal hormones which affect the reproductive system directly are oestrogen and progesterone, produced mainly by the ovaries, and in a lesser proportion by the adrenal glands.

Oestrogen is inactivated by the liver; if there is a failure in liver function, the oestrogen activity may be greatly increased.

The actions of the ovarian hormones upon their

Table 3.1 The menstrual cycle
The cycle can be divided into four phases:
menstrual — 4 days approx. secretory — 11 days
proliferative — 10 days approx. regressive — 3 days

Pituitary gland	Ovary	Uterus (endometrium)
Menstrual phase FSH released	Follicles start to ripen	Endometrium is shed, except for the basal layer
Proliferative phase FSH continues to be released; level of FSH drops 24 hours before ovulation; LH is released; the LH 'surge'	Follicles continue to ripen, one much more than the others—the graafian follicle; produces oestrogen and some progesterone; graafian follicle grows, distends ovarian capsule, and it ruptures, releasing its ovum	Repair and rebuilding of the endometrium
Culminates in ovulation 14 days before next menstruation due		
Secretory phase LH continues to be released for a few days then level drops rapidly	Corpus luteum develops from ruptured follicle and produces progesterone and some oestrogen	Endometrium thick and highly vascular; glands of endometrium become enlarged, secrete and store glycogen, mucus and other substances which can nourish a fertilised ovum
Regressive (or premenstrual) phase Low levels of oestrogen stimulate production of FSH	Corpus luteum degenerates (limited lifespan); therefore levels of progesterone and oestrogen fall	Endometrial growth and secretion ceases → ischaemia of surface layers → cells die → bleeding below surface → gradual stripping off of whole functional surface → menstruation

Table 3.2 Actions of the ovarian hormones

Oestrogen	'Target organ'	Progesterone
Proliferation of endometrium stimulates growth of myometrium	Uterus	Enlargement of stromal cells and glands; mucus and glycogen secretion
Growth of cervical glands; abundant secretion of clear thin mucus	Cervix	Changes secretion to scant but thick mucus
Growth of cells of vaginal epithelium; glycogen appears in cells	Vagina	Maturation of cells of epithelium ceases; surface cells degenerate and are shed → release of glycogen
Growth and health of vulval tissues	Vulva	
Growth of duct system; enlargement and pigmentation of nipple and areola	Breasts	Growth of breast alveoli

various target organs, i.e. those organs which are especially designed to respond to these hormones, are show in Table 3.2.

Oestrogen brings about the body changes of puberty. Together with androgens, it is responsible for the growth and pattern of pubic and axillary hair. In addition, there is some evidence to suggest that oestrogen plays a part in the retention of calcium in the bones.

Progesterone acts upon all the organs of the reproductive tract but only if they are being, or have been, acted upon by oestrogen. With oestrogen, it contributes to fluid retention in the tissues. Progesterone also affects other body tissues, leading to the deposition of fat, and is thermogenic, i.e. it raises the basal body temperature by about 0.5°C.

4

CONCEPTION

Chapter outline
Fertilisation
Chromosomes and genes
Development before implantation
Implantation

Key words

blastocyst
chromosome
decidua
fertilisation
gamete
implantation
morula
trophoblast
zygote

FERTILISATION

Fertilisation is the union of the sperm from the male with the ovum from the female.

Spermatozoa are minute cells with a long tail which enables them to move in a fluid medium (Fig. 4.1). They are believed to retain their fertilising ability for 2–4 days.

Ova live for a maximum of 48 hours after ovula-

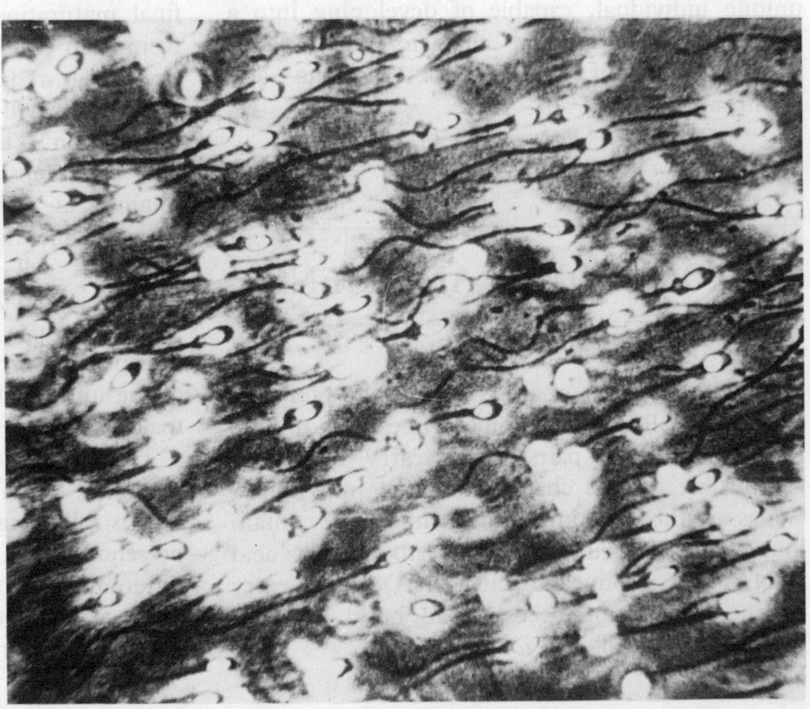

Figure 4.1 Spermatozoa

tion, so for fertilisation to be successful, intercourse must take place during the 5 days around the time of ovulation.

During intercourse as many as 300 million spermatozoa are deposited in 3 ml of seminal fluid. A large number are destroyed by the acidity of the vagina, and several more die on the journey to the fallopian tubes. They travel under their own power by lashing their tails, and at the time of ovulation their passage is assisted by the easily penetrable cervical mucus. Their journey through the cervix and the body of the uterus and into the fallopian tubes is believed to take about 20 minutes.

At ovulation, the ovum is expelled from the graafian follicle and picked up by the embracing fimbria of the fallopian tube on the side. The spermatozoa meet the ovum near the fimbriated end of the tube. Only one sperm will fertilise the ovum, but several (millions) are necessary to supply their substance *hyaluronidase*, which softens the corona radiata (the cells surrounding the ovum).

One spermatozoa penetrates the ovum by burrowing its head through the wall of the ovum which is then immediately rendered impenetrable to all other sperm. The two cells fuse; they unite to form one single cell. This one cell is a new and unique individual, capable of developing into a baby with its sex and characteristics already decided, and of forming the placenta and membranes.

CHROMOSOMES AND GENES

Within the nucleus of every cell of the body are structures called chromosomes. These are minute rods arranged in pairs which carry the genes responsible for the characteristics of individuals. Genes are the basic unit of heredity. They contain long-chain molecules of deoxyribonucleic acid (DNA) and ribonucleic acid (RNA) which carry all the information necessary to build each individual body cell.

A human gene is made up of approximately 1000 molecules of DNA. Each chromosome contains about 25 000 genes, and in the nucleus of each human cell there are 46 chromosomes. This number (46, arranged in 23 pairs) is constant and characteristic for humans, and is retained in each new cell that is formed by simple cell division (mitosis).

Sex determination

Of the 46 chromosomes, 44 are called autosomes and are responsible for the characteristics of the person as a whole, i.e. the hereditary physical and intellectual potential of the person (Greek: *soma*—the whole person). The remaining two chromosomes are concerned with the sex of the individual. These sex chromosomes are not given a number but are called either X or Y. The female cells always contain two X chromosomes (XX) and the male cells contain one X and one Y chromosome (XY).

The division of the germ cells (the ovum and the spermatozoon) differs from mitosis, because they bring only 23 chromosomes each when they ultimately conjoin to form a new combined cell or zygote. To achieve this, the germ cells undergo a form of reduction known as *meiosis* during their final maturation, half of the chromosomes (one from each pair) being retained and the other half becoming redundant and disintegrating. The ovum then will contribute one X chromosome at fertilisation. The sperm will carry either an X or a Y chromosome, depending on which was retained at meiosis. If the sperm carried an X chromosome, its union with the ovum will produce a human cell containing 46 chromosomes—44 autosomic and 2 sex chromosomes, X plus X (46 XX)—a female zygote and a female individual. If the sperm contributes a Y chromosome, the result of the union will be 46 XY—a male zygote and a male individual (Fig. 4.2).

The embryo develops initially as neuter or bipotential, with the rudimentary reproductive organs following the basic female pattern. It is the presence of the Y chromosome that stimulates the differentiation of the male gonads (testes) which produce androgens and thus cause the embryo to develop as a male. It is the absence of the Y

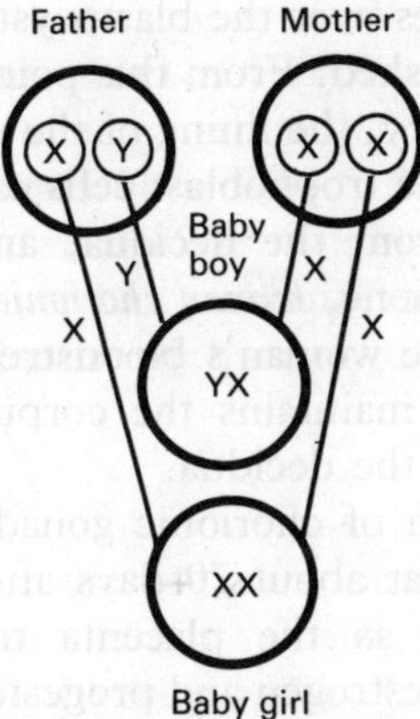

Figure 4.2 Sex determination at the time of conception

chromosome which allows the female (XX) embryo to differentiate with female gonads (ovaries) and so develop along female lines. Differentiation becomes apparent at about the 7th week after fertilisation, and chorion villus sampling can reveal the sex of the embryo as early as the 10th week.

DEVELOPMENT BEFORE IMPLANTATION

The fertilised ovum (zygote) spends 6–8 days travelling to the uterus. Its passage along the fallopian tubes is assisted by the peristaltic action of the tubes, the sweeping action of the cilia lining them, and the fluid produced by the ciliated epithelium.

During its journey to the uterus, the zygote develops by simple cell division every 12–15 hours, but does not increase in size. When it reaches the uterus it is a mass of cells and is referred to as a morula (Fig. 5.3). The morula then separates into two layers, the outer cell mass and the inner cell mass, fluid is formed and fills the space between the layers, and the structure is then termed the blastocyst. The outer cell mass is called the trophoblast; this will attach the ovum to the decidua and will develop into the placenta and outer (chorionic) membrane. The inner cell mass will develop into the embyro, cord and inner (amniotic) membrane.

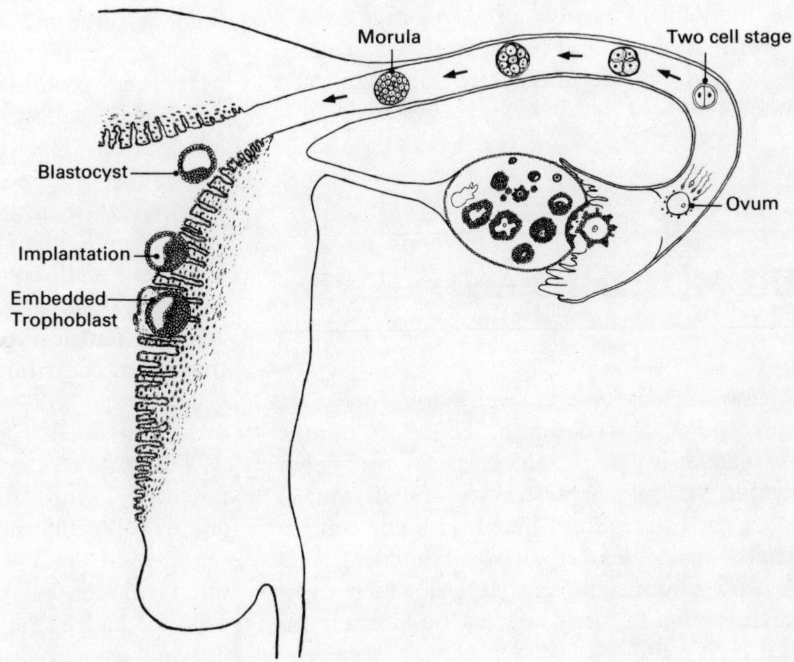

Figure 4.3 Ovulation, fertilisation, passage to the uterus and implantation.

IMPLANTATION

About 10 days after fertilisation of the ovum, the blastocyst implants or 'sinks to rest', in the endometrium (Fig. 4.3). Implantation (also called embedding or nidation) normally occurs in the upper body of the uterus.

The outer cells of the blastocyst secrete a substance, *proteolytic enzyme*, which breaks down the surface of the endometrium, thus enabling the blastocyst to embed. Uterine muscular activity is low at this time because of the relatively high level of progesterone in the bloodstream.

Once implantation has occurred, the lining of the uterus closes over the blastocyst and the pregnancy is established. From this point on, until the end of pregnancy, the lining of the uterus is called the *decidua*. The trophoblast cells can then absorb nourishment from the decidua, and can secrete their own hormone, *human chorionic gonadotrophin* (HCG), into the woman's bloodstream. Chorionic gonadotrophin maintains the corpus luteum and thus maintains the decidua.

The secretion of chorionic gonadotrophin rises rapidly, peaks at about 70 days after conception, then decreases as the placenta takes over the production of oestrogen and progesterone from the corpus luteum. The measurement of the urinary products of HCG is usually the first test done to establish the presence of pregnancy.

5

PLACENTA AND FETUS

Chapter outline
Development of the placenta
The placenta at term
Placental circulation
Functions of the placenta
Development of the fetus
Viability
Membranes, liquor and the cord
Fetal circulation
Temporary structures
Adaptation to extrauterine life
Hazards of fetal development

Key words

amnion
chorion
embryo
fetus
liquor
placenta
viability

DEVELOPMENT OF THE PLACENTA

The outermost cells of the trophoblast develop finger-like projections (villi). These primitive villi project into the maternal capillaries to enable the exchange of oxygen, nutrients, and waste products. In the centre of each villus, tiny blood vessels from the embryo ultimately form. Four distinct layers of tissue develop between the fetal and maternal capillaries. The layers are very close together and are collectively termed the placental membrane. Because of this barrier, the fetal and maternal bloodstreams do not mix.

The decidua completely lines the uterus. Where the pregnancy implants, the decidua splits. The decidua directly beneath the blastocyst is called the *decidua basalis*, and the decidua superficial to the blastocyst (i.e. that portion which closed over after implantation had occurred) is called the *decidua capsularis*. The rest of the decidua lining the uterine cavity is called the *decidua vera* (Fig. 5.1).

The ovum capsule grows until the decidua capsularis meets the decidua vera. They fuse and the uterine cavity is obliterated by the end of the 12th week of pregnancy.

The villi surrounding the ovum increase in number, with each villus developing a core with blood vessels. The villi in contact with the decidua capsularis (chorion laevae) soon atrophy and eventually become the outer membrane (the chorion). The villi in contact with the decidua basalis do not atrophy; they develop to form the chorion frondosum.

The chorion frondosum (the ovum's contribution) and the decidua basalis (the maternal contribution) together form the placenta. This process is complete by the end of the 3rd month. The placenta continues to grow throughout the pregnancy until term (40 weeks). Figure 5.2 shows the placenta in cross-section.

THE PLACENTA AT TERM

By term, the placenta weighs about one-sixth of the baby's weight, and is usually about 20 cm in diameter and 2–3 cm thick. It is mainly fetal in

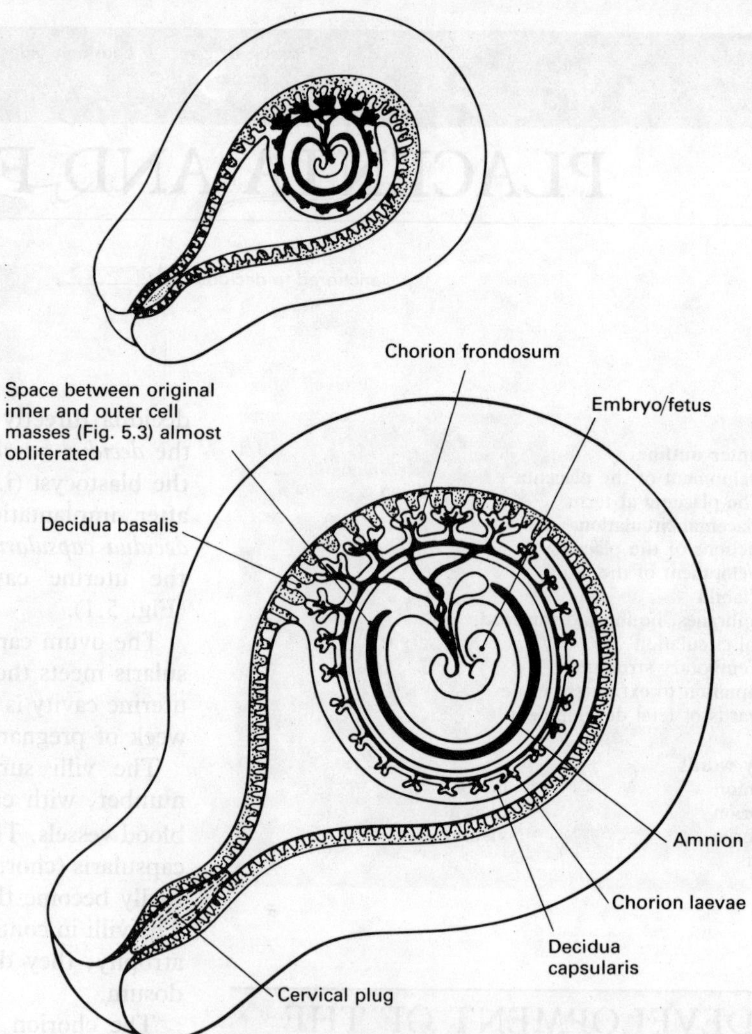

Figure 5.1 Development of the placenta at 5 weeks and 10 weeks.

origin, but the rough red surface is maternal in origin.

Fetal surface

The membranous cover can be seen on the fetal surface with the cord usually arising from the centre. The surface is smooth and glistening. Many large blood vessels are visible, radiating from the cord outwards.

Maternal surface

The maternal surface is dark red in colour. It is divided into cotyledons (lobes). The mature placenta often has gritty patches–areas of calcification; sometimes dark solid areas–evidence of old haemorrhage; and occasionally pale solid areas–placental infarctions.

PLACENTAL CIRCULATION

Blood is pumped through the fetus by the fetal heart. It leaves the fetus through the arteries of the

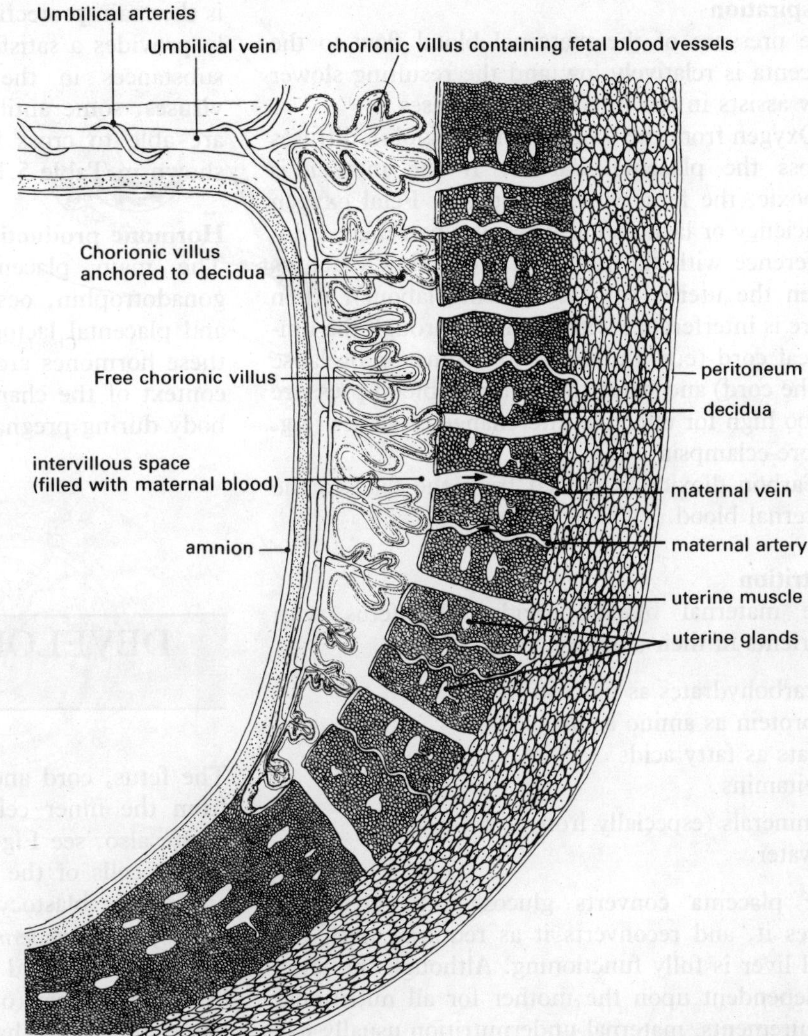

Figure 5.2 The placenta — cross-section.

umbilical cord and travels to the placenta. The umbilical arteries branch over the surface of the placenta, subdivide, and terminate in the chorionic villi.

The villi are bathed in maternal blood, but there is no direct connection between the fetal and maternal blood. Carbon dioxide and any waste products are given off, and oxygen and nutrients are taken in across the placental barrier. The replenished blood returns to the fetus via the umbilical vein.

FUNCTIONS OF THE PLACENTA

The functions of the placenta are:

- respiration
- nutrition
- excretion
- protection
- hormone production.

Respiration

The pressure of the maternal blood flow to the placenta is relatively low and the resulting slower flow assists in the interchange of gases.

Oxygen from the mother's haemoglobin diffuses across the placental barrier. If the mother is hypoxic, the fetus will be hypoxic. Fetal oxygen deficiency or lack will also result when there is interference with the placental blood flow (such as when the uterus contracts during labour), when there is interference with the flow through the umbilical cord (e.g. thinning, stretching or prolapse of the cord) and when the maternal blood pressure is too high for effective interchange of gasses (e.g. in pre-eclampsia).

Carbon dioxide is passed from the fetal to the maternal blood.

Nutrition

The maternal blood provides the fetus with nutrients in their simplest form:

- carbohydrates as glucose
- protein as amino acids
- fats as fatty acids
- vitamins
- minerals (especially iron)
- water.

The placenta converts glucose into glycogen, stores it, and reconverts it as required until the fetal liver is fully functioning. Although the fetus is dependent upon the mother for all nutritional requirements, maternal undernutrition usually has to be of a severe degree for intrauterine growth to be affected.

Excretion

The placenta excretes any waste products. These are minimal because all nutrition is in an available form; the emphasis is on building-up.

Protection

The protective function of the placenta is achieved in two ways–chemical and physical.

By its enzyme function, the placenta inactivates some of the toxic factors that pass through the placental barrier and with which the immature fetal liver cannot cope.

The physical barrier (the placental membranes) is the main protection for the fetus, and it normally provides a satisfactory defence against harmful substances in the mother's blood. But many viruses, some antibodies and a number of drugs are able to cross the barrier; these hazards are shown in Table 5.1.

Hormone production

The main placental hormones are chorionic gonadotrophin, oestrogens, progesterone, relaxin and placental lactogenic hormone. The effects of these hormones are discussed on page 55, in the context of the changes occurring in the mother's body during pregnancy.

DEVELOPMENT OF THE FETUS

The fetus, cord and amniotic membrane develop from the inner cell mass of the blastocyst (see p. 30; also, see Fig. 5.3).

The cells of the inner cell mass collect at one end of the blastocyst and form into two distinct layers, the *ectoderm* and the *endoderm*. Between these layers a third layer, the *mesoderm*, will form.

The ectoderm (outer layer) will develop to become the skin, hair, nails, brain and nervous system.

The endoderm (inner layer) will develop to form the intestines, internal organs, germ cells of the ovaries or testes, and the respiratory system.

The mesoderm will develop to form the circulatory, lymphatic, skeletal, muscular, and renal systems, and most of the reproductive tract.

As the layers of cells differentiate, a cavity appears above the ectoderm–the amniotic cavity. The lining of this cavity will become the amniotic membrane, and will secrete fluid which will make up part of the liquor (see below).

The amniotic cavity gradually enlarges and folds around the developing embryo, so that eventually the embryo is suspended by a body stalk (the umbilical cord) in a closed bag of fluid (liquor).

Table 5.1 Development of the fetus and possible hazards

Ovum **5 weeks gestation** **(weeks after LNMP)** complete sac 1 cm in diameter covered with chorionic villi, no human characteristics recognised *Embryo* **6 weeks gestation** sac—2.3 cm in diameter, 1 g weight; head enlarges; arm and leg buds forming; primitive heart beginning to function; heartbeat audible electronically, circulation in primitive form; connections made between vessels in chorion and those which have grown out through body stalk **10 weeks gestation** embryo 4 cm long, external genitalia appear, anal membrane breaks down, hands and feet recognisable, human origin apparent *Fetus* **12 weeks gestation** fetus 8 cm long, 15 g weight; fingers and toes, eyes and ears, circulation and kidneys developed; nasal septum and palate have fused; endocrine glands and nervous system (reflex responses) begin to function **16 weeks** fetus 16 cm long, 110 g weight; sex easily identifiable; fingernails visible; good heartbeat; fetal movements felt	**Hazards to fetal development in early pregnancy** chemical or mechanical contraceptives (which have failed in their function) may leave the ovum alive but damaged in some way; maternal age extremes (under 17 years or over 40 years) have a higher incidence of genetic defects; exposure to radiation may inhibit cell division; pesticides and other chemicals may be dangerous; infections, specifically rubella, cytomegalovirus, toxoplasmosis, syphilis, pelvic (e.g. from attempted abortion) and infection via innoculations, e.g. smallpox and rubella vaccine; cytotoxic drugs may kill embryo; teratogenic (e.g. causing malformation) drugs include phenytoin, excessive alcohol, quinine, warfarin, lithium; carcinogenic effects have resulted from silboestrol; corticosteroids can upset whole endocrine balance; androgens and progestogens can cause virilisation of a female fetus; thyroid drugs can cause fetal goitre; radiation exposure increases likelihood of leukaemia and cancer in childhood; ectopic implantation—no room to grow; malformation from teratogenic drugs should no longer be a hazard after 12 weeks, but caution is still advised until after 16 weeks
Basic *development* *is now complete*—the fetus now has to *mature*	
20 weeks 22 cm long, 300 g weight; vernix on skin; lanugo (fine hair) on body, eyebrows; fetus now legally viable (see below) **24 weeks** 30 cm long, 600 g weight; wrinkled skin, fat deposited, brain development continues **28 weeks** 35 cm long, 1000 g weight; if born, moves energetically and cries **32 weeks** 42 cm long, 1700 g weight; skin red, wrinkled **36 weeks** 46 cm long, 2500 g weight; nails reach fingertips **40 weeks** 50 cm long, 3400 g weight; baby well covered with fat; skin red, not wrinkled; all organs are functioning with the exception of the lungs	**Hazards to maturation and well-being in later pregnancy** from now on dietary deficiencies or extremes, maternal diseases (e.g. diabetes, hypertension, renal disease, anaemia, severe infections) and obstetric complications may be hazardous; cervical incompetence may cause premature labour from 18 weeks onwards; drugs of addiction, including nicotine and alcohol, cause growth retardation; antibiotics are given cautiously, tetracyclines can cause yellow discoloration of the teeth, retarded bone growth and cataracts; sulphonamides can disturb fetal liver function pre-eclampsia may arise and cause fetal deprivation and growth retardation pre-term labour may arise before the fetus is mature; induction may be necessary for Rh incompatibility, low oestriol levels, pre-eclampsia, diabetes depressant sedatives, analgesics or anaesthetics administered during labour, traumatic or precipitate delivery; post maturity

The embryo continues to develop by a process of bending and folding. The cells grow and develop extremely rapidly, with different body parts developing more quickly than others, e.g. the first to develop is the head, the arms grow more quickly than the legs. Figure 5.4 shows an embryo of 8 weeks gestation.

VIABILITY

20 completed weeks gestation is currently the legal definition of viability in all Australian States with

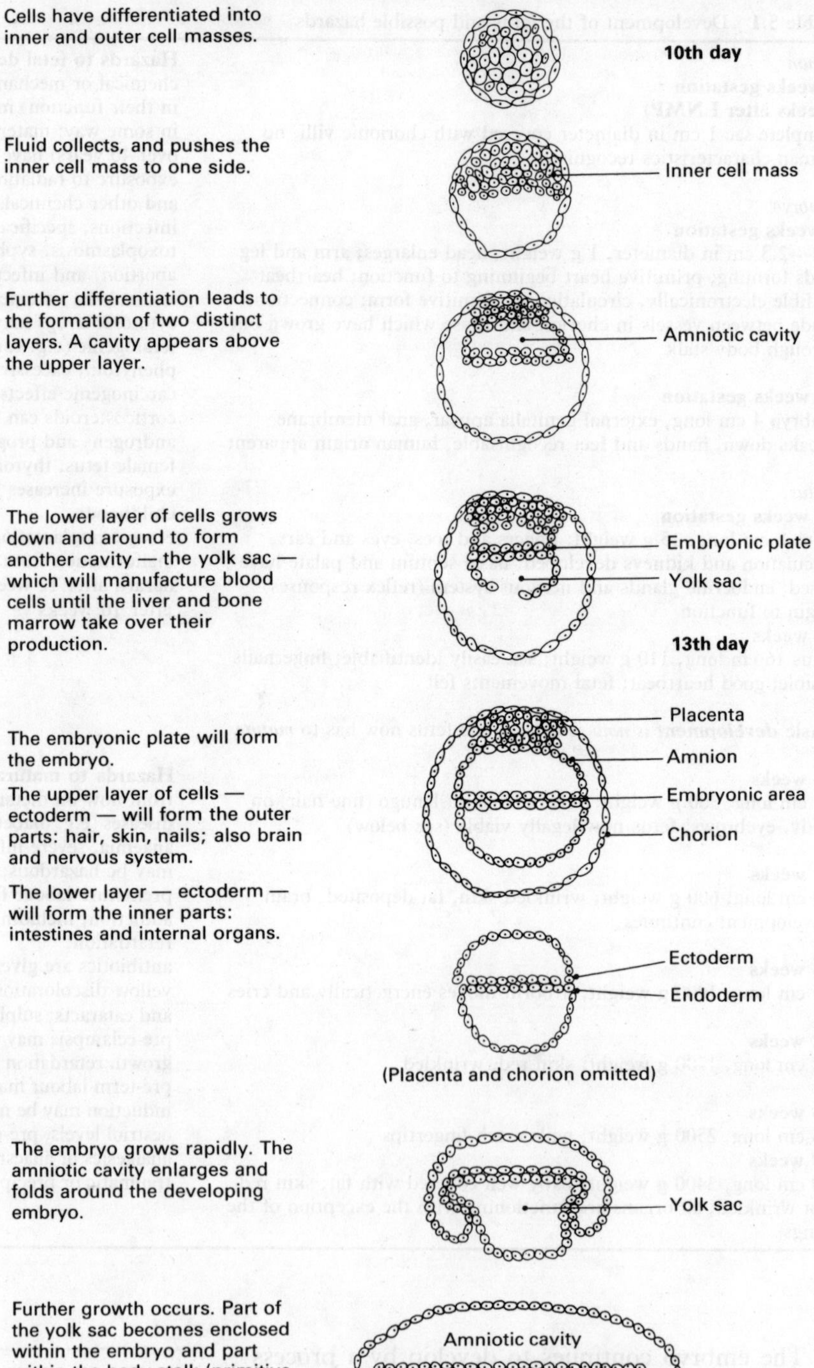

Cells have differentiated into inner and outer cell masses.

10th day

Fluid collects, and pushes the inner cell mass to one side.

Inner cell mass

Further differentiation leads to the formation of two distinct layers. A cavity appears above the upper layer.

Amniotic cavity

The lower layer of cells grows down and around to form another cavity — the yolk sac — which will manufacture blood cells until the liver and bone marrow take over their production.

Embryonic plate

Yolk sac

13th day

The embryonic plate will form the embryo.

The upper layer of cells — ectoderm — will form the outer parts: hair, skin, nails; also brain and nervous system.

The lower layer — ectoderm — will form the inner parts: intestines and internal organs.

Placenta

Amnion

Embryonic area

Chorion

Ectoderm

Endoderm

(Placenta and chorion omitted)

The embryo grows rapidly. The amniotic cavity enlarges and folds around the developing embryo.

Yolk sac

Further growth occurs. Part of the yolk sac becomes enclosed within the embryo and part within the body stalk (primitive cord).

Amniotic cavity

Figure 5.3 Development of the embryo (Sources: Sheehan J M 1970 Embryology made easy-3. Nursing Times 3 (10 December): 1548, 1645).

At this stage the embryo appears as a hollow tube, sealed at both ends. Later, cells at the head and tail ends disappear and thus the mouth and anus are formed.

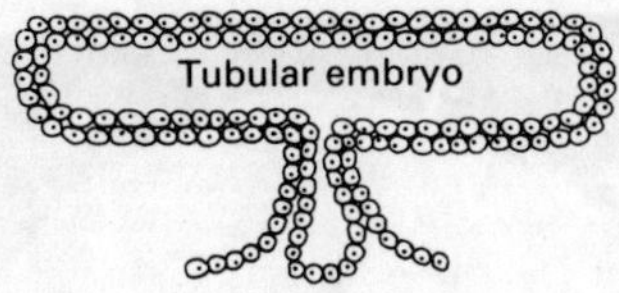

A third layer of cells has appeared between the ectoderm and endoderma. This third layer — the mesoderm — will form the muscles, skeleton, heart and blood vessels, and connective tissue.

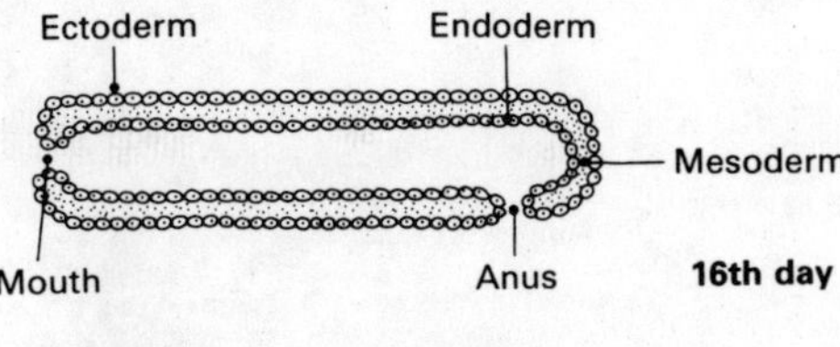

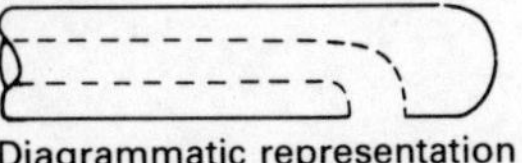

Diagrammatic representation

The head develops greatly on the dorsal (back) aspect of the embryo.

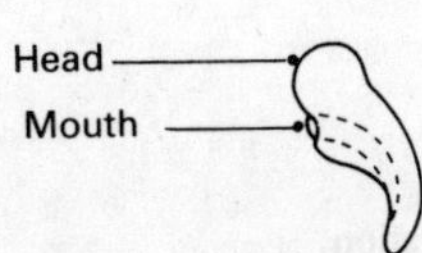

The brain enlarges and overhangs the head, and the mouth becomes smaller.

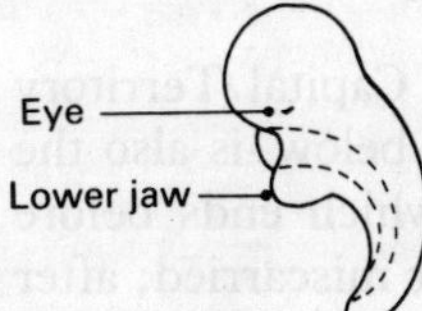

Limb buds appear at approximately five weeks (the embryo is 6 mm in length).

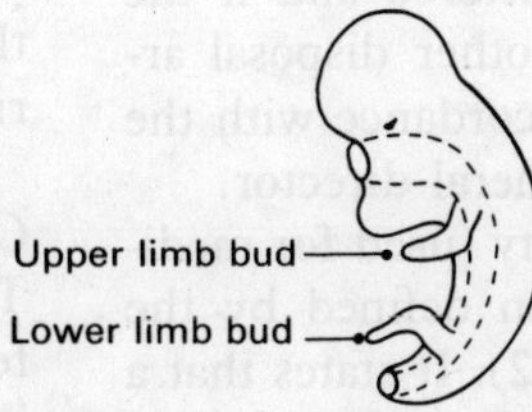

By the end of the second month the embryo has developed to resemble a miniature human. It measures 30 mm, and from now on is called a fetus.

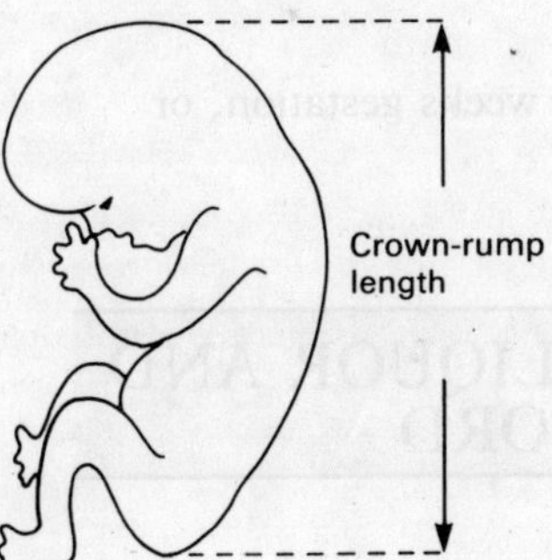

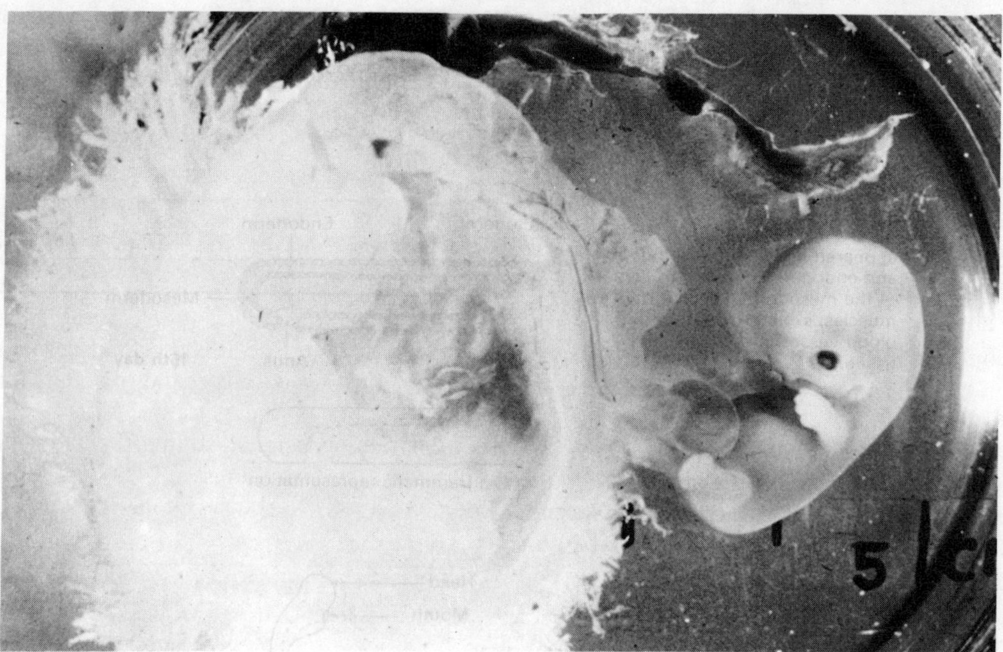

Figure 5.4 An embryo of 8 weeks' gestation.

the exception of the Australian Capital Territory (where the WHO definition–see below–is also the legal definition). A pregnancy which ends before 20 weeks is said to be aborted or miscarried; after 20 weeks it is defined as a birth. All births after 20 weeks are require to be registered and if the baby should die, the burial or other disposal arrangements must be made in accordance with the law, in most cases through a funeral director.

The criteria for *medical* viability (used for medical statistical purposes) has been defined by the World Health Organization (1982). It states that a baby is potentially capable of independent existence if it:

- is known to be over 22 weeks gestation, or
- weighs 400 g or more.

MEMBRANES, LIQUOR AND THE CORD

Membranes

Two separate membranes are attached to the placenta–the amnion and the chorion.

Amnion

The amnion is the inner membrane, enclosing the fetus and liquor. It is smooth, thin, tough and transparent. It is closely applied to the chorion (although it can easily be peeled away). It covers the fetal surface of the placenta up to the insertion of the cord, then continues as the cover of the cord right up to the umbilicus of the fetus.

Chorion

The chorion is the outer opaque membrane formed from those villi of the ovum which were in contact with the decidua capsularis. It is continuous with the margin of the placenta and is adherent to the uterine lining.

Liquor

Liquor amnii (amniotic fluid) is the pale, clear, straw-coloured fluid surrounding the fetus in the amniotic sac. It is 99% water, plus mineral salts, and is derived mainly from the secretions of the cells of the amniotic membrane. Some of the liquor is derived from the fetal urine.

Liquor has a characteristic odour which is quite distinct from the odour of maternal urine. This is useful to know in an emergency or when there is doubt about whether or not the membranes have ruptured. At term, in a normal pregnancy, the amniotic cavity contains about 1000 ml of liquor.

Functions

The amniotic fluid helps to:

- maintain an even temperature in utero
- enable free movement of the fetal parts
- protect the fetus from injury–it acts as a shock absorber
- 'flush out' the lower genital tract when the membranes rupture.

Umbilical cord

The umbilical cord (Fig. 5.5) extends from the fetal umbilicus to the fetal surface of the placenta and measures 50–55 cm. It encloses the two umbilical arteries which transport deoxygenated blood from the fetus, and the single umbilical vein which carries replenished blood from the placenta to the fetus.

The umbilical vessels are embedded in a thick gelatinous substance known as Wharton's jelly; this protects the vessels from compression and helps to prevent kinking of the cord. Wharton's jelly swells upon exposure to the air.

The force of the blood flow (approximately 400 ml per minute) through the cord helps to keep the cord relatively straight and prevents the cord from becoming tangled as the fetus moves about.

FETAL CIRCULATION

During intrauterine life the fetal respiratory system is not functioning and oxygenation of the blood occurs in the placenta. Therefore the fetal circulation is designed so that the major blood flow bypasses the fetal lungs.

THE TEMPORARY STRUCTURES

There are four temporary structures in the fetal circulation. These are the:

- ductus venosus (venous duct) (1)
- foramen ovale (2)

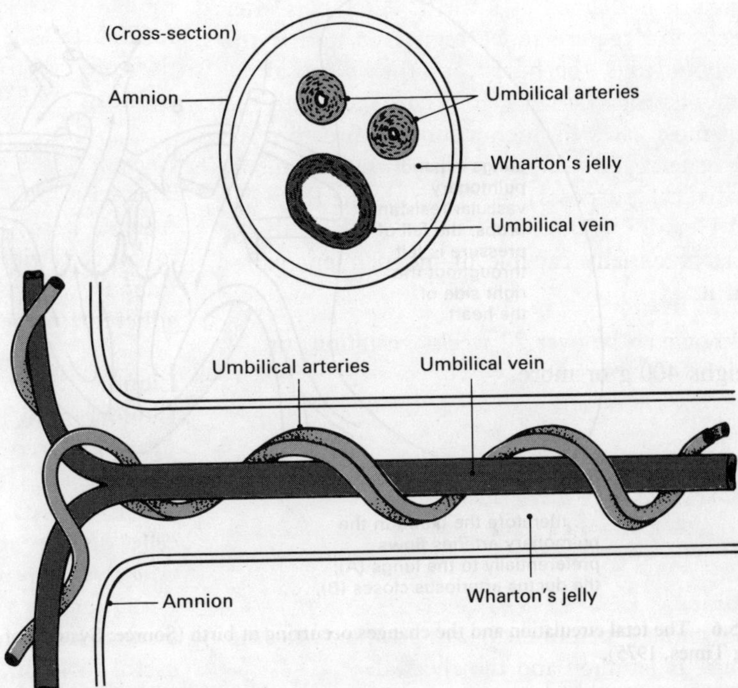

Figure 5.5 The umbilical cord.

- ductus arteriosus (arterial duct) (3)
- hypogastric arteries (4).

The understanding of the fetal circulation will be assisted by studying Figure 5.6. (The numbers in parentheses refer to Fig. 5.6.)

Ductus venosus

The ductus venosus (1) runs from the umbilical vein to the vena cava. It carries replenished (oxygenated) blood to the heart, for circulation through the fetus.

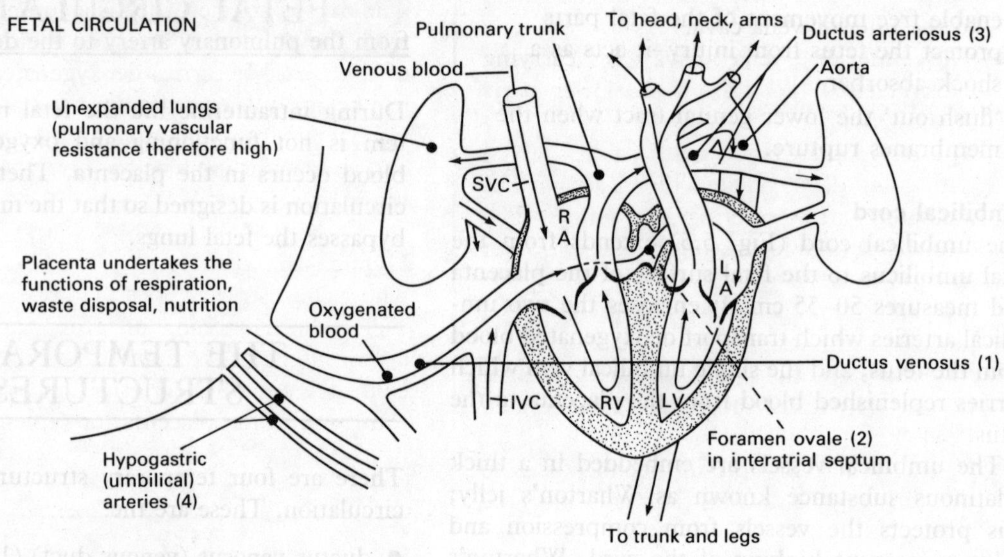

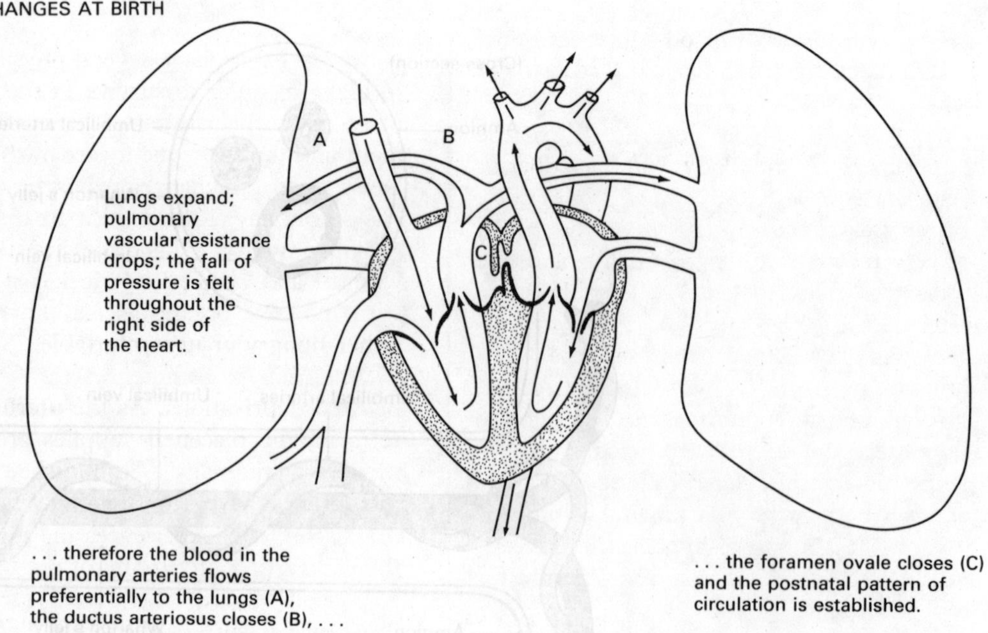

Figure 5.6 The fetal circulation and the changes occurring at birth (Source: Systems of Life No. 10, Cardiovascular system — 2, Nursing Times, 1975).

SUMMARY OF THE FETAL CIRCULATION

- Oxygenated blood enters the fetus via the umbilical vein.
- The umbilical vein goes straight to the liver, but has a large branch (ductus venosus) which carries most of the blood to the inferior vena cava.
- The inferior vena cava is carrying deoxygenated blood from the lower parts of the fetus.
- The oxygenated blood is, therefore, mixed with some deoxygenated blood almost immediately after entering the fetus. (The fetus has a high haemoglobin concentration to cope with this.)
- The inferior vena cava empties its blood into the right atrium.
- The main volume of blood passes straight to the left atrium, through the foramen ovale.
- From the left atrium, the blood passes to the left ventricle, and then out into the aorta.
- Most of the blood goes through branches of the aorta to supply the brain and upper limbs.
- A limited amount of blood continues down the descending aorta to supply the lower parts of the body.
- Deoxygenated blood returns from the upper part of the body via the superior vena cava.
- From the superior vena cava the blood travels through the right atrium and the right ventricle to enter the pulmonary artery.
- Most of the blood bypasses the non-functioning lungs by being directed, through the ductus arteriosus, straight to the descending arch of the aorta.
- Some blood is circulated to the lower parts of the body, but the main volume is diverted, through the hypogastric arteries, to the cord, and thence to the placenta for replenishment.

Foramen ovale

The foramen ovale (2) is an oval-shaped opening which allows blood to flow from the right atrium directly to the left atrium, thus bypassing the right ventricle and therefore the fetal lungs.

Ductus arteriosus

The ductus arteriosus (3) is a communicating duct from the pulmonary artery to the descending arch of the aorta. It carries deoxygenated blood which has been returned from the head and upper limbs via the superior vena cava and the right ventricle, and so most of the blood is diverted from the fetal lungs.

Hypogastric arteries

The hypogastric arteries (4) are two vessels, one each side, branching off from the internal iliac arteries to enter the umbilical cord. There they become the umbilical arteries, and carry the blood returning to the placenta for replenishment.

ADAPTATION TO EXTRAUTERINE LIFE

Newborn babies have several physical adjustments to make in order to survive in the outside world. Most of the principles of the immediate management and the subsequent care of the new baby are based upon the changes which he experiences.

Without any effort on his part the fetus has been provided with all his necessities: oxygen, food, warmth and protection. He has not had to cope with infective organisms and he has never been either hungry or uncomfortable.

When labour commences the fetus experiences his first deprivations. As the uterus contracts and retracts, the placental supplies are gradually (although minimally) diminished. After the membranes have ruptured and liquor begins to drain, the fetus experiences the direct pressure of the contracting uterus and of the birth canal as he is pushed towards the outlet. He also feels the resisting pressure of the pelvic floor. Labour is a strenuous ordeal for the fetus as well as for the mother.

As soon as he is born, the baby must cope with a dramatic reduction in oxygen and often a significant reduction in temperature. He will also experience the shock of light (often very bright light) and what may be to him very loud sound. Within a comparatively short time he has to adapt to the process of obtaining and digesting food for himself. As well, he may encounter infective organisms with which he will have a limited ability to cope.

Thus the initial and continuing care of the newborn infant as he adjusts to his changed environment is an important factor in the achievement of good quality life.

Respiration

The initiation of respiration is the most urgent physiological adjustment for the baby. It is achieved in response to the stimulation of the respiratory centre in the medulla by a high level of carbon dioxide. Other factors assist the onset of respiration: the chest wall, previously compressed by the birth canal, suddenly expands, allowing the air to rush in, and the changed temperature or the shock of being handled may cause the baby to gasp.

The first breaths are probably the hardest in life. It has been calculated that the first few breaths take five times the effort normally required for breathing. Air must be drawn in to expand the many thousands of tiny uninflated air-sacs (alveoli) of the formerly solid lungs to oxygenate the blood and thus the brain. A mature baby's lungs contain a detergent-like substance called surfactant, which prevents the alveoli walls from adhering.

After the first initial efforts, the baby will usually gasp, then will probably cry for a short time. Crying does cause good lung inflation and so is not really discouraged; on the other hand it is no longer prolonged deliberately by vigorous stimulation and handling.

The newborn baby breathes quickly, usually at a rate of just over 40 breaths per minute, and uses his abdominal muscles for assistance. The respiratory rhythm is usually irregular for several hours after birth.

Circulation

The temporary structures of the fetal circulation have to close to provide effective circulation for extrauterine existence. The closure of the structures is dependent upon the beginning of respiration.

The lungs expand with the onset of respiration, and this lung expansion opens up the pulmonary capillary bed, creating a negative pressure. The blood now flows from the pulmonary artery through to the lungs (to balance the pressure) for oxygenation. The ductus arteriosus contracts as the lungs expand, and it eventually becomes a supporting ligament in the thorax.

The increased blood flow to the lungs reduces the pressure on the right side of the heart and increases the pressure on the left side. Now that the pressure within the heart has been equalised the valve-like foramen ovale is no longer being forced open, so it closes.

The umbilical vessels contract at birth. Blood clots in the umbilical vein and arteries and in the ductus venosus and hypogastric arteries. These structures remain as fibrous bands.

Heat regulation

The newborn baby has a limited ability to regulate his body temperature in relation to the environment, and he is in danger of hypothermia unless preventive measures are taken. Important factors to consider in the newborn are that:

- heat production is poor, because of the low metabolic rate
- there is usually a dramatic change in the temperature of the baby's surroundings—especially if he is born into a delivery room conditioned for the comfort of the labouring mother
- he is born wet, and so loses heat by evaporation
- he has a large body surface in proportion to his weight
- his hypothalamic temperature-regulating centre is not fully mature, and so the processes of shivering and sweating are poorly developed.

The newborn baby is dried as soon as it is practical to do so, and the time of his exposure to the cooler environment is minimised. Warmth is provided by wrapping, or by overhead heat lamps or warm air-conditioning, with the aim of keeping the baby's axillary temperature at about 36.5°C.

Digestion

Before birth, the fetus received adequate nourishment in the simplest form. After the birth, the baby's digestive system must be able to digest and absorb food as well as eliminate wastes.

The food designed by nature to introduce the baby's digestive system to the process of digestion is called colostrum. It is secreted by the breasts during pregnancy and for the first 2–3 days after delivery, before the milk supply 'comes in' (usually on the 3rd day).

Colostrum is thicker and yellower than true breast milk, and probably because of its appearance was once thought to be bad for the baby and was discarded. In fact it is highly nutritive, very easily digested (with its protein in the form of lactoglobulin), contains vitamins and immune bodies, and functions as a laxative.

In order to obtain colostrum, the new baby must be able to suck and swallow. These are reflex actions which are present in the mature baby at birth.

The processes of taking in and digesting food stimulates peristalsis of the bowel and results in the passage of meconium. Meconium is the dark green tarry substance which has formed in the intestine from about the 16th week of gestation.

Immunity

The mature baby has received antigens and passive immunity to certain infections from the mother in the last 6 or so weeks before birth. However he does leave a sterile environment to meet many micro-organisms and other antigens suddenly. It may take some weeks for active immunity to these to develop.

The process of birth itself, from the breaking of the sealed amniotic sac onwards, exposes the fetus to new organisms. *Candida albicans* (thrush), the *gonococcus* and *herpesvirus* may be encountered in the vagina. In the case of known herpesvirus infection, vaginal delivery would not be allowed. Once born (especially if born in a hospital), the baby is likely to encounter *Staphylococcus aureus*, an organism to which he may have little resistance.

To compensate for the poorly-developed immunological status of the newborn baby, careful antenatal supervision and exclusion or treatment of all possible infections, delivery techniques aimed at the non-introduction of organisms, and extreme care exercised in all aspects of the new baby's management, are vital.

HAZARDS TO FETAL DEVELOPMENT

Much of maternity care is preventive care. A knowledge of the hazards to fetal development, maturation and well-being, can be applied by everybody who has contact with any pregnant or potentially pregnant woman. For example, any female in the years from puberty to menopause *could* be in the vital early days of pregnancy even before a period is missed. This is why the rule for exposure to X-rays of any sort is the 'first 10 days of menstrual cycle only'. The date of the first day of the last normal menstrual period should always be ascertained unless the X-ray is an emergency investigation.

The woman should always be warned of the possible dangers with drugs and inoculations should pregnancy occur during the course of treatment or during the active effect of the inoculation. It is important that the pregnant woman be aware of the hazards of taking any medication or treatment that has not been prescribed by a doctor who knows that she is pregnant.

Table 5.1 shows the possible hazards to the development, maturation and well-being of the fetus. In summary, the major hazards are substances or events which:

- *destroy developing cells*–radiation, pesticides, cytotoxic drugs
- *raise the fetal temperature*–infections, especially those caused by viruses
- *cause malformations* to developing cells–teratogenic drugs, alchohol, certain viruses
- *disturb attachment or security* of the pregnancy–decidual breakdown due to hormone imbalance; ectopic pregnancy, cervical incompetence

- *interfere with oxygenation and nutrition*–anaemia, hypertension, renal disease, pre-eclampsia, diabetes, very poor maternal nutrition, nicotine, alcohol.

Although the basic development of the fetus is complete at 12–16 weeks, and the protective functions of the placenta are in action, all possible hazards should be avoided *throughout* pregnancy. Fetal oxygenation and nutrition must be maintained at their highest in order for the baby to cope well with the stresses of labour and for successful adaptation to extrauterine life.

6
COMPLICATIONS OF EARLY PREGNANCY

Chapter outline
Abortion
Ectopic pregnancy
Hydatidiform mole

Key words

abortion	ectopic
carneous mole	oxytocin
choriocarcinoma	prostaglandins
curettage	Shirodkar suture

The complications of early, non-viable (before 20 weeks gestation) pregnancy—abortion (miscarriage), ectopic pregnancy and hydatidiform mole—are conditions which are often managed in a general, as distinct from maternity, hospital or unit. Whether or not a nurse enters the field of midwifery, it is important for her to be able to recognise and understand these conditions and to be able to observe and care for the woman experiencing them.

The threat to the continuation of a pregnancy can have profound effects upon a woman and her family. What might have been a longed-for, and perhaps widely advertised and celebrated, pregnancy is now in danger. There is little that the parents can do. They will look for causes, for faults in themselves or their actions. The mother-to-be is bleeding and perhaps in pain, and it has all happened suddenly. On the other hand the pregnancy might not have been acknowledged, maybe not even diagnosed, or there may have been mixed or negative feelings.

Whatever the situation, the couple are in need of accurate and truthful information and compassionate care. The woman may be rushed into hospital and, in the case of an incomplete abortion or ruptured ectopic pregnancy for example, be taken straight to an operating room in order to prevent further blood loss or other complications. Her husband or partner may be left quite stunned by the urgency of it all and may not know how to cope with this crisis. On the other hand, there may be a situation of anxiety drawn out over many days, wondering if a threatened pregnancy will settle or miscarry, or over many months following a hydatidiform mole while waiting to be declared free of serious complications.

After the couple leaves our care they must face other people who are also grieving that this pregnancy has ended. It can prove very hard to resume normal relationships with these people, or with others in whom fertility and pregnancy success seems to come so easily. A number of the points made in Chapter 21 of this book relate also to these conditions of early pregnancy and are worth some reflection in this context. There may be an appropriate occasion to emphasise that, although not part of its title, the Stillbirth and Neonatal Support group (SANDS) includes those whose pregnancies ended early and sadly, and the group shows a deep interest in, and concern for, them.

ABORTION

Abortion is the termination or ending of a pregnancy before the fetus is viable (in this context, 20 weeks). It is believed that between 10 and 20% of pregnancies end in spontaneous abortion, most of them during the first 12 weeks.

Causes of spontaneous abortion

- abnormality of the embroyo or fetus is the most common cause of early abortion and is often due to chromosomal defects
- abnormalities of the uterus, resulting in a distorted uterine cavity or restriction of growth and expansion of the uterus, e.g. fibroids, congenital malformations, uterine prolapse or retroversion
- damage to the cervix, from deep tearing during childbirth or surgical procedures (dilation, amputation)
- maternal diseases and ingestion of drugs: diseases include acute viral infections, high fevers, and inoculations, e.g. against smallpox. Chronic nephritis and heart failure may result in fetal anoxia. Errors in the metabolism of folic acid, which is necessary for fetal development, will result in fetal death. Certain drugs, especially cytotoxic agents, will interfere with the normal process of rapid cell division. Prostaglandins will cause abortion by stimulating uterine contractions
- trauma, but usually only when applied directly to the uterine cavity. Sexual intercourse, especially when orgasm occurs, might be associated with abortion in a woman who has a history of repeated miscarriages
- hormonal factors, e.g. reduction in the output of progesterone, may be blamed for abortion occurring at 10–12 weeks, the time when the placenta takes over hormone production from the corpus luteum
- psychosomatic causes: stress and strong emotions are known to affect the uterine functioning, working through the hypothalamic-pituitary system. Many obstetricians can quote case histories of stress-related spontaneous abortions, and they can usually also tell of successful pregnancies occurring (in women with previously bad histories) after anxieties have been removed.

Types of spontaneous abortion

Four types are shown in Figure 6.1.

Threatened abortion

Bleeding from the uterus is noticed. In 50% of cases the bleeding is slight, gradually ceasing after a few days, and the pregnancy proceeds normally. Even so, the woman may continue to worry about the effect of the bleeding on the baby. She can usually be assured that were the fetus damaged, the pregnancy would generally not continue; it is wise to ask the doctor to add his reassurance. The treatment is bed rest and sedation for at least 48 hours, with careful observation of the colour and type of all vaginal loss. Enemas and laxatives should not be given. An ultrasound scan of the uterine contents is performed at this stage, and may be repeated 2 weeks later. The couple are advised against having intercourse for this period.

The woman in hospital should use pans rather than go to the toilet, and all pads should be kept for inspection before disposal. If the bleeding persists and is accompanied by pain and cervical dilatation, the abortion is then classified as 'inevitable'.

Inevitable abortion

Ineviable abortion is characterised by moderate to severe blood loss, uterine contractions causing lower abdominal cramping pains, and cervical dilatation. Its management consists of:

- complete bed rest
- careful measurement and observation of all matter passed vaginally. Forceps should be used to separate any clots to see whether or not they contain fetal tissue. All matter passed is saved and sent off for laboratory examination.
- frequent and accurate recording of vital signs (temperature, pulse, respirations, blood pressure)
- relief of pain
- food should be withheld, possibly fluids as well, because a general anaesthetic may be necessary
- ergometrine may be ordered, to contract the uterus
- a specimen of blood is taken for Hb, typing and cross-matching.

If abortion does not occur within 24 hours, the

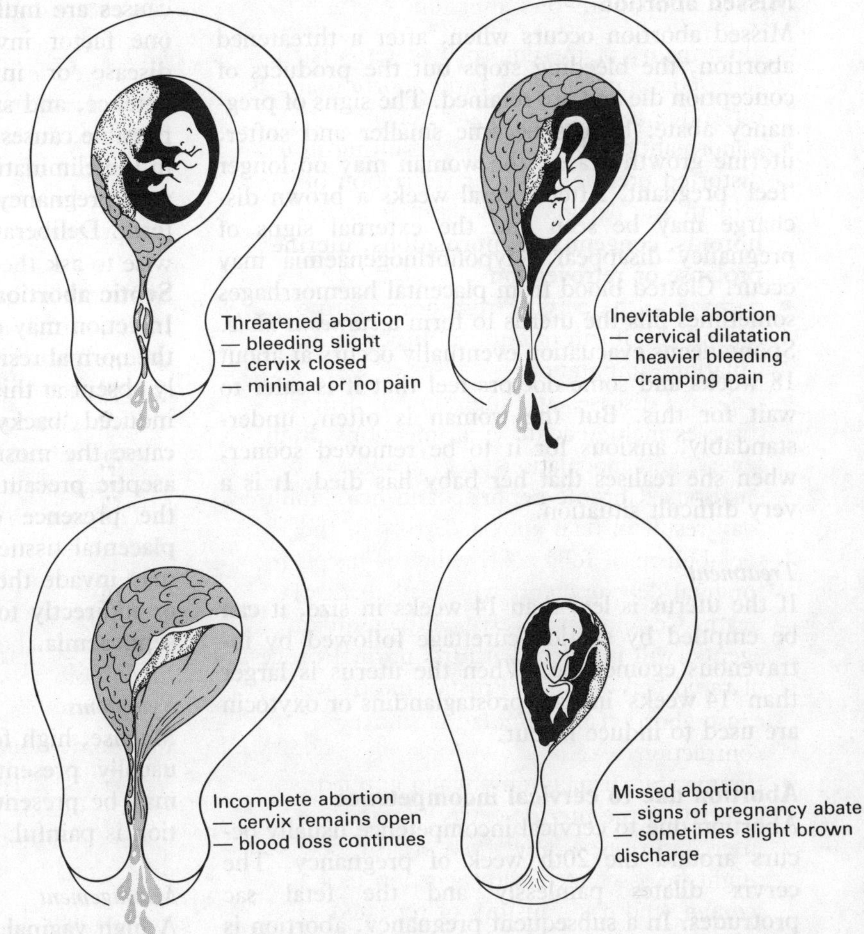

Figure 6.1 Types of abortion.

uterus is evacuated, using ovum forceps, a curette or a suction cannula; all material obtained is sent away for histological examination. Antibiotics are frequently prescribed at this stage.

While attending to all of these important physical aspects of care, consider the emotional needs of both the woman and (usually) her partner are not forgotten. Privacy and some flexibility in the hospital routine should be arranged to allow them to be together during this difficult time.

Complete abortion

Complete abortion has occurred when all the products of conception—the fetus, membranes, and placenta—have been expelled. Bleeding and pain will then cease, the cervix closes, and the uterus involutes.

Incomplete abortion

Incomplete abortion refers to the retention of part of the products of conception, almost always the placenta, which does not separate as readily in early pregnancy as it does at term. The bleeding does not progressively decrease and the cervix remains open.

Treatment, nursing care and observation are as described for inevitable abortion. The evacuation of the uterus, however, is performed immediately after diagnosis to prevent further blood loss. The woman is usually kept in hospital for a further 2 days to be observed for bleeding. Special attention is given to vulval hygiene. In some cases, suppression of lactation may be necessary. Anti-D gammaglobulin would be given to an Rh-negative woman.

Missed abortion

Missed abortion occurs when, after a threatened abortion, the bleeding stops but the products of conception die and are retained. The signs of pregnancy abate: breasts become smaller and softer, uterine growth ceases, the woman may no longer 'feel' pregnant. After several weeks a brown discharge may be seen and the external signs of pregnancy disappear. Hypofibrinogenaemia may occur. Clotted blood from placental haemorrhages sometimes fills the uterus to form a *carneous mole*. Spontaneous evacuation eventually occurs at about 18 weeks and some doctors feel that it is safer to wait for this. But the woman is often, understandably, anxious for it to be removed sooner, when she realises that her baby has died. It is a very difficult situation.

Treatment

If the uterus is less than 14 weeks in size, it can be emptied by suction curettage followed by intravenous egometrine. When the uterus is larger than '14 weeks' in size, prostaglandins or oxytocin are used to induce labour.

Abortion due to cervical incompetence

Abortion due to cervical incompetence usually occurs around the 20th week of pregnancy. The cervix dilates painlessly and the fetal sac protrudes. In a subsequent pregnancy, abortion is prevented by the insertion (under anaesthesia) of a purse-string suture around the cervix at the junction of the vaginal rugae and the smooth cervix (Shirodkar's suture). This suture is left until the 38th week of pregnancy, when it is divided and the onset of spontaneous labour anticipated. The success rate is up to 80% in cases of genuine cervical incompetence.

Where this treatment is not successful or is unsuitable, a more complicated ligature, using a polyvinyl suture, may be inserted at the level of the internal os, at a time when the woman is not pregnant. The suture is non-recoverable, and so the woman will need a caesarean section for delivery of any subsequent fetus.

Habitual abortion

This term is used when a woman has had three or more consecutive spontaneous abortions. The causes are multiple and often there is more than one factor involved. General ill-health, chronic disease or infection, anxiety, cervical incompetence, and states of hormonal imbalance are all possible causes. When careful investigation results in the elimination of even one of these factors, the next pregnancy will often continue successfully to term. Deliberate rest has some of the best results.

Septic abortion

Infection may complicate any type of abortion, as the normal resistance of the genital tract is virtually absent at this time. Criminal abortions (illegally induced 'backyard' abortions) although rare still cause the most serious infections due to lack of aseptic precautions. The other factor involved is the presence of products of conception, dead placental tissue, within the uterus. The infection may invade the endometrium and spread directly or indirectly to cause peritonitis, salpingitis, and septicaemia.

Symptoms

Malaise, high fever, tachycardia and headache are usually present. An offensive vaginal discharge may be present, but not always. Pelvic examination is painful.

Management

A high vaginal swab is taken for culture, and antibiotic therapy is commenced. Retained products are evacuated by curettage (or, if after 12 weeks, by oxytocin infusion) but, unless there is severe bleeding as well, curettage is delayed for 12–24 hours to allow the antibiotics to act. This lessens the risk of organisms entering the bloodstream and possibly causing bacteraemic (endotoxic) shock or disseminated intravascular coagulation (DIC). Both are serious and often fatal complications of septic abortion.

ECTOPIC PREGNANCY

Ectopic pregnancy occurs when a fertilised ovum embeds in a site other than the uterine cavity. The

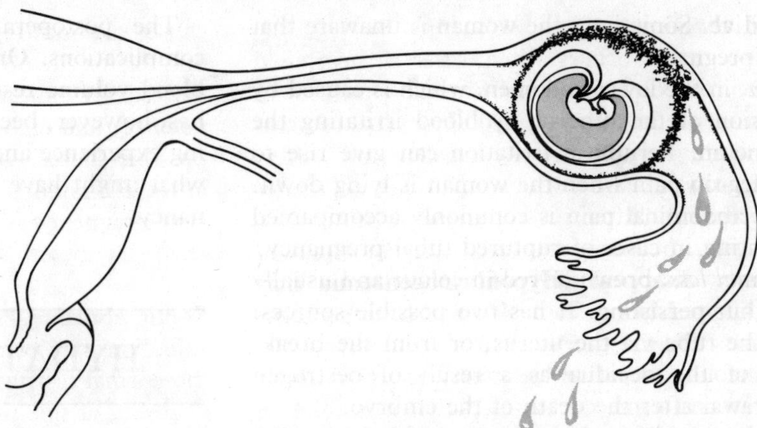

Figure 6.2 Tubal ectopic pregnancy.

pregnancy is rarely able to survive for longer than 6–10 weeks, either because the site is unsuitable for satisfactory development of the placenta, or because there is insufficient room to accommodate the growing pregnancy (Fig. 6.2).

Sites of ectopic implantation

The site may be:

- a fallopian tube
- the cervix
- the abdominal cavity
- an ovary
- a broad ligament.

Tubal pregnancy is by far the commonest of these, and so is the only one discussed here in detail; the others are rare. Abdominal pregnancies very occasionally go to term to be delivered by laparotomy; the placenta has attached itself to whichever organs would supply its needs, and so its removal poses great problems, especially the danger of haemorrhage.

TUBAL PREGNANCY

Tubal pregnancy will result in one of three outcomes:

Death of the ovum in the early stages; it then is either completely absorbed or remains as a tubal mole.

Tubal abortion, the most common outcome, with the ovum (and possibly blood) being expelled from the tube into the uterus or out into the peritoneal cavity. This usually results in its death; very occasionally it implants again and develops as a secondary abdominal pregnancy.

Tubal rupture: erosion and finally rupture of the tube occurs when the ovum continues to grow past the stretching ability of the muscular tube. The rupture of the tube is usually accompanied by rupture of one or more large arterioles, so there can be considerable blood loss which drains to the pouch of Douglas to form a pelvic haematocele.

Causes

- partial obstruction of the tube. There is enough room for the passage of spermatozoa, but not enough for the fertilised ovum. Obstruction is most often the result of old inflammation, tuberculous or other salpingitis, but is also caused by diverticuli, previous tubal surgery, kinking and pressure or adhesions from outside
- tubal endometriosis
- delay in the passage of the ovum to the uterus, e.g. unilateral development of the Mullerian system combined with ovulation from the opposite ovary.

Signs and symptoms

Pregnancy: amenorrhoea, early breast changes, uterine enlargement (due to hormonal influence) and the other signs of early pregnancy are usually present; the pregnancy may have been confirmed as positive. Sometimes the woman is unaware that she is pregnant.

Pain, in the lower abdomen, which is caused by distension of the tube or by blood irritating the peritoneum. Peritoneal irritation can give rise to shoulder-tip pain when the woman is lying down. Severe abdominal pain is commonly accompanied by fainting in cases of ruptured tubal pregnancy.

Vaginal loss, brown or red in colour and usually slight but persisting. It has two possible sources: from the tube via the uterus, or from the breakdown of the decidua as a result of oestrogen withdrawal after the death of the embryo.

Evidence of internal blood loss: the slow bleeding that follows tubal abortion or the leakage prior to rupture may cause anaemia but it is the severe bleeding that can follow tubal rupture that gives rise to collapse and shock. The abdomen is extremely tender and is distended.

Management

The woman is admitted to hospital. Shock, if present, is treated, and intravenous fluids commenced while waiting for blood cross-matching. In those cases where there is real doubt about the diagnosis, a laparoscopy may be performed. Otherwise the treatment is immediate laparotomy, excision of the affected tube, and removal of clots from the pelvic cavity. Sometimes considerable efforts are made to conserve the tube, especially where the other tube is absent or known to be damaged.

The postoperative period is usually without complications. Once the bleeding has ceased and blood volume restored, the danger has passed. It has, however, been a sudden, urgent and frightening experience and it has resulted in the ending of what might have been a very much wanted pregnancy.

HYDATIDIFORM MOLE

Very occasionally and for no known reason, an early pregnancy develops abnormally and the uterus fills with a mass of grape-like vesicles (see Fig. 5.3) which produce enormous quantities of the hormone *chorionic gonadotrophin*. The vesicles grow from the chorionic villi, which project from the outer cell mass of the blastocyst and which are normally destined to become the placenta. The embryo dies and disappears.

The uterus is larger than normal for the period of gestation, and is soft and rounded. The fetal heart is not heard, nor are fetal parts felt. Hyperemesis may occur and pre-eclampsia appears early. There may be episodes of slight, dark vaginal bleeding and, rarely, grape-like vesicles are passed vaginally. The urine pregnancy test is strongly positive.

Diagnosis is aided by ultrasonography (which

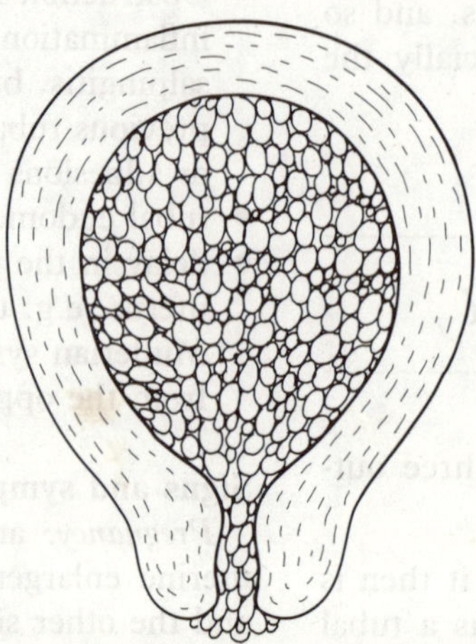

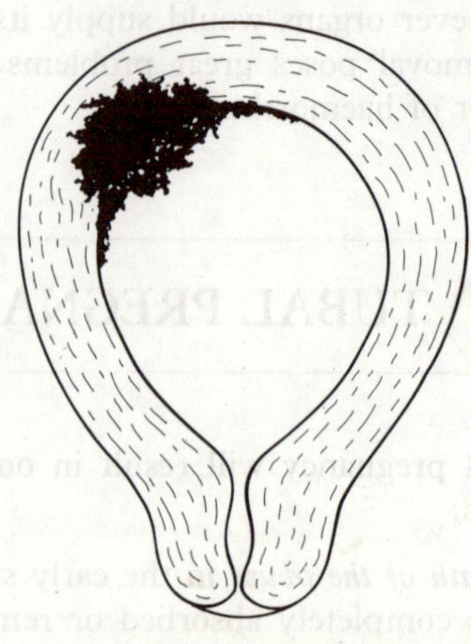

Figure 6.3 Hydatidiform mole and choriocarcinoma.

can be used as early as 8 weeks), the use of diluted urine for pregnancy tests, and X-ray of the abdomen to confirm the absence of a fetal skeleton.

Hydatidiform mole occurs on an average in about 1 in 750 pregnancies in Australia. Its incidence in South-East Asia and in the Far East, however, is far greater. It occurs more frequently in the older age group (over 35 years) and in women who have had more than one baby, although it can happen in any pregnancy.

Treatment

Once hydatidiform mole is diagnosed, it must be removed immediately because some (5%) of these moles develop into malignant trophoblastic disease—choriocarcinoma. Spontaneous delivery does occur in some cases, but may not be complete. The uterus has to be *emptied* and this is most often done by careful suction curettage. Hysterectomy is usually performed when the woman is over the age of 40.

Follow-up

After discharge from hospital, frequent (at first, weekly) follow-up examinations are essential. These will continue for 2 years, their frequency depending on the findings at each visit. The couple is warned against starting another pregnancy during this time, and family planning advice or referral is usually necessary. The doctor will observe for persistent bleeding which may indicate retained products, and for the return of normal menstruation which would be suppressed by elevated levels of HCG (human chorionic gonadotrophin). Chest X-rays are performed regularly until the urinary HCG levels are normal, to exclude pulmonary metastases of choriocarcinoma.

The routine pregnancy test cannot be used for follow-up as it is not sufficiently accurate. Precise measurements of the urinary excretion of HCG over 24 hours are performed weekly until the levels are within the normal range for the non-pregnant woman. After this the levels are measured monthly for 12 months or longer. HCG levels drop very rapidly after a normal pregnancy, usually within 2–3 days. Following a hydatidiform mole the return of these levels to normal can take from 2–6 months. If a progressive decline does not occur (or if the decline is followed by a rise), courses of methotrexate are given. Methotrexate is a folic acid antagonist, and trophoblastic (placental) tissue has high folic acid requirements. The treatment is given in hospital and daily white cell counts are performed.

7

THE PHYSIOLOGY OF NORMAL PREGNANCY

Chapter outline
Actions of hormones
Weight gain
Changes in the uterus
Changes in the vagina
Changes in the breasts
Changes in the alimentary tract
Changes in the respiratory system
Changes in the skin
Changes in the skeleton and joints
Changes in the metabolism
Changes in the cardiovascular system
Calculation of confinement date

Key words

Braxton-Hicks contractions	oestriols
chloasma	operculum
colostrum	uterine isthmus
hyperemesis	

Pregnancy affects the whole of the mother's body, causing physiologic changes in virtually all organ systems. The mother's body has to:

- protect the developing embryo/fetus
- provide all of its necessities
- adapt to make room for it as it grows
- prepare to feed it when it is born.

Most of the changes in the mother's body are temporary, and most are caused by the action of hormones. (The usual management of the minor disorders caused by the physiological changes can be found in Table 8.2.)

ACTIONS OF HORMONES

During the first weeks, the corpus luteum in the ovary produces oestrogens and progesterone. Their main function at this stage is to maintain the growth of the decidua and to prevent it breaking down and being shed. The trophoblast cells produce chorionic gonadotrophin, which maintains the corpus luteum until the placenta is fully developed and has taken over the production of oestrogens and progesterone from the corpus luteum.

When the placenta takes over, there is a marked increase in the output of oestrogens and progesterone. The levels of these hormones remain high until just before term, when the placenta, which has a limited lifespan, starts to decline in its function. When this occurs, the placental hormone levels begin to fall.

Oestrogens

Oestrogens are an influencing factor in:

- uterine growth
- breast growth
- water and sodium retention
- pituitary hormone release.

Oestriol, the main oestrogenic hormone of pregnancy, is a product resulting from the interaction of the placenta and the fetal adrenal glands. Oestriol levels can be measured in the urine and the blood, and are an important indication of placental function and fetal well-being, especially in later pregnancy.

Progesterone

Progesterone affects the mother's body by the:

- relaxation of smooth muscle (with widespread effects, see Fig. 7.1)
- relaxation of connective tissue
- elevation of temperature
- development of the lactiferous ducts and alveoli
- secretory changes within the breasts.

Other placental hormones

In addition to chorionic gonadotrophin, oestrogens and progesterone, the placenta produces two other specific hormones–*placental lactogenic hormone* and *relaxin*.

Placental lactogenic hormone promotes growth, stimulates development of the breast and is important in maternal fat metabolism. Levels of placental lactogenic hormone can be measured to assess fetal and placental functioning.

As its name implies, relaxin has a relaxant effect, especially upon connective tissue.

Other endocrine changes

The pituitary gland secretions are generally increased, and this in turn causes increased secretion

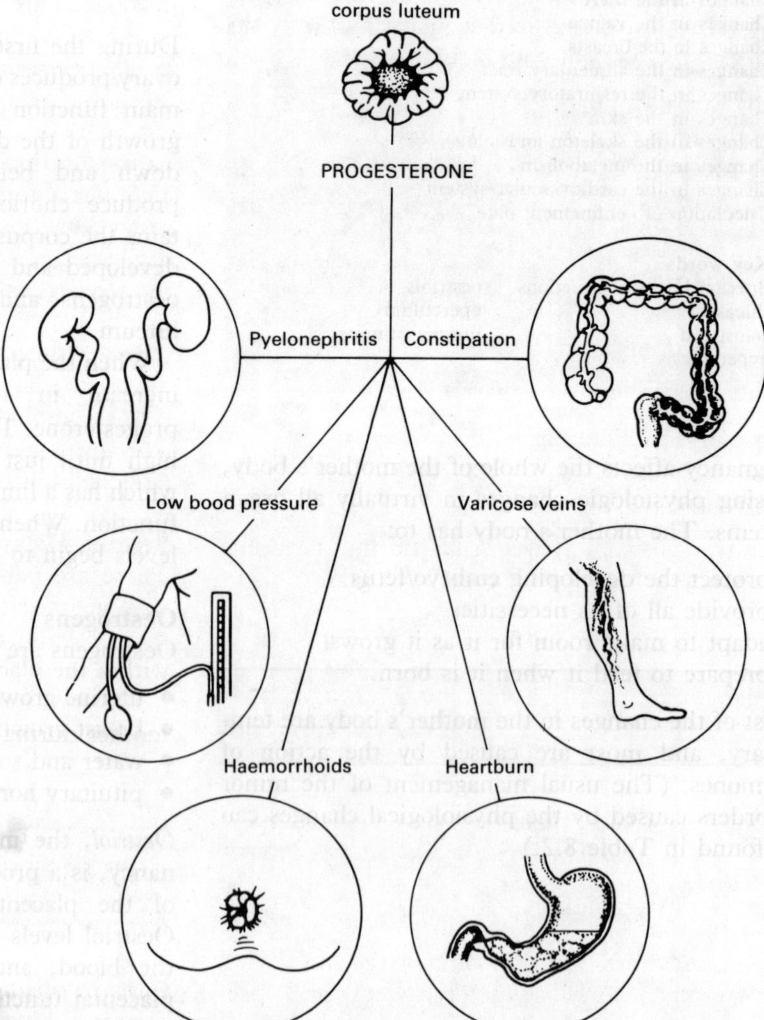

Figure 7.1 Diagrammatic representation of the effect of progesterone on plain muscle fibres during pregnancy.

from all endocrine glands (especially the thyroid, parathyroid and adrenal glands). Levels of the pituitary hormone, *prolactin*, increase gradually towards the end of pregnancy, but prolactin's function of initiation of lactation is suppressed until after the placenta is delivered and the level of oestrogen has fallen.

WEIGHT GAIN

The increase in the mother's weight is normally equivalent to 25% of her pre-pregnant weight. The main increase is in the second half of pregnancy. In an average-sized woman, by term, the breakdown of weight gain is as follows:

- the uterine contents:

the fetus	3.5 kg
liquor	1.0 kg
placenta	0.5 kg

- the growth of:

the uterus	1.0 kg
the breasts	0.5–1.0 kg

- maternal storage of fats and protein — 3.0 kg
- increase in maternal blood volume and interstitial fluid — 2.0 kg

The average total weight gain during a normal pregnancy is between 11 and 12 kilograms.

CHANGES IN THE UTERUS

Size:	non-pregnant	8 × 5 × 3 cm
	at term	30 × 22 × 20 cm
Weight:	non-pregnant	50 g
	at term	1 kg

The muscle fibres multiply, grow large and stretch due to the stimulus of oestrogens and progesterone, and because of the mechanical pressure from within–the fetus, placenta and liquor all taking up more room.

The *uterine wall* gets thinner and softer as the uterus enlarges. At term the wall is less than 0.5 cm thick. Uterine blood vessels dilate enormously to supply a greatly increased volume of blood to the placenta.

Cervix

The cervix is mainly fibrous. In preparation for labour, oestrogens and the placental hormone relaxin cause it to become softer.

A plug of mucus, the operculum, is formed by the 8th week from the secretions of the cervical glands. It remains in the cervix until labour commences, when cervical dilatation causes it to dislodge. This 'show' of cervical mucus can be one of the early signs of labour. The operculum acts as a physical barrier, sealing off the uterus from ascending organisms.

Lower uterine segment

The uterus forms into two segments during pregnancy. The lower uterine segment develops from the upper part of the cervical canal at the level of the internal os, together with the uterine isthmus (see p. 17). The lower segment is thinner than the upper segment and becomes soft and dilated during the last weeks of pregnancy, thus allowing it to accommodate the presenting part of the fetus. The lower part of the cervix is not thinned and stretched until labour occurs.

Braxton-Hicks contractions

These are painless, irregular contractions of the uterine muscle occurring throughout pregnancy; they probably assist in the circulation of the blood within the placenta.

Braxton-Hicks contractions are felt by the mother during the last few weeks of pregnancy.

CHANGES IN THE VAGINA

Early in pregnancy, the vagina and cervix become almost a blue colour (they are normally a pink colour in the non-pregnant woman). This blueness is caused by venous dilatation due to the action of progesterone. The normal acidic vaginal secretions increase significantly.

Thrush

Thrush, or monilial vaginitis, is common in pregnancy. It is due to the overgrowth of a fungus, *Candida albicans*. Although this fungus is normal flora for the bowel, and not the vagina, *Candida albicans* can exist in the vagina without causing problems unless there are conditions which favour its growth.

Pregnancy, with its high levels of both oestrogen and glucose in the circulation, supplies these favourable conditions and *Candida albicans* increases to cause local irritation, a scant, white, cheesy discharge, occasionally red raw patches on the vaginal walls, and intense pruritus.

CHANGES IN THE BREASTS

The changes in the breasts leading to lactation are caused by the increased levels of oestrogens, progesterone, placental lactogen and prolactin. This hormonal stimulation leads to the proliferation of the breast tissue, dilatation of the blood vessels and secretory changes. Slight enlargement of the breasts, increased sensation and tingling may be experienced, especially by the primigravida, as early as the 4th week of pregnancy. A clear fluid is present in the breasts at 4 weeks, and colostrum can be expressed at 16 weeks.

Appearance

The breasts grow throughout pregnancy, increasing in size and weight by about 500 g each. Surface veins are visible at about 8 weeks. The nipples become larger, more erect and darker in colour. The areolae become darker and are surrounded by prominent sebaceous glands (Montgomery's tubercles), which appear at about 12 weeks (see Fig. 7.2).

CHANGES IN THE URINARY TRACT

Changes in the urinary tract have both hormonal

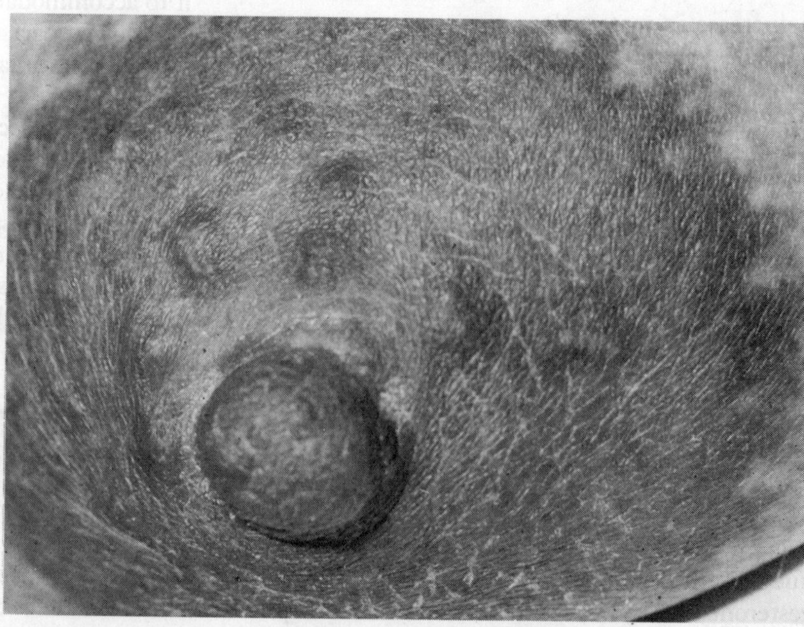

Figure 7.2 Nipple changes during pregnancy: darkening of the areolae and prominence of the sebaceous glands (Montgomery's tubercles).

and mechanical causes, and give rise to urinary problems. Although there is an increased blood flow to the kidneys, extra urine is not produced, because the retention of sodium and water is increased.

Urinary tract infection
Progesterone, with its relaxant effect on all smooth muscle fibres, causes the ureters to become dilated, elongated and kinked (Fig. 7.3). Pooling of urine occurs in the lower ureters, and loss of muscle tone in the bladder may lead to incomplete emptying. Both of these factors make the woman prone to urinary tract infection or to the resurgence of previous infection. Pyelonephritis can occur, and for this reason catheterisation during pregnancy is avoided unless absolutely necessary.

Frequency of micturition
As the uterus enlarges in the early months of pregnancy it occupies more of the pelvis. Thus there is less room for the bladder to enlarge and bladder pressure is felt more frequently. After 3 months the uterus has risen out of the pelvis and bladder function returns to normal. Frequency occurs again near term when the presenting part of the fetus enters the pelvis.

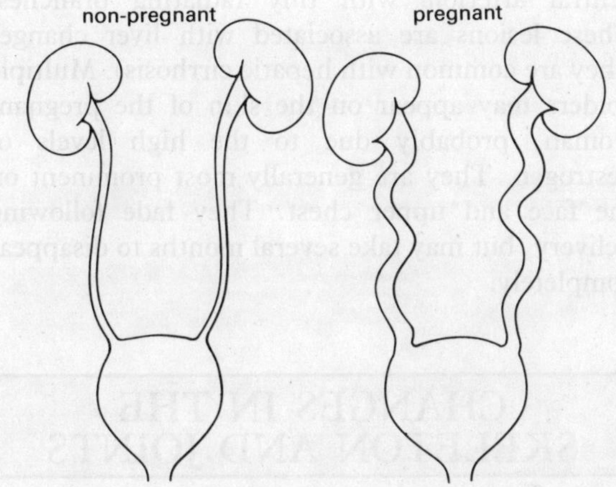

Figure 7.3 Dilatation, elongation and kinking of the ureters during pregnancy.

Stress incontinence
Inability to control the flow of urine, especially under the stress of sudden increased intra-abdominal pressure (such as when laughing or sneezing), may occur towards the end of pregnancy. This is due to the reduction of muscle tone in the pelvic floor (due to progesterone) and to the increased pressure from the weight of the uterine contents.

CHANGES IN THE ALIMENTARY TRACT

The changes in the alimentary tract are also due to both hormonal and mechanical causes.

Morning sickness
Nausea or vomiting occurring in the early months of pregnancy (and usually only on rising) is common and is usually mild. Its exact cause is not known, but it is most likely a reaction to the suddenly increased hormonal levels. If morning sickness persists beyond the 14th week, or if it is severe (hyperemesis), it is regarded as abnormal and requires active treatment.

Gastric acid reflux
Gastric acid reflux ('heartburn') is caused by regurgitation of stomach contents into the lower end of the oesophagus. Progesterone has caused both relaxation of the cardiac sphincter of the stomach and reduced stomach motility thus delaying gastric emptying. Also, the mechanical pressure of the enlarged uterus from below displaces the stomach upwards.

Heartburn usually appears only in the last month or two of pregnancy. It can be most unpleasant.

Constipation
Constipation is common, and is due to the reduced motility of the intestines, allowing more time for fluid to be absorbed. There is also 'crowding' of the intestines by pressure from the enlarged uterus.

CHANGES IN THE RESPIRATORY SYSTEM

The enlarging uterus pushes the diaphragm upwards, changing the shape of the thorax, but not reducing lung capacity. The respiratory rate is increased in order to obtain the higher amount of oxygen necessary; this can result in slight hyperventilation.

CHANGES IN THE SKIN

Pigmentation
The anterior pituitary gland, stimulated by the high levels of oestrogen, increases its output of melanophore stimulating hormone (MSH). The effect of this varies according to the natural colour of the woman's skin. Darker pigmentation occurs:

- in the nipples and areolae (Fig. 7.2)
- on the face (chloasma–the 'mask of pregnancy') (Fig. 7.4)
- on the abdominal midline (from above the umbilicus to the pubic hair)–the *linea nigra*.

Pigmentation usually fades following delivery, but the nipples of a parous woman always remain brown.

Stretch marks
Striae gravidarum, commonly called stretch marks, may appear on the abdomen (Fig. 7.5), breasts and buttocks.

The skin in these areas becomes very stretched, and the collagen fibres may rupture. The marks are red initially, but fade to a silvery appearance following delivery. Stretch marks are not caused by stretching itself, but are associated with increased secretion from the adrenal cortex. They also appear as a prominent symptom in disorders associated with the adrenal gland, e.g. Cushing's syndrome.

Spider naevi
Spider naevi is a bright red skin lesion with a central arteriole with tiny radiating branches. These lesions are associated with liver changes (they are common with hepatic cirrhosis). Multiple spiders may appear on the skin of the pregnant woman, probably due to the high levels of oestrogen. They are generally most prominent on the face and upper chest. They fade following delivery, but may take several months to disappear completely.

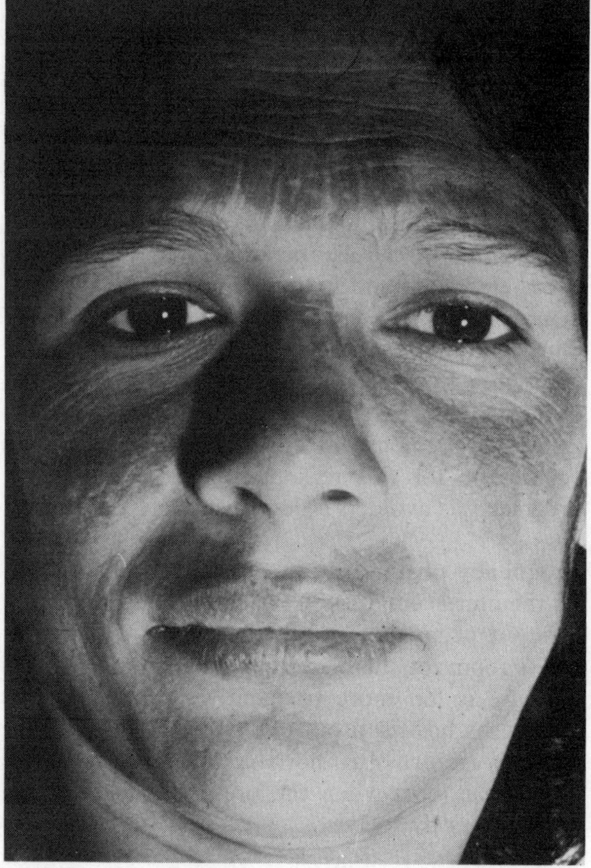

Figure 7.4 Brown pigmentation on the skin: chloasma, the 'mask of pregnancy'.

CHANGES IN THE SKELETON AND JOINTS

The weight of the uterus and its contents causes an alteration in the centre of gravity and in the

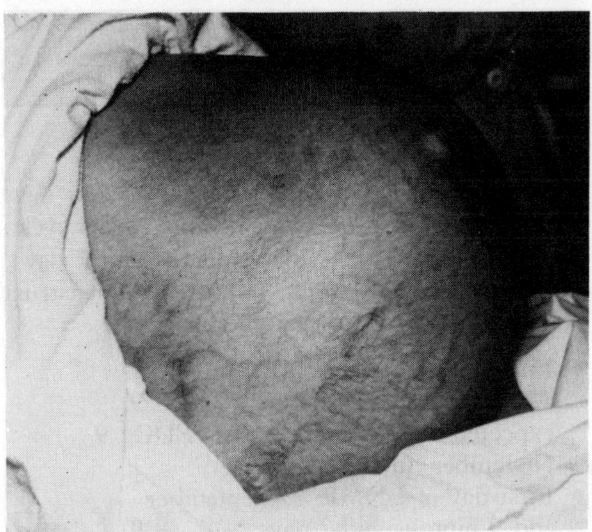

Figure 7.5 Abdominal striae.

contour of the body. The spinal curvature is changed to compensate for the abdominal enlargement and, towards the end of pregnancy, many women adopt a typical posture (called lordosis), standing and walking with the back arched and the shoulders held backwards.

As well, the connective tissue in the pelvic joints softens in preparation for labour. The symphysis pubis and sacro-iliac joints become slightly mobile, and the pelvis becomes wider.

These changes can give rise to rolling, unstable movement when walking, and to backache.

CHANGES IN THE METABOLISM

The body of the healthy pregnant woman is functioning at its maximum efficiency. The basal metabolic rate is 15–25% higher than usual in the second half of pregnancy, thus the woman's dietary intake must be sufficient to cope with the extra physiological activity.

Carbohydrate metabolism

The causes of the radical changes in carbohydrate metabolism during pregnancy are not fully understood.

The woman's blood sugar level is higher than in the non-pregnant state, possibly due to an insulin-antagonist produced by the placenta. The result is that more sugar is present in the maternal blood for a longer time, enabling more to be passed to the fetus.

Glycosuria is common, and is due to both the higher blood sugar levels and the increased amount of blood (see below) being circulated through the kidneys. The renal threshold is lowered, and a blood sugar level of about 6.7 mmol/litre is normal.

Gestational diabetes, i.e. diabetes which manifests for the first time during pregnancy, is discussed on page 94.

Protein and fat metabolism

Protein tends to be built up during pregnancy because of the demands of both fetal and maternal growth. Nitrogen storage occurs (also not fully understood) in anticipation of milk production; therefore the blood urea concentration is reduced.

Fat stores are increased, and there are high blood levels of lipoids and cholesterol, with less fat being converted to glycogen for storage. Fat may be metabolised for use more readily than in non-pregnant women, and there is therefore a tendency to ketosis, especially when the need for energy is greater than that which can be supplied by the limited glycogen stores.

CHANGES IN THE CARDIOVASCULAR SYSTEM

Haemodilution

The blood volume increases during pregnancy by about 40–50% to meet the requirements of the placental circulation.

The plasma volume is increased more than the red cell volume (which increases by approximately 30%); therefore there is a state of haemodilution, with the haemoglobin lowered to about 80% of its normal level. This situation is called *physiological anaemia of pregnancy*, and is probably responsible for the episodes of tiredness and fainting that some women experience.

Blood pressure
Cardiac output is increased because of the increased blood volume. The heart has to pump with more force, especially near term, and it dilates slightly. Progesterone relaxes the smooth muscles and causes dilatation of the blood vessel walls which compensates for the increased force from the heart; so the blood pressure should remain at, or close to, the prepregnant reading. Even so, the woman is prone to supine hypotension when she is lying on her back, because of the pressure of the heavy uterine contents on the inferior vena cava.

Blood coagulability
The coagulability of blood is slightly increased during pregnancy. If it failed to increase, there would be danger of excessive bleeding at the time of delivery. Because coagulability *does* increase, the danger of venous thrombosis is present. Therefore careful observation and education (about immobility, garters, and so on) are important aspects of preventive care during pregnancy, labour and the postnatal period.

CALCULATION OF CONFINEMENT DATE

Calculating by dates
The average duration of pregnancy is 266 days after fertilisation of the ovum or (in a 28-day cycle) 280 days, or 40 weeks, or 9 months and 7 days, from the first day of the last normal menstrual period (LNMP). Two examples are:

- First day of LNMP: 2 February
  add 9 months and 7 days: + 7, + 9
  expected date of confinement (EDC): 9 November (in the same year)
- First day of LNMP: 27 September
  add 9 months and 7 days: + 7, + 9
  expected date of confinement: 4 July (in the following year)

Quickening
There are times when the menstrual history is uncertain: when the woman does not remember her dates, when she has recently ceased oral contraceptives, or when the pregnancy occurred before menstruation had returned following a pre-

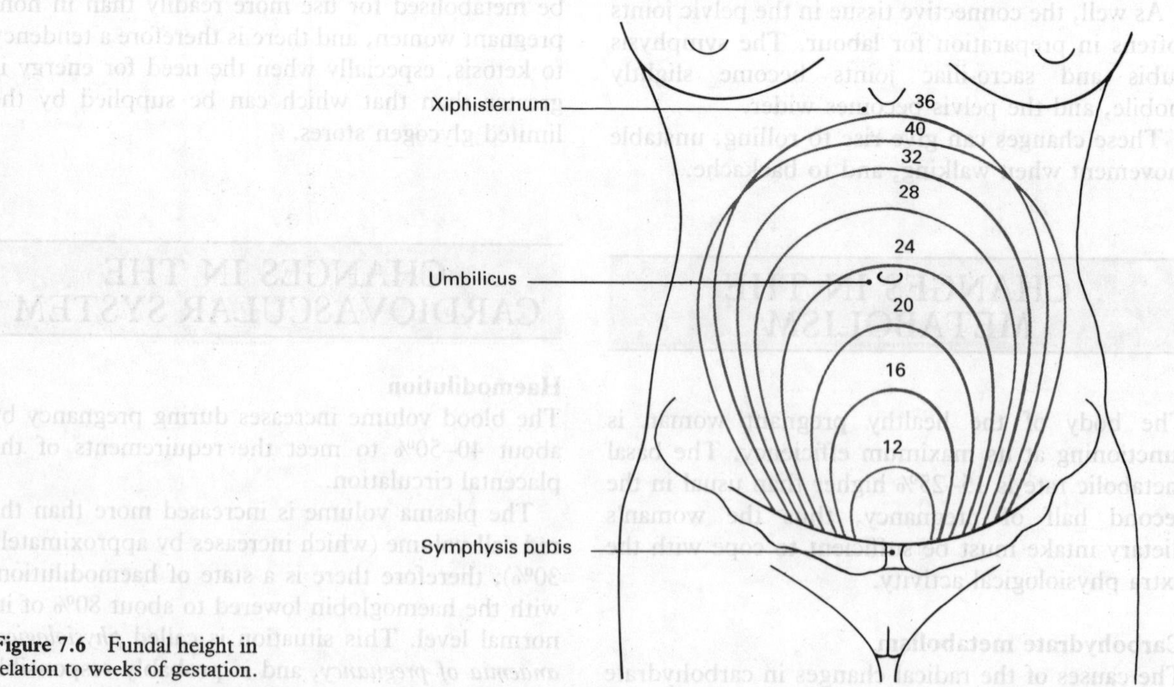

Figure 7.6 Fundal height in relation to weeks of gestation.

vious pregnancy. In such cases she would be asked to be alert for quickening (the first fetal movements she feels) and to record the date on which it happens. 5 calendar months are added to the date of quickening to arrive at the expected date of confinement.

Fundal height

The height of the uterine fundus, in relation to various landmarks (Fig. 7.6), is measured at each visit. The uterus grows steadily and predictably and fundal height is generally a good guide to gestation. Variations from normal (as may happen with multiple pregnancies or where there is an excess of amniotic fluid) are indications for further investigation.

X-ray evidence

X-rays will show the ossification of various parts of the fetal skeleton from as early as 16 weeks, but are almost never used to assess gestation because of the hazards involved.

Ultrasound

The fetal sac can be seen as early as 6–7 weeks and the fetal head measured by 13 weeks using ultrasound–high frequency, short wavelength, sound wave reflections. Ultrasound is a non-invasive method of investigation.

Ultrasound has now virtually replaced X-rays in the assessment of fetal maturity.

Table 7.1 The principal signs and symptoms of pregnancy

	0–4	4–8	8–12	12–16	16–20	20–24	24–28	28–32	32–36	36–40
Pregnancy is possible										
Absence of menstruation		✓	✓	✓	✓	✓	✓	✓	✓	✓
Tingling of breasts		✓								
Morning sickness		✓	✓							
Enlargement of breasts		✓	✓	✓	✓	✓	✓	✓	✓	✓
Frequency of micturition		✓	✓							✓
Nipple pigmentation			✓	✓	✓	✓	✓	✓	✓	✓
Colostrum in breasts					✓	✓	✓	✓	✓	✓
Quickening					✓					
Pregnancy is probable										
Pregnancy test positive		✓	✓	✓	✓	✓	✓	✓	✓	✓
Uterus felt abdominally				✓	✓	✓	✓	✓	✓	✓
Braxton-Hicks contractions						✓	✓	✓	✓	✓
Pregnancy is positive										
Fetal heart heard (aurally)							✓	✓	✓	✓
Fetal movements felt (by an observer)						✓	✓	✓	✓	✓
Fetal parts felt							✓	✓	✓	✓
X-ray evidence					✓	✓	✓	✓	✓	✓
Ultrasonic evidence			✓	✓	✓	✓	✓	✓	✓	✓

Table 7.2 Minor disorders related to the physiology of pregnancy

Symptom	Occurs (usually)	Common causes	Specific management	Nursing aspects and advice
Morning sickness (nausea and vomiting)	Early	Response to hormones, psychological influence as well	Dietary, if vomiting persists anti-emetics may be ordered	Advice on nutrition, small but more frequent meals, something solid before rising; to report of it persists or worsens; warn that anti-emetics may cause drowsiness
Food cravings	Any time	Taste bud response to hormones; may be attention-seeking in some	Advice and reassurance	Ensure (without preaching) that a proper diet is not affected by wrong foods
Heartburn	Later months	Progesterone and pressure	Dietary, antacids sometimes	Advice about nutrition, small meals, plenty of milk, avoid spicy, fried or fatty foods, raise head of bed
Constipation	Later months	Progesterone and crowding of bowel, iron tablets	Dietary, occasionally mild laxatives	Advice—high-fibre diet, bran, fruits, vegetables, extra fluids; encourage deliberate exercise
Haemorrhoids	Later months	Progestrone and impeded venous return	Dietary; haemorrhoid creams or suppositories; digital replacement, occasionally surgery if thrombosed	Advice on avoidance of constipation, application of ice packs may help
Varicose veins	Mid to later months	Progesterone and impeded venous return	Elastic stockings	Advice—avoiding long periods of standing; elevation of legs when possible; teaching application of elastic stockings with legs elevated; warning about garters
Vulval varicose veins	Later months	Progesterone plus impeded venous return	If very painful may be injected, otherwise firm pressure to area; care during delivery (avoiding cutting episiotomy near varicose veins)	Advice on application of firmly held perineal pad, stretch pants
Fainting	Early and late	Vasodilation, hypotension, haemodilution	Reassurance, sometimes iron supplements, lying down when giddy; exclusion of serious causes, cardiac, pre-eclampsia, hypoglycaemia, anaemia	Advice on avoiding situations which make it worse (e.g. heat), explanation of causes, avoid long periods between taking food, avoid constrictive clothing
Insomnia	Early and late	Pressure on bladder, pruritus, worry, fetal movements, cramps, heartburn	Investigation and treatment of cause; rarely, sedation; milk drink before going to bed may help	Reinforcement of medical advice; ensuring that simple ways of relieving symptoms are understood; referral to social worker if appropriate
Muscle cramps	Late	Not understood; transient local ischaemia, calcium demands	Calcium, vitamins, sometimes prescribed, their value still uncertain	Advice—not to use proprietary medicines without medical permission; symptomatic relief—heat, massage, pulling upwards on toes
Frequency of micturition	Early, then late	Progesterone and pressure	Exclusion of infection	Advice—decrease fluid intake after evening meal, avoid drinks containing caffeine
Stress incontinence	Later months	Progesterone and pressure, plus multiparity	Physiotherapy; reviewed after pregnancy	Advice—on pelvic floor exercises, protective pads and hygiene; skin care if indicated

Table 7.2 (*contd*)

Symptom	Occurs (usually)	Common causes	Specific management	Nursing aspects and advice
Vaginal discharge	Any time	Physiological (oestrogen); thrush common, glycosuria, antibiotics, infection: trichomonas, gonorrhoea	Reassurance, exclusion (or treatment) of infection; thrush—antifungal medication, creams or suppositories; oral antifungals to prevent reinfection from bowel; acidic vaginal jelly, yoghurt, gentian violet, may be prescribed	Advice—explanation of physiological increase in vaginal secretions; care with hygiene, laundry; avoidance of tight jeans, pantyhose and synthetic underwear; no soap; management of pruritus
Pruritus	Any time	Generalised—drugs, liver dysfunction; vulval—poor hygiene, thrush or trichomonas, diabetes,	Antipruritic skin applications; sedation if associated insomnia is serious	Advice—cool baths rather than hot showers, no soap, light cotton underwear, hygiene, avoidance of proprietary preparations without doctor's permission
Backache	Late	Progesterone and relaxin (softening connective tissue) and altered posture	Exclusion of serious causes, physiotherapy, local heat, analgesia, rest	Advice—posture, sensible (low-heeled) shoes, ways to achieve rest, advantages of wearing a maternity girdle, board under mattress if necessary

8

SOCIAL AND EMOTIONAL ASPECTS OF PREGNANCY

Chapter outline
Responses to pregnancy
Social effects of being pregnant
Reaction to physical changes
The prospect of labour
Subsequent pregnancies
Psychological problems during pregnancy

RESPONSES TO PREGNANCY

Everybody responds differently to the diagnosis of pregnancy: there are probably as many different responses to the diagnosis of pregnancy as there are babies conceived. But one fact remains constant and that is that life, for the parents, from this moment will never be the same. There may be delight at the achievement of a much-wanted and planned pregnancy, or there may be shock, even to the point of near despair, at the news and the anticipation of huge social and financial problems.

Ambivalence

Sometimes the woman's response may be ambivalent, even when the pregnancy was planned. Now that it is a fact a number of the wider implications of being pregnant have to be faced. These can include the effect upon career plans, financial considerations, relationships with others, especially with family members, the inevitable physical progress of pregnancy with its body changes and discomforts, and the prospect of labour and delivery. There is, as well, the realisation of forthcoming responsibility for the child which will be born, and the expectations of other people in the parents', particularly the mother's, ability to manage in what might be to her an entirely unfamiliar area and one in which, until now, she has had little interest. So even when all around her show their excitement and joy at the news of the pregnancy, the mother-to-be may herself take longer.

Acceptance

Mixed or ambivalent feelings normally resolve as the pregnancy progresses and the mother's body begins to adapt to the changes. As her abdomen begins to enlarge, and as certain positive events such as seeing ultrasound pictures, feeling fetal movements or hearing the amplified fetal heart beat occur, she begins to accept the fetus as a potential child and so begins to prepare herself for the coming baby. In some cases the mother's feelings may turn in upon herself for a period. If this quite normal and usually brief introspective phase is prolonged or is misunderstood by her husband or partner, the couple's relationship may be strained.

Emotional lability

Emotional lability, feeling happy and feeling miserable—sometimes almost feeling both at once, is also common and also can strain relationships. Most people allow a pregnant woman some margin for her emotional state, acknowledging the hormonal changes and physiological demands that are being made upon her body, but to the woman herself such mood swings are upsetting and may make her feel inadequate.

SOCIAL EFFECTS OF BEING PREGNANT

The effects of pregnancy upon a woman's daily life depend, very much, upon her social support framework. To go into pregnancy knowing that this baby is wanted by herself and her husband, and will be welcomed by their parents, wider families and friends is ideal. It helps, too, to know that the pregnancy will not cause a great financial burden, that she can give up her paid employment for the time being at least, that their housing will be suitable and that they can afford to buy the good food that she should be eating.

Not all mothers-to-be have this ideal set of circumstances. Not every pregnant woman is in a stable relationship or has a close or good relationship with her own parents or family. Or she may feel the disapproval of friends or companions when they hear about the pregnancy. She may have very few people to turn to for company and help. Some may urge her to terminate the pregnancy and, when she refuses to do that, might withdraw their support. Or perhaps she is pushed towards a marriage that she or her partner do not want, and again, if she or they do not co-operate, she could be left to cope very much on her own.

Career

A woman's career prospects or advancement can certainly be limited by pregnancy, despite the usually generous conditions of maternity leave (where it applies). The effect of pregnancy upon her work and work upon her pregnancy depends to a large degree upon the type of work the mother does and the people with whom she works. In many cases she is able to remain working well into the pregnancy, especially if the work is not physically demanding and she is able to rest well at night. Leaving work may be welcomed at first, but quite often leaves a gap in a pregnant woman's life as she misses both her work companions, the discipline of a daily routine, and (possibly) the feeling of having a 'function in life'. If her husband is away from home all day, she may find the time drags and loneliness can become a problem.

On the other hand, the woman may find that she now has time and opportunity to resume or take up personal interests, hobbies, activities, or further education which can be continued after the baby is born.

Financial aspects

Financial aspects can became critical when a pregnancy occurs unexpectedly and where commitments (e.g. mortgage, car, bank loan repayments) are beyond the means of a single income. Or, in the case of a woman on her own, there may be no prospect of income apart from the supporting parent's benefit. If the mother has to leave work she may no longer be able to afford the accommodation she has now, and may have to find cheaper housing, perhaps in an area or type of dwelling where she feels vulnerable. She may be unable to keep up hire purchase or credit card commitments and may well need skilled financial advice to prevent her getting behind in payments. To save money, she may start to deprive herself of the very nutrition she needs, eating cheaper starchy foods instead of the protein and calcium-rich fresh foods important both for her body and her baby. The financial considerations arising when an unexpected pregnancy occurs in a family which had decided to have no more children can also be significant. There may need to be extensions made to a house, or perhaps even a move made to a larger house to accommodate an extra child, perhaps just as the mother was about to or had even started paid work again.

Relationships with others

Relationships with others will inevitably change because of a pregnancy. No longer will the couple be quite as free to continue with their former social or wider family activities, or even responsibilities, in quite the same way. The anticipation of a new family unit, and the financial and physical preparations involved will consume some of their interest, energy, enthusiasm and money, thus displacing their former activities to some degree. They may find themselves drawn to the company of others who have recently had children and discussing matters to do with childbirth and baby care and the relative merits of various items of baby equipment, rather than being available to join groups who (for example) are planning ski-ing holidays.

Jealousy, sometimes from quite unexpected sources, is another problem with which expectant parents may have to cope. It can come from those who cannot, for whatever reason, have babies or further babies, or from those who envy the couple their current happiness, stage of life, youth and prospects for the future. Jealousy can be hard to deal with and very hurtful.

Family relationships may be affected when the couple's parents are made to feel left-out, even offended, when their advice and related experiences are ignored or countered with the 'new' ideas learnt at antenatal classes or from younger friends. Where relationships have been fairly satisfactory until now, differing opinions about the conduct of pregnancy or planning for the baby may cause tension and stress. Sometimes the daughter or daughter-in-law is not able to cope with criticism or direction until she is more confident in herself and more secure with her pregnancy.

Most relationship problems sort themselves out during pregnancy, especially if others allow the couple time to adapt to their changed status. By the end of pregnancy the majority of couples find themselves surrounded by a circle of supportive and concerned people who have subsumed their personal ideas and lessened their pressures upon them.

Fears and worries

The pregnant woman and her husband may suffer from fears, worries and emotional responses which she or they may feel unable to share with their family and friends. They may be ashamed to be seen as weak or irrational when pregnancy and birth are such normal and widespread occurrences and ones which other people seem to take in their stride.

REACTION TO PHYSICAL CHANGES

The common disorders and discomforts of pregnancy such as nausea, constipation, insomnia, backache, to name a few, arise as a result of physiological changes, but do not affect all women to the same degree. If they are not easily managed or controlled they can make life miserable, no matter how much the pregnancy and baby are welcomed and wanted. Most women do not want to be seen as, the 'complaining type', or may fear that if they cannot cope with these discomforts in silence they will not be very successful in the larger task, of labour, which lies ahead.

Body image is another aspect of pregnancy which can take some time to adapt to. Changes in the size and shape of the breasts and abdomen, deposition of fat, stretch marks and skin pigmentation, and perhaps becoming generally awkward, can be of significance to a woman whose ideal image of herself is one of neatness in shape and presentation and who is competent and in control. She may also fear that she is less attractive to her husband or partner. Generally these worries and fears are ill-founded but some women do need to bring them to the surface and need reassurance.

THE PROSPECT OF LABOUR

Antenatal care and education are planned to bring to labour a woman who is physically and emotionally well prepared to undergo this normal event. These days her husband or partner is also included in the antenatal programme so that he, as a well-informed labour companion, can share the experience, the stresses and the joys, and they can both be involved in the initial and powerful bonding with their baby.

Deep in all of us is the knowledge that labour is a very hard job of work. From earliest times it has been described as 'travail'–as painful, tedious and wearying–which it certainly can be. It also is not entirely risk-free for either the mother or the baby. Antenatal and obstetric care has minimised the risks of childbirth, but sometimes this has been achieved by using unnatural or interventive management which the couple may not fully understand or appreciate.

Antenatal preparation should dispel fear and ignorance and, in most cases, does. Anticipating a first labour is, however, contemplating the unknown and there are many influences apart from formal antenatal education upon the couple. They will find themselves to be the target for well-meant but often confusing information from family and friends, whose experiences may have been coloured as time has passed, or who have been influenced by the personalities of caregivers that this mother-to-be is unlikely to encounter. The couple is likely to hear not only long-labour horror stories, but also about personal labour triumphs, analgesia-free beautiful birth experiences, and the mother may worry that she will be unable to 'perform' so well or that she will be a 'failure' in the challenge of natural childbirth. A further concern is when her husband is all fired up at the prospect of his success as a labour 'coach', and she is not as confident as he is about the experience.

The best way for the fears and worries about labour to be minimised or dispelled is for the couple to have trust–trust in the ability of her body to function normally, in her doctor and midwives as being experienced professionals in this area, and in the hospital which she has chosen to be a suitable setting for her experience of childbirth. With such trust the couple will have the ability to relax, thus giving her and her body the best chance of labouring well.

SUBSEQUENT PREGNANCIES

The concerns of a couple who have already had a child are usually quite different from those of first-time parents. There are certain assumptions made by others about the mother who has already experienced pregnancy and labour, and she is much less likely to have to suffer unsolicited advice and opinions. On the other hand, this next pregnancy will probably attract less in the way of sympathy, attention and advice. She is usually expected to be very business-like about this pregnancy, in managing her child or children and not allowing the physical discomforts to interfere with daily life. In most cases the mother does adapt well and with far less evidence of emotional and social effects, her first experience having prepared her for this time.

Where the first child or children are still small, daily life has most likely been dominated by them and their needs. The mother's response to another pregnancy will often be not so much one of concern for the effect upon herself but upon the changes it will mean for her existing child or children. She will wonder how she will have both time and energy to devote to another child when the present one takes so much out of her. She may also wonder if she has the capacity to share her love between more than one baby. She may doubt her ability to keep up high or even moderately good standards in household matters when she remembers how tired she was during the early months at home with the first baby.

The mother may also worry about how her existing child will fare during her time in hospital. It is not always easy to find satisfactory child carers to cover the whole hospital stay and, if her husband is not able to have time off work, the child might have to stay with other people. This may have to be away from his or her familiar surroundings and out of normal routine for sleeping, eating and activity. Another problem may be to find someone who will stand by to take over at short notice when the labour starts, at any time of night or day.

Small children do react to the sudden absence of their mothers, and this can take the form of regressional behaviour in such areas as toilet training and speech progress, and the child may show jealousy and become generally naughty and difficult to handle. As much preparation for the event should be given as is appropriate to the child's age and understanding, but parents can be assured that if they keep things in perspective the family unit will certainly survive the addition of another baby.

PSYCHOLOGICAL PROBLEMS DURING PREGNANCY

Psychological, as distinct from social and emotional, problems are uncommon during pregnancy, although depression is known to occur in susceptible women. Pre-existing psychological disorders can either improve or become worse, and it is important that the woman's antenatal history-taking covers her previous psychological as well as physical medical history.

Continuity of care is an important factor in maternity care and even in the busiest of clinics an attempt is made to allow the woman to be seen by the same doctor whenever possible. An objective assessment of the woman's psychological state is made throughout pregnancy and any departure from her previous (or the 'normal') attitude or behaviour is noted. Appropriate help is given after referral to a specialist in psychiatric medicine.

9

ANTENATAL CARE

Chapter outline

First visit
- History-taking
- Physical examination
- Discussion and advice
- Subsequent visits

Antenatal education
- General lifestyle
- Nutrition
- Alcohol
- Smoking
- Drugs and medications
- Exercise
- Employment
- Intercourse
- Hygiene
- Clothing
- Dental care
- Breast care
- Travel
- Immunisations

Preparation for childbirth
- Antenatal classes
- Elective caesarean births

Signs to report at once

Signs of labour

Key words

amniocentesis	chorion villus sampling
bimanual	epidural analgesia
caesarean	parity
cardiotocograph	speculum

The expected outcome of pregnancy is survival of the mother and her baby. The aim of antenatal care is more; *not just survival*, but *good quality life*, for both.

Antenatal care includes:

- supervision of the pregnancy, to see that all remains normal, to detect and treat any abnormalities that arise, and to anticipate problems during labour, delivery and the postnatal period
- education about the pregnancy and how to cope with its symptoms, about diet, dental care, and lifestyle; almost every contact with the pregnant woman (and her husband) brings an opportunity for education in one form or another
- preparation (both physical and psychological) for labour and delivery, and instruction in aspects of infant care
- support where there are social or psychological difficulties.

In relation to the outcome of a pregnancy, 'good quality life' means a healthy mother with a healthy baby that she knows how to care for. Most centres now include the father-to-be in their educative and preparatory programmes. These programmes are both successful and very popular.

FIRST VISIT

The woman suspecting pregnancy goes to a doctor or hospital to have her suspicions confirmed. It is often rather a big occasion for her and a lot can depend upon her experiences during this first visit. A regular pattern is usually followed, beginning with history-taking, followed by full physical examination, discussion of any problems, advice about nutrition and other matters, prescription of any necessary medications, information about further visits and booking into the place of confinement.

HISTORY-TAKING

A comprehensive history is taken at the first visit. With the findings of the physical examination it provides the basis for planning individual care during pregnancy. After the usual recording of name, address and date of birth, information is gathered under five headings: the menstrual, present pregnancy, obstetric, medical (including surgical and family) and social histories. Table 9.1 shows the kind of information that is sought at the first visit.

The history-taking can sometimes reveal private and emotional matters. For this reason, some doctors prefer to have this interview alone with the woman. If her husband is present he is usually encouraged to stay; he may be able to contribute additional information. The presence of even one observer such as a nurse or medical student *could* inhibit the conversation and prevent the establishment of a good rapport.

The nurse should be sensitive to this. Even if it is the usual practice of the place in which she is working (or observing) for the nurse to remain during the history-taking, she can stand there quietly, away from the woman's direct line of vision. She can also leave quietly if she feels that it would be better to do so, especially if she senses that the woman is hesitating or is reluctant to answer a question or if she catches the woman looking at her before replying to something.

On the other hand, some women do not have difficulties with the presence of a third person. Indeed, some welcome the nurse as an ally, as another female (when her doctor is male), as someone who might have experienced some of her symptoms and concerns.

Table 9.1 History taken at the first antenatal visit

Information sought	Rationale
Menstrual history	
Date of last normal menstrual period	Base for calculation of expected date of confinement
Description of last menstrual period, and of usual menstrual experience	Variation in volume, duration or accompanying symptoms may make calculation wrong; also, may indicate gynaecological disorders
Present pregnancy	
Signs and symptoms that the woman has noticed	May give an early indication of the woman's response to her pregnancy; may need treatment for early symptoms or investigations if they are abnormal
Whether she is taking any medications or treatments (prescribed or unprescribed), alcohol or smoking or drug habits	Elimination of hazards to fetal development; discovering reasons for undergoing treatments or medication; opportunity for education about addictions
Obstetric history	
Number of previous pregnancies and their outcomes i.e. abortions, stillbirths, live births, whether still living, and whether in good health)	Management of first pregnancy and first labour differs considerably from that of subsequent pregnancies; all influence the woman's response to this pregnancy
Whether any complications or interventions in any previous pregnancy, labour or puerperium, and whether aware of cause(s)	Prevention of (if possible), or being alert for, recurrence of complications

Table 9.1 (*contd*)

Information sought	Rationale
Past medical history	
All important illnesses, injuries, responses to treatment, hospitalisations, known allergies, blood transfusions; all operations, but especially those involving pelvic structures; fractures	Guide to management of pregnancy and labour; special investigations may be indicated, to predict or prevent possible complications in labour
Family history, especially diabetes, tuberculosis, heart disease, hypertension; obstetrically significant are histories of multiple pregnancy, congenital abnormalities and hereditary conditions, in either the mother's or the father's family	Pregnancy involves physiological changes to, and stress on, most body systems, these conditions may emerge under such stress; special investigations can be performed, to give earlier diagnosis
Ethnic origin	
Country of birth and ethnic origin: religion	To anticipate cultural and religious practices associated with pregnancy, birth and acceptance of medical treatments; to be alert for racially-linked conditions such as Tay-Sachs and sickle-cell disease, and neural tube defects and thalassaemia
Social history	
Marital status: if married, whether first marriage; whether marriage 'happy'; if unmarried, whether there is any supportive relationship	Support of a marital partner often presumed (unless in obvious cases); possibility of problems in attitude towards pregnancy
Security of financial situation	If financially insecure or disadvantaged, may not be able to comply with suggested diet, rest or other ideals of pregnancy
Whether employed; type of occupation	Fatigue from employment could exaggerate symptoms; deliberately becoming pregnant to remove the stigma of unemployment does occur; alternatively, being forced to give up satisfying work can be resented.
Knowledge about, and attitude to, sex, reproduction, parenthood	Pregnancy involves body exposure which often causes extreme embarrassment; special consideration of this is important in those who are very shy of the subject; education is best when it is tailored to individual needs
Awareness of supportive services, social welfare, community facilities	Referral to such agencies early may make the pregnancy easier to cope with, can often extend the knowledge of the woman and her husband, and can encourage co-operation with pregnancy ideals

PHYSICAL EXAMINATION

The physical examination at the first visit of a pregnant woman is sometimes the first thorough examination of her body that the woman has had since childhood. Those looking after her should have this in mind, and help her accordingly. Occasionally symptomless but serious conditions (such as tuberculosis, breast tumours, cardiovascular disease, anaemia) may be discovered for the first time. Other less serious problems can be recognised and treated early, before their effects are felt. An empty bladder makes the examination more comfortable for the woman and more informative for the doctor.

General observation

General observation involves the following points:

- height (measured at first visit)
- weight (weighed at first visit)
- way of walking—any limping, stiffness
- body build and posture
- skin colour and texture
- general animation and vitality.

General examination

The following areas are examined in a general examination:

- blood pressure, pulse, hands and nails
- mouth—teeth, tongue, lips, gums
- neck—thyroid
- chest—heart and lungs listened to, breathing observed
- abdomen inspected and palpated; scars, hernias, masses; whether the uterus can be felt abdominally
- general condition of feet.

Breast examination

The breasts are examined as follows:

- appearance of breasts
- palpation for lumps or thickenings
- appearance of nipples—normal, flat inverted, puckering.

Pelvis (vaginal) examination

The vaginal examination covers the following:

- vulval inspection—inflammation, varicosities, lumps, other abnormalities, signs of previous childbirth
- speculum examination (Fig. 9.1) to observe cervix and vagina; previous childbirth, cervical lacerations
- cervical smear obtained; also, if indicated, swabs for culture

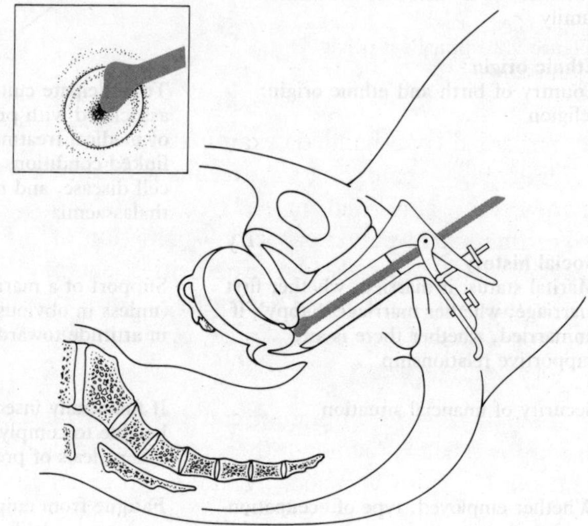

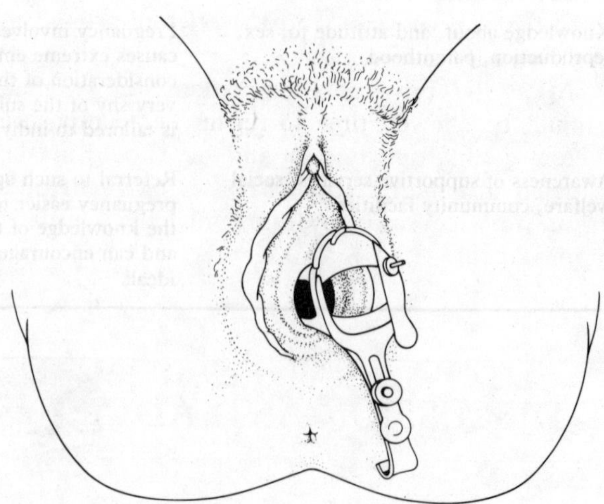

Figure 9.1 Speculum examination during which a cervical smear is obtained.

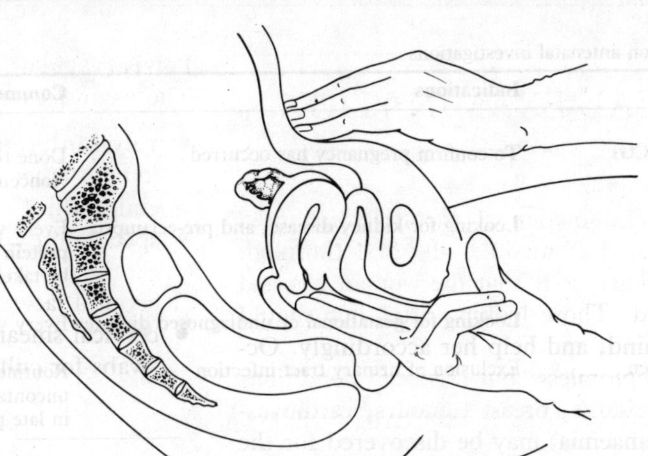

Figure 9.2 Bimanual pelvic examination.

- bimanual (two-handed) examination (Fig. 9.2)—palpating for uterine size, softness of cervix, abnormal masses
- estimation of pelvic capacity—palpation of bony landmarks (ischial tuberosities, sacral promontory and tip of sacrum)
- inspection of perineum—size, evidence of previous repairs.

The physical examination can be embarrassing and, for a short while, rather uncomfortable for the woman. This is especially likely if it is her first such experience. She can be helped by attention to draping, minimising exposure, advice on relaxation ('flopping' knees, slow breathing during the bimanual palpation—having the breathing done *with* her if necessary), and the offer of a hand to hold on to if she wants one.

After the physical examination, the woman should be allowed time to regain her composure before getting up to dress, and she should not be hurried in her dressing. The offer of swabs or a tissue to wipe away any lubricant jelly is usually appreciated.

DISCUSSION AND ADVICE

The questions asked during the history-taking, the responses given, and the findings of the physical examination, will determine the type of discussion that follows. Once again the nurse may sense that she should quietly withdraw. It is at this time that the woman may wish to express her response to the diagnosis of pregnancy. If her husband is nearby, she may want him to join her.

The woman (or the couple) will often now have questions to ask, perhaps some worries or misunderstandings as well. Although all aspects of antenatal care and education cannot be dealt with at one sitting, the basic principles are discussed, and the importance of continuing with antenatal care is emphasised. Immediate worries and simple problems are dealt with immediately; others are deferred (if possible), or referred for specific advice from experts.

After this, the woman will complete having any routine specimens collected for examination (Table 9.2) and will make arrangements for her hospital stay—'booking in'. Because of the problem of availability of beds, and difficulties with administration of institutions such as hospitals, the couple will need to decide early in pregnancy where they want their baby to be born.

SUBSEQUENT VISITS

For the rest of the pregnancy the woman visits every 4 weeks until 28 weeks, then every 2

Table 9.2 Common antenatal investigations

Test	Indications	Comments
Urine tests		
Pregnancy tests (HCG)	To confirm pregnancy has occurred	Done routinely at first visit; early morning (concentrated) specimen is best
Protein	Looking for kidney disease, and pre-eclampsia	Every visit, routine, urine is boiled if protein found, and mid-stream specimen may be taken
Glucose	Looking for gestational or undiagnosed diabetes	Every visit, routine
Mid-stream specimen	Exclusion of urinary tract infection	Routine at first visit, then when indicated; uncontaminated specimen may be difficult to get in late pregnancy
Glucose tolerance test	To exclude diabetes	Routine in many centres at 32 weeks
Oestriol collection	To assess placental function and fetal well-being	Routine in some centres at 30 and 36 weeks; 24-hour specimen
Blood tests		
Group and Rh	Knowledge of blood Group and Rh important in case of need for urgent transfusion; Rh negative blood tested for antibodies	Routine at first visit; if Rh antibodies positive, titres may be repeated at 16, 24, 28, 32 and 36 weeks
Haemoglobin	To exclude anaemia	Routine at first visit, at 32 weeks, and as indicated
Rubella antibody titre	Establishment of immune status	Routine at first visit
USR (unheated serum reagin) or VDRL	To exclude syphilis	Routine at first visit, may be repeated if indicted during pregnancy
Serum oestriol levels	To check placental functioning	Done as indicated.
Swabs		
Cervical smear	To exclude cervical malignancy	Routine at first visit
Vaginal swab	Any vaginal discharges, and to exclude gonorrhoea and Group B streptococcal infection	As indicated for vaginal discharges; routine exclusion of gonorrhoea and Group B streptococcal infection in some centres at first visit.

weeks until 36 weeks, then weekly until she delivers. If there are complications or risk factors she will be seen more frequently. She is encouraged to contact the doctor or hospital if she is worried or if she notices abnormalities, rather than wait until her next appointment.

At these subsequent visits, the following points are recorded:

- weight
- urinalysis—protein, sugar, ketones
- blood pressure
- presence of oedema—ankles, feet, hands (wedding ring 'tight')
- legs checked for calf tenderness
- fundal height
- fetal lie and movements
- fetal heartbeat
- after 36 weeks, fetal position in detail—lie, presentation, position, attitude, engagement.

Table 9.3 Less common antenatal investigations

Test	Indications	Comments
Chorion villus sampling (removal of some of the villi surrounding the pregnancy sac—Fig. 9.3)	To exclude chromosome disorders in women at risk; to diagnose certain genetic diseases	Performed under ultrasound at 8–10 weeks, most results available within 2 weeks; risk to pregnancy about 5%; occasionally false positive results
Amniocentesis (removal of sample of amniotic fluid — Fig. 9.4)	Suspected fetal abnormalities, familis with sex-linked diseases, to exclude neural tube defects. Later, in Rh negative women with antibodies, to assess fetal lung maturity (L/S ratio)	Done under ultrasound: about 5% danger of damage to pregnancy; not done before 14 weeks, results can take 4 weeks
Ultrasound scanning	Evidence of pregnancy, gestation, and size, location of placenta, exclusion of multiple pregnancy and some abnormalities	Non-invasive; becoming fairly common
Serum alphafeto protein	To exclude neural tube defects such as anencephaly and open spina bifida	Blood test; done if indicated and condition not excluded by amniocentesis
Amniscopy	To exclude meconium in liquor, overdue baby, poor history	Not done before 37 weeks; metal tube with light source inserted through cervix; may bring on labour
Fetal monitor (cardiotocograph)	To exclude abnormalities of fetal heart beat; to note fetal response to contractions; low oestriols, reduced movements, high risk pregnancies	Non-invasive; not routine but becoming more common
X-ray (pelvic)	Persistent breech; to measure pelvis (pelvimetry); to confirm gestation (rare)	Not routine; done as late as possible; never before 16 weeks.

General enquiries are made (and questions answered) about:

- general health, well-being and home life
- minor disorders
- taking of prescribed medications
- referral, as necessary, to dietitian, social worker, other medical specialties
- progress of pregnancy education and childbirth classes.

Investigations are done or repeated as indicated (Tables 9.2 and 9.3), and the reasons for doing them are explained.

ANTENATAL EDUCATION

Antenatal education is a significant part of maternity care, and everybody involved in this care has a responsibility to further this education. Almost every contact with the pregnant woman and her husband provides opportunities to do this.

It would not be unreasonable to presume that having been through at least one pregnancy, the woman undergoing a second or subsequent pregnancy has less need for formal (or informal) instruction and advice. In many cases this is so, but not in all. The first pregnancy may have been some years ago; trends, ideas, investigations and management methods change quickly enough in general medicine, in midwifery they seem to change even more often. As well, if the woman has changed from the public to the private system (or vice versa) or has become involved with community or specific-interest groups, her educational needs will be different. It must be remembered as well that each pregnancy is a unique experience, and with second or subsequent pregnancies the symptoms, minor disorders and risks will be different.

Every pregnant woman will therefore have some

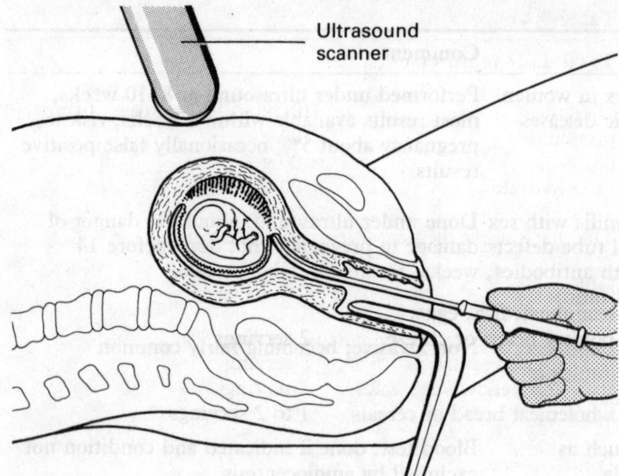

Figure 9.3 Chorion villus sampling.

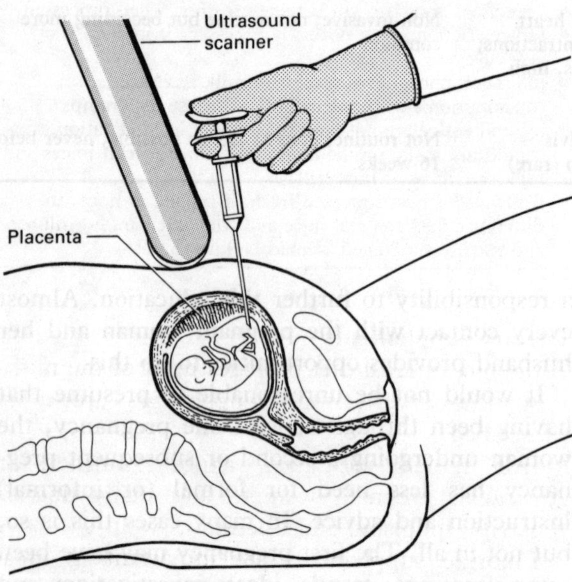

Figure 9.4 Amniocentesis.

educational needs. But whether this is her first or fifth pregnancy, she should be given credit for some intelligence and general knowledge, for her reading, discussion with others, and specific learning (perhaps previous employment in the health field).

Whatever the situation, nobody responds well to the sort of patronising, domineering, 'baby talk' that often used to be associated with formal instruction. Nowadays, explanation, advice and reassurance are all based on continual assessment of the woman's understanding. Many hospitals arrange classes as small discussion groups, in order to promote participation and to allow for questioning of all aspects of pregnancy; community health centres and childbirth education groups do likewise. These are available both during the day and in the evenings to allow participation of employed women, husbands and others; some centres offer play-groups or child-minding facilities as well.

GENERAL LIFESTYLE

Pregnancy does demand some curtailment of frenetic activity, although the fact of being pregnant ought not to be used as an excuse to get out of everything that the woman does not like doing! She should be advised to consider her lifestyle in relation to her own health and that of the expected baby. Late nights, a heavy social life, parties in smoke-filled rooms, her consumption of alcohol, intense study for non-urgent qualifications—all of these should be considered and minimised where possible.

One problem that may not be obvious (even to the woman) is that of the demands of conscience and her 'contribution to society'. In the case of a first pregnancy, where the woman has just stopped her outside employment to become a full-time 'housewife' for the first time, she may feel a need to prove to her husband (and to the world) that she is worthy of his support. Whereas before it did not really mater if there was the occasional scratched-together meal or if the cupboards under the sink were a bit of a jumble, she now may feel she has to make every meal almost a dinner party, that she cannot sit down if there is dust on top of the piano—that she should be a perfect housewife. As well as often being more tiring than going out to work, such a newly acquired perfectionism can sometimes cause a strain in the marriage relationship and could later make the woman feel guilty for not maintaining such high standards after the baby arrives. It is a common problem, and one which husbands are often very eager to discuss.

Simple questioning about lifestyle and what the woman does with her time is an important aspect of antenatal care. Boredom can be as big a problem as over-activity; suggestions to resolve both are important for the enjoyment of the pregnancy and the well-being of the family unit.

NUTRITION

Nutrition advice during pregnancy comes from four sources: the doctor or midwife, antenatal classes, family and friends, and when indicated, a dietitian.

Most doctors can tell from observation whether or not a woman's nutritional intake is satisfactory for the demands of pregnancy. Questioning will find out any variations from the ideal (Table 9.4), and those at risk will be referred to a dietitian. Most doctors and hospitals routinely provide literature which outlines the basic nutritional needs of a pregnant woman and often includes menu suggestions, recipes and shopping advice.

Those at risk, of poor nutrition, are those with:

- social-economic problems
- persistent nausea or vomiting
- young children (the mother can become too tired or bored to cook properly for herself)
- strict vegetarian diets (especially if taking no first-class protein)
- alcohol, cigarette or other drug problems
- pre-existing disorders relating to nutrition—diabetes, malabsorption problems, gastro-intestinal disorders.

The very young (still growing herself) mother-to-be, the underweight woman, and the woman who has a low weight gain during pregnancy are also in need of special dietary education and management.

Table 9.4

Total daily requirements:

kilojoules	10 500 (2500 calories) from:
protein	100 g
fat	100 g
carbohydrate	300 g

The diet should include at least the following

milk	$\frac{3}{4}$ to 1 litre
lean meat, fish, eggs, poultry beans or cheese	2 servings
leafy green vegetables	1 serving
fruit and yellow vegetables	2 servings
wholemeal bread or cereals	1 to 2 servings

Points to note:

- milk may be taken in several forms (e.g. custards, junkets, drinks, yoghurt)
- some fats and vegetables oils should be taken (for source of fat soluble vitamins)
- vegetables and fruit are better fresh than when processed.
- salt restriction is not normally necessary if intake is not excessive
- too much phosphorus (excessive milk and meat consumption and supplements) can cause leg cramps
- tea and coffee are not harmful if taken in moderation, but should not make up the entire fluid intake (fruit juices and milk should be at least half)
- fruit juice is best squeezed fresh; if buying as juice, the difference between real juice and fruit juice *drinks* (diluted and usually sweetened) should be known.

Dietary supplements

Although an ideal diet provides most of the nutrition necessary, certain supplements are often prescribed.

Iron tablets are given almost routinely to Australian pregnant women, and many doctors prescribe folic acid and calcium as well.

Fluoride supplements are important in areas where the water is also 'hard' (e.g. Adelaide), some people never use the tap water for drinking or cooking; the woman should be asked about this and fluoride supplements given in the second half of pregnancy if they are necessary.

Vitamin supplements are not usually prescribed if a good diet is assured. The woman is warned against taking excessive or unprescribed extra vitamins or minerals, as these will pass through the placental barrier and the fetal liver may not be able to cope with them. Herbal and naturopathic medicines should also not be taken without the obstetrician's knowledge as these are in fact drugs, the effects of which may be unknown.

ALCOHOL

Alcohol consumption in normal pregnancy is permitted if it is minimal. Wine taken with meals is less harmful than at other times. It is probably best to limit alcohol intake to one glass of wine with the occasional special meal.

Other forms of alcohol—spirits, fortified wines and beer—are usually high in calories and this may upset the woman's appetite for proper foods. Excess alcohol can cause fetal malformation, growth retardation and later mental retardation.

SMOKING

Smoking is potentially harmful to the pregnancy. Mothers who smoke more than 10 cigarettes a day have higher rates of abortion, perinatal death, and intrauterine growth retardation.

The woman should stop smoking cigarettes as soon as the pregnancy is diagnosed. This is particularly important where other risk factors (e.g. uncertain nutrition) are present, or when the woman's smoking is associated with chronic respiratory irritation or gastric symptoms.

The mother is referred for professional help in giving up smoking if the positive-health aspects of stopping either do not convince her, or are not sufficient to help her stop. She should be warned not to take anti-smoking medications without her doctor's permission.

Fortunately, the nausea of early pregnancy helps some women to find cigarettes distasteful, and when the nausea phase is over, their bodies have lost their dependence on the habit.

DRUGS AND MEDICATIONS

Many medications that have been taken regularly under prescription before pregnancy can be continued, but the obstetric doctor must know what the woman is taking. It may be necessary for the medications or dosages to be varied.

The woman is told of the importance of never taking any drug (the word is *explained*) without telling her doctor *first*. Most drugs do pass the placental barrier and could harm the fetus, especially in the early stages of its development. The woman is cautioned against departing from instructions given about prescribed drugs, and is encouraged to contact the hospital or doctor first if she wishes to vary any medication regime.

Drugs of dependence are a different problem. If a drug addiction is admitted or discovered during the antenatal period, education and assistance is given in an attempt to overcome the habit. This may involve hospital admission and close medical attention, and can be very difficult for the woman. In many cases serious (e.g. heroin) addiction is not discovered during the antenatal period, because the addicts are not usually very good at seeking antenatal care. They may be seen first when they present in labour and give birth to a heroin-addicted baby. In those who smoke marijuana, there has been an increased incidence of fetal abnormality.

EXERCISE

Deliberate exercise is encouraged during pregnancy. A lot of people believe that they get enough exercise in their very busy daily lives; they get tired enough without seeking to use more energy.

Deliberate exercise is different. It involves a conscious decision to do it. A daily walk or swim at a certain time will exercise the whole body, aid in relaxation, inflate the lungs more completely, improve the circulation, and will perhaps even help to organise the daily routine. It is also a good time for the woman to get out of the house.

Some activities are not suitable for pregnant women in the later months, nor for those who have a history of abortion, premature labour or placental insufficiency. Waterskiing, complicated gymnastics, vigorous athletics and squash are advised against. Anything dangerous in the normal course, or in which there is not full control of body balance at all times, is foolish in pregnancy. Swimming is a really good form of exercise, but even then caution must be given against swimming out in ocean beaches or fast-flowing rivers, as there may be lowered ability to cope with difficulties.

EMPLOYMENT

When to give up outside employment depends very much on the work involved, what dangers it may bring, and the mental and physical energy needed for the job. The doctor always asks about the woman's present and previous employment in case it could have affected the pregnancy already or in the future. Radiographers, for example, are advised to leave their field of work several months before they contemplate a pregnancy.

If the work is not too demanding and if it does not matter whether or not the pregnancy shows, the woman is usually advised to continue working for as long as she enjoys the work. She is usually told that a full month's rest from work, before the baby is born, would be of advantage to both of them.

The woman is usually advised to tell her employer that she is pregnant. It is responsible behaviour and common courtesy to do so. The employer will then be able to plan for her absence or replacement, and may also be able to adjust the work situation to her benefit. Some employers also require that the woman submit a signed statement acknowledging her pregnancy and accepting liability for any related problems or accidents. As well, some aspects of compensation for work-related injury may be affected.

INTERCOURSE

If the woman has a history of spontaneous abortion or premature labour, intercourse is advised against for the first 2–3 months and again in the last month. Otherwise, the couple are advised to continue to enjoy their usual sexual activity. They should be advised that:

- hormonal effects can sometimes alter interest in intercourse—generally it is greater during the first and last months
- the physical demands of the baby can make the woman a lot more tired than usual
- emotional lability is common, and allowance must be made for this
- they may need to try various different ways of lying or sitting to make intercourse comfortable.

It is one of the advantages of the relatively recent 'sexual revolution' that most people can now discuss sex fairly openly. Before this, the pregnant woman who had not been advised (and who had not had the courage to ask) about intercourse during pregnancy, did not know that was allowed, what might harm the baby, or what to do instead.

HYGIENE

A daily shower or bath is recommended. Bath water does not enter the vagina and so does not harm the fetus. Showering is usually recommended in the last 2 or 3 months, because getting out of a bath can be awkward. Whether she takes baths or showers, the pregnant woman is advised to leave the bathroom door unlocked. If she slips because of awkwardness, becomes stuck in the bath, or faints when in the bathroom, someone can come to her assistance. The same is recommended for when she goes to the toilet. If she feels uncomfortable about leaving the door unlocked, she could make an 'occupied' sign to hang on the door so that she will not be disturbed.

General hygiene is important. Skin infections should be cleared early: the woman is advised to report immediately any rashes, nail-bed infections, cold-sores and boils. Toenails should be kept short (she may need help with cutting them in the later months), and fingernails should not be allowed to grow too long. It is tempting for the woman to grow long nails especially if she has had a job that required nails to be short, but she will soon be handling a newborn baby with delicate skin and limited resistance to the type of infection that long nails can harbour. She will also probably be wanting to hold someone's hand when she is in labour or delivering.

Vaginal hygiene measures are usually unnecessary and douching should be avoided in pregnancy. Douching can upset the normal defence mechanism of the vagina, and *forceful* douching (especially with a bulb syringe) could cause air or fluid embolism. Simple washing of the vulval area during the daily bath or shower and after intercourse is usually sufficient. Vaginal 'feminine' deodorants should not be necessary, they might, in fact, cause allergic dermatitis. If there seems to be an offensive smell, the woman should find out what is causing it, and have the cause treated. If there is no cause and the smell is in fact no more than a natural body odour, the woman may be hypersensitive about sexual matters and may benefit from further discussion on the subject.

CLOTHING

Clothing for the pregnant woman is nowadays a big business and the expectant mother has a wide range of attractive garments to choose from. Clothing should be comfortable, with no constricting bands at the waist or wrists, or tightness at the neck. Leg garters are still being worn by some, especially certain migrant groups. These should be forbidden as they can impede circulation.

Clothing should be light in weight and attractive—this makes a great deal of difference when the figure grows large and awkward. Although money is not always available for a large maternity wardrobe, the woman should be encouraged to get at least one 'good' maternity dress, so that she can go out and *feel* good.

Shoes should be sensible and safe. High heels and pointed toes are bad for feet at any time, but are especially bad during pregnancy when body stability is uncertain and when oedema of the feet is common. Flimsy shoes and thongs are often unsafe as well.

Maternity bras

These are designed to support the breasts as they grow, and to open to allow easy access to the breasts and nipple during suckling. They have wide straps to prevent cutting into the shoulders. They are recommended to be worn from the 4th or 5th month. After the woman has become used to the sight of herself in them, especially if she had formerly used the tiniest bras available or no bra at all, she finds them very comfortable.

There is usually a choice between plain cotton and lacy maternity bras. The lacy ones are fine for special occasions, but the plain bras wash better, last longer and rarely cause irritation. Maternity bras should be a priority in the pregnant woman's budget. They should be properly fitted by a trained person by the end of the 5th month.

Maternity girdles

These help to give relief from dragging lower abdominal and back pains. They are designed to give support just above the symphysis pubis in front and just each side of the middle of the waist at the back. They do not put any pressure (other than gentle firm support) on the growing abdomen, and are recommended if the woman can afford to buy them, especially if she has poor abdominal muscle tone. Antenatal exercises for muscle control are important whether or not a girdle is worn.

Girdles that are not designed for pregnancy can cause discomfort and pressure on the uterus. Pregnant women should be told about this and advised against wearing them.

DENTAL CARE

Teeth and gums should be given extra preventive care during pregnancy. The gums are affected to some extent (hypertrophied) by the circulating hormones, and irritation and infection of the gum margins can result if they are neglected. New eating habits and cravings may predispose to tooth decay.

The old saying 'for every child, a tooth' *is* an old wives' tale. The calcium content of the mother's teeth is not affected by pregnancy; it is always easier to blame some factor over which one has no control than to admit to neglect of dental care.

The importance of dental health as part of general good health is stressed, and the woman is advised to have her teeth examined early in pregnancy. She is asked to tell the dentist that she is pregnant so that he can plan any necessary treatment, including medications involved, for the most suitable time during the pregnancy.

BREAST CARE

Most women in Third World societies manage to feed their babies with no formal breast preparation at all. The trouble with our society is that female breasts are covered. This brings about two problems: firstly, the nipples are protected from the sun and air, and so become soft; and secondly, the breasts have sexual connotations, so that handling and exposure may cause embarrassment and even aversion to breast feeding in the woman who is not confident about her own sexual feelings.

Antenatal education and advice about breast care is simple to give to the woman who is keen to breast feed.

Nipple shape

The breasts and nipples are examined at the first visit. If the nipples are depressed or inverted (Fig. 9.5) nipple shields may be prescribed, to be worn from the 12th week onwards. One form of nipple shield is the Woolwich shield (Fig. 9.6); it aims to lengthen the nipple by depressing the areola while allowing the nipple itself to extend. In some cases of severe nipple inversion, it may take several months for extension to occur, but it is worthwhile persevering with the use of nipple shields.

No special preparation is necessary, however, in the majority of women whose nipples are simply flat. They can be reassured that following delivery there is usually an improvement in nipple shape, with the nipples becoming more protractile. Some mothers may need extra assistance in ensuring that the baby is correctly positioned at the breast, particularly for the short period of natural venous breast engorgement which occurs on about the third day after delivery.

Nipple care

Nipple care is simple. It consists of washing away any crusting of dried colostrum during the daily bath or shower, then gently pulling out and rolling the nipples between the fingers (Fig. 9.6). During the last month, a few drops of colostrum may be

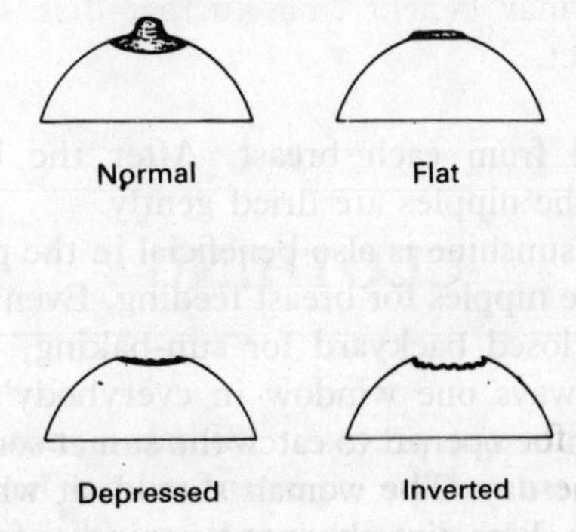

Figure 9.5 Types of nipples.

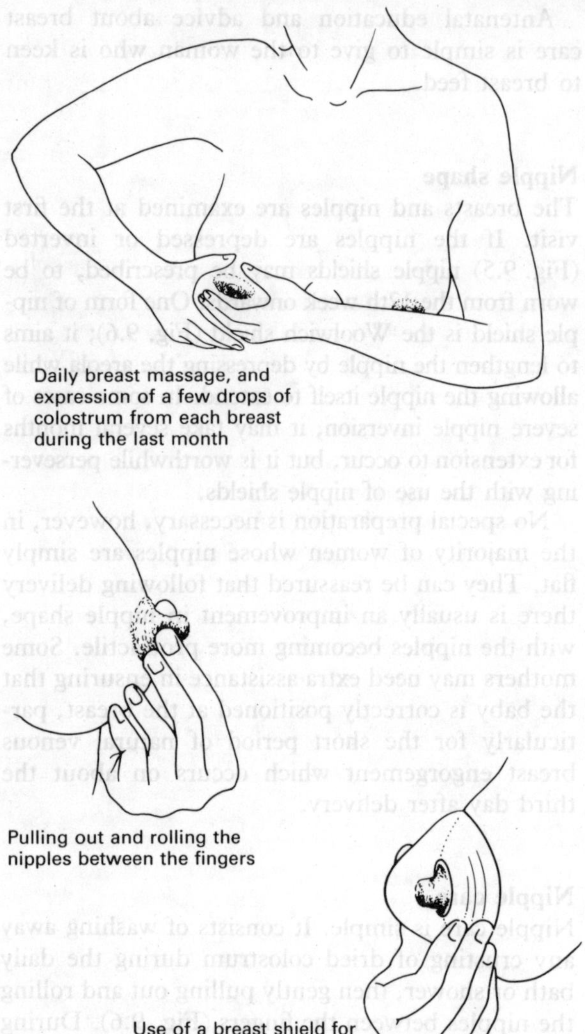

Figure 9.6 Antenatal preparation for breast feeding.

expressed from each breast. After the bath or shower, the nipples are dried gently.

Direct sunshine is also beneficial in the preparation of the nipples for breast feeding. Even if there is no enclosed backyard for sun-baking, there is almost always one window in everybody's house which can be opened to catch the sun at some time during the day. The woman should sit where the sun's rays shine directly onto her nipples for about 10 minutes each day but should take case to protect her breasts and other areas not normally exposed to the sun.

There are two old wives' tales about nipple care and they crop up continually. They are that methylated spirits makes nipples tough and that scrubbing with a nail brush does the same thing. These methods actually cause the nipple skin to become dry and often damage it. Some women, wanting to do the very best to prepare for breast feeding, do everything they have heard about, as well as what has been recommended by the doctor or midwife. It is therefore important that the woman be *asked* what she is doing about nipple preparation, to make sure that her practices are not ultimately damaging.

Breast preparation
The breasts are massaged gently for a short time as part of the daily bath of shower. This helps to improve their circulation. They may become uncomfortable from physiological (venous) engorgement, especially in early and late pregnancy. At these times it is wise to wear a well-fitted maternity bra. As well, cold compresses for limited periods or bathing the breasts in cold water can help to relieve the soreness.

Negative attitudes to breast feeding
Disinterest and aversion to breast feeding are not easy to overcome. Women who have these attitudes need a lot more than a lecture on the advantages of breast feeding. Where there is real aversion to the idea—'it's revolting'—there has probably been insidious pressure from many sources over the years. One source of pressure is from women who defend their own failure with breast feeding when they are probably jealous of another's ability or potential to succeed.

Disinterest, on the other hand, may mask all sorts of psychological or social problems: there may be little interest in the coming baby, or the woman may not be allowing herself to become interested, perhaps because she suspects that life is likely to be difficult after the baby is born. It is very rare for a woman who is interested in her future baby's welfare to be completely disinterested in how he is to be fed, unless there is something drastically wrong.

If the reply to the question, 'Are you planning

to breast feed?' is anything less enthusiastic than 'yes' or 'if I can; I do want to', discussion should proceed carefully. If there are definite medical or social contra-indications, there may be real disappointment, and the woman could feel a deep hurt if the subject is pushed too hard. In any case, she should be asked if she minds 'if we talk about it for a minute'. If she agrees, the various reasons for her attitude can be explored and problems can be resolved or at least referred. She can sometimes be given courage to overcome other people's opposition to her breast feeding her baby. Where it is opposition from the husband this can be difficult, but he can at least be invited to come and talk about it. If it is simple innocence or ignorance about breast feeding, then a programme of education and encouragement can be commenced. Referral to an expert (some hospitals have specialist 'breast care' midwives or lactation consultants) or to a community group such as the Nursing Mothers' Association may be advisable; in most cases it ought to be encouraged.

Breast feeding is terribly important, and it is ridiculous that there is even a need to have to promote it. Good antenatal education about breast feeding as the normal and natural follow-on from pregnancy, without making it seem an outstanding challenge at which the woman must succeed if she is not to be a total failure, is one of the most important aspects of maternity care.

TRAVEL

The pregnant woman should be careful in making plans for any travel which is likely to be long or tiring. Sitting still for long periods can be very uncomfortable and can lead to circulatory problems and dependent oedema. Seat belts should be worn with the lap belt under, and the sash belt over, the prominent abdomen. Most States require a certificate of exemption for a doctor to avoid prosecution for failing to wear a seat belt.

If possible, air travel is best when long distances are involved. Modern aircraft are pressurised and a high-altitude should not affect the pregnancy. Many airlines are reluctant to carry pregnant women after they have reached 35 weeks gestation; some airlines refuse to carry them, others require a statement from the woman's doctor to the effect that the woman is not likely to come into premature labour and that she is fit to travel.

Travelling has other problems. It is usually very tiring, food and fluid intake are likely to be different from usual, constipation or diarrhoea commonly occur and there is the uncertainty of access to satisfactory medical care.

On the other hand, the couple may feel that this time is their last opportunity for many years to travel freely, without the restrictions and paraphernalia associated with a baby. There is not doubt that the sort of holiday which is quiet, involves clean air, good food, pleasant exercise and plenty of rest is of very great benefit to expectant parents.

IMMUNISATIONS

Pregnancy is not the time to begin programmes of immunisation against preventable diseases. Any substance (or any encounter with organisms) which is likely to cause a sharp rise in the woman's temperature is to be avoided. Rubella, typhoid and influenza vaccinations are not given during pregnancy because of possible damage to the fetus. Smallpox vaccination should only be given if the woman is going to live in a known-risk area, and is then never given before the end of the 16th week.

Polio protection, either Salk or Sabin, can be given if the woman has not been vaccinated already.

PREPARATION FOR CHILDBIRTH

Childbirth education and relaxation techniques are conducted individually by physiotherapists or in

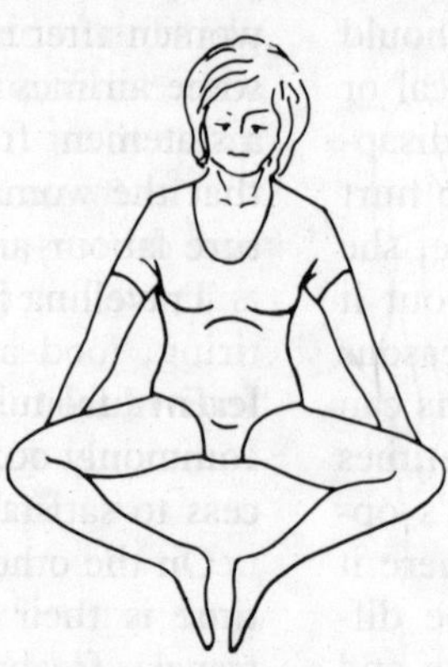

Pelvic floor exercises

Sit with soles of feet together and press knees down, also sit cross-legged

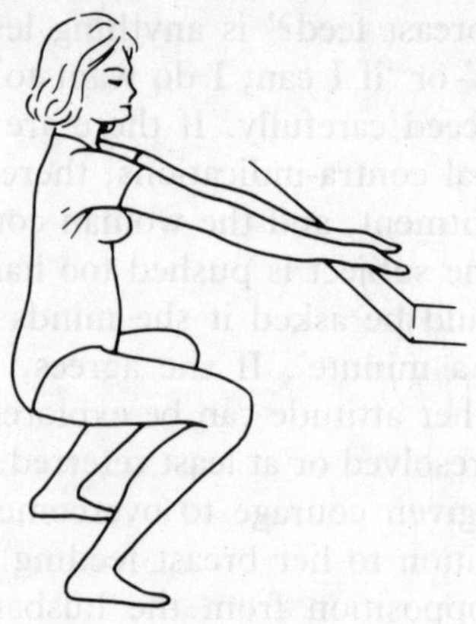

Squat and stand, tightening and relaxing pelvic floor

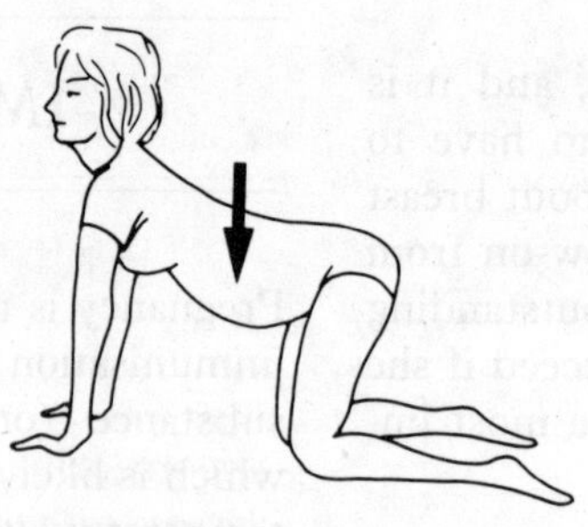

Abdominal muscle exercise

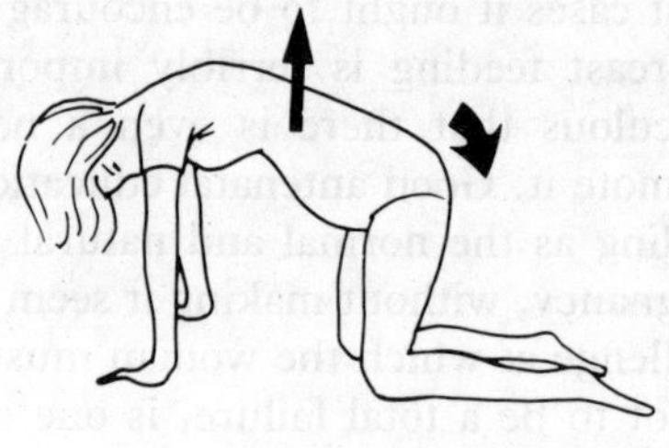

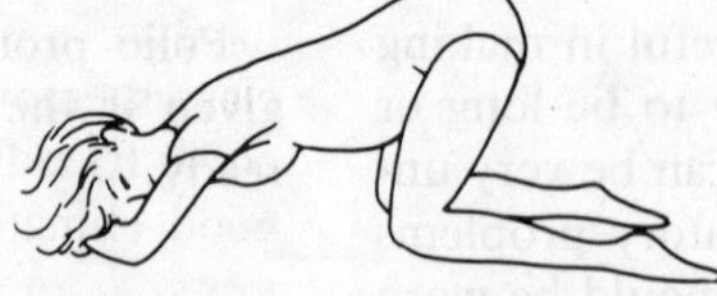

Resting position

Not to be maintained for long periods; helps to relieve back pain

Figure 9.7 Antenatal exercises.

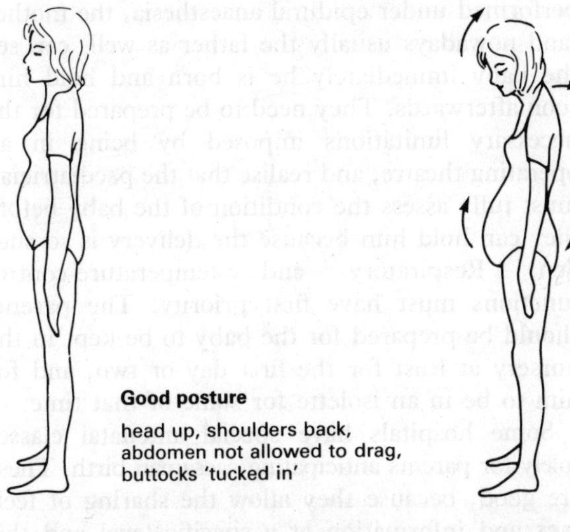

Good posture

head up, shoulders back, abdomen not allowed to drag, buttocks 'tucked in'

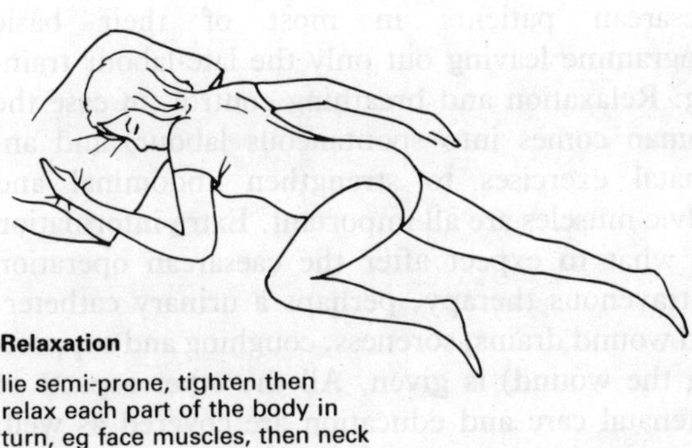

Relaxation

lie semi-prone, tighten then relax each part of the body in turn, eg face muscles, then neck muscles, then shoulder muscles, etc

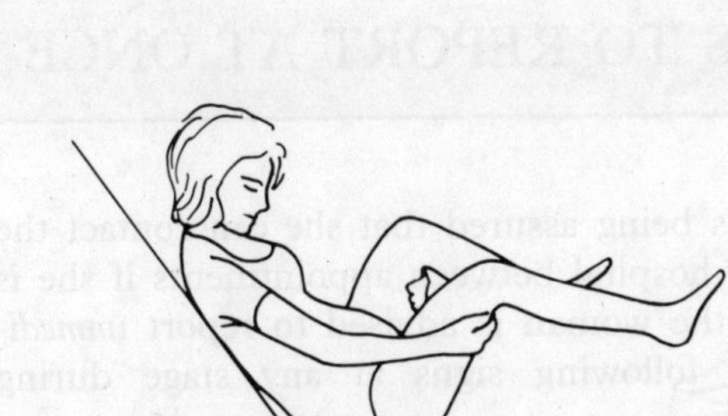

Labour 'pushing' position

bend head forward, chin on chest, lift knees up and wide apart, use hands to pull on backs of thighs

groups or classes by a team of people including physiotherapists and midwives. In some centres, where childbirth education is structured to include most of the other facets of antenatal instruction, the team includes dietitians, parentcraft teachers and doctors. Figure 9.7 illustrates some common antenatal exercises.

Individual tuition

Individual tuition is right for some people, particularly if there are special medical or social needs. The physiotherapist who has usually undergone extra obstetric training, prepares the woman and possibly her husband as well in basic anatomy, the anticipated events of pregnancy, techniques of relaxation, breathing patterns for labour (see p. 132), pushing positions and techniques, and posture and muscle control methods. The physiotherapist will sometimes attend the delivery to encourage and revise the use of the learned techniques.

ANTENATAL CLASSES

The majority of expectant parents attend antenatal classes rather than become private patients of physiotherapists. The classes are ideally in the form of small groups, and are organised so that the women in each group are likely to be at about the same stage of pregnancy. The women are therefore likely to meet each other again when they are in hospital if the classes are hospital-based. As they have a common interest and almost always find the classes enjoyable, the parents soon relax and become friendly with each other and this provides a good climate for questions, answers and suggestions. A lot of interest is expressed in the previous experiences of any women there who have already had babies. Misconceptions about those experiences can be cleared through discussion in the presence of the midwife.

The classes are taken through the same basic teaching programme that those under individual care receive. But there are usually extras such as the following:

- a film of delivery followed by discussion
- a guided tour of the hospital, with introductions to the midwives of the delivery suites, the nurseries and the postnatal floors (usually with opportunities to see into these areas)
- advice on nutrition, not only for pregnancy but for the future, when time for food preparation must be fitted around the care of a new baby
- advice on baby care, what to buy before the baby is born, and what to leave until later
- how to handle newborn babies
- how to cope with visitors (in hospital and later on)
- where to go for specialised help
- advice on sexual activity during pregnancy, and forward-thinking about family planning afterwards.

The presence of husbands at all of these classes is welcomed and encouraged in most places. The informed and understanding husband is a great support at those times during pregnancy when everything seems to go wrong at once, and during labour when it seems that *nobody* could ever before have had such a bad backache or had such an urgent desire to push. Understanding and participation helps to make the experience of being present at the birth of their child far more meaningful for the father.

ELECTIVE CAESAREAN BIRTHS

The parents who know in advance that they will not experience normal vaginal delivery have only slightly differing needs for antenatal education. They may be disappointment at first because labour and delivery are not going to be normal, but in most cases the woman will understand the reasons (see p. 145) for having her baby this way.

Now that many caesarean section operations are performed under epidural anaesthesia, the mother (and nowadays usually the father as well) can see the baby immediately he is born and hold him soon afterwards. They need to be prepared for the necessary limitations imposed by being in an operating theatre, and realise that the paediatrician must fully assess the condition of the baby before they can hold him because the delivery is so sudden. Respiratory and temperature-control functions must have first priority. The parents should be prepared for the baby to be kept in the nursery at least for the first day or two, and for him to be in an isolette for some of that time.

Some hospitals have special antenatal classes solely for parents anticipating caesarean birth. These are good, because they allow the sharing of feelings and information at a specific level and this can be very reassuring. Other centres involve caesarean patients in most of their basic programme leaving out only the late-labour training. Relaxation and breathing control (in case the woman comes into spontaneous labour) and antenatal exercises to strengthen abdominal and pelvic muscles are all important. Extra information on what to expect after the caesarean operation (intravenous therapy, perhaps a urinary catheter, and wound drains, soreness, coughing and supporting the wound) is given. All the other aspects of antenatal care and education are covered as well.

SIGNS TO REPORT AT ONCE

As well as being assured that she can contact the doctor or hospital between appointments if she is worried, the woman is advised to report *immediately* the following signs at any stage during pregnancy:

- any bleeding from the vagina
- draining of fluid (smelling different from urine) from the vagina
- any severe pain
- any definite abdominal or 'period-like' pain
- excessive or unusually rapid fetal movements
- absence of fetal movements

- high temperature, fever, shivering
- excessive vomiting (keeping nothing down)
- severe frontal headache
- blurring of vision
- very little urine passed (over several hours)
- difficulty or burning when passing urine
- swelling of hands, feet or face.

SIGNS OF LABOUR

As well as knowing the importance of seeking advice for possible problems, the woman should clearly understand and be able to recognise the signs of the onset of labour. She should contact the hospital if she has the following symptoms:

- regular contractions, occurring every 10 minutes (or more frequently)
- any vaginal 'show' or blood loss
- evidence of rupture of the membranes or unexplained fluid draining.

Obviously these points are only guidelines and depend on such factors as the woman's parity (the number of babies she has already had), and how far away she lives. Most hospitals ask the woman to phone when she suspects that she is in labour; they will then be able to advise her on what to do and when to come, and the staff will be able to prepare for the woman's admission when she does come.

10

HEALTH COMPLICATIONS DURING PREGNANCY

Chapter outline

- Pre-existing diseases
  - Cardiac disease
  - Diabetes
  - Urinary tract infection
  - Anaemia
  - Essential hypertension
- Sexually transmitted diseases
  - Syphilis
  - Gonorrhoea
  - Genital herpes
  - HIV (AIDS)
- Rhesus incompatibility
- Pre-eclampsia
- Eclampsia
- Hyperemesis
- Multiple pregnancy
- Antepartum haemorrhage

Keywords

binovular, breech, eclampsia, fibroids, gestational, phototherapy, physiological anaemia, pre-eclampsia, primigravida, Rh factor, transverse, uniovular

PRE-EXISTING DISEASES

Although her body is ideally functioning at maximum efficiency, the pregnant woman is not immune to the diseases of the non-pregnant state. A pre-existing health problem requires additional care and supervision because of the extra physiological stress caused by the pregnancy. In such a case the woman should be cared for by specialist physicians, as well as obstetricians, at a centre which is equipped to cope with any possible complications.

The woman also needs to be looked after by nurses who understand both her medical condition and her pregnancy. Those conditions (e.g. diabetes and cardiac disease) which are dramatically affected by pregnancy, are often managed until late pregnancy in a special unit or a medical ward in a general hospital. Thus, the general nurse should frequently revise her knowledge of the physiology of pregnancy and the effects of pregnancy upon the various body systems. Pre-existing cardiac disease, diabetes, urinary tract infection, anaemia and venereal disease are discussed in this section.

CARDIAC DISEASE

Cardiac disease affects about 1% of all pregnant women. It is usually due to either previous heart damage from rheumatic fever or (most commonly now) congenital heart disease.

Cardiac disease is classified into four groups (I to IV) according to how active a person can be without symptoms arising. Pregnancy places extra demands upon the heart (p. 61) and almost always causes the woman to be graded into a higher risk classification.

Serious complications can arise as a result of the increased demands upon the weakened or diseased heart unless preventive measures are taken. Heart failure can occur in the mother, and the baby is in danger of intrauterine hypoxia, fetal growth retardation, premature labour and birth asphyxia.

Pregnancy
The basis of medical and nursing management of the pregnant woman with heart disease is the reduction of all possible extra stresses. This is to ensure satisfactory oxygenation of the fetus and prevent worsening of the condition. The woman is usually examined fortnightly (instead of monthly) during early pregnancy, and weekly from 28 weeks, so that any signs of early heart failure can be detected as soon as they appear. She must have extra and deliberate rest periods during the day as well as at least 9 hours of sleep each night. A detailed allowed-activity plan should be drawn up, and this should be adjusted each visit after a discussion of its suitability to her responsibilities and her health. Extra help in the home should be considered especially when there are other children in the family; a social worker will have access to the various supportive services.

Admission to hospital may be necessary if it is difficult for the woman to rest at home. Between 28 and 34 weeks is often the time of greatest physical stress when exact administration or adjustment of cardiac medications (e.g. digitalis) is needed.

Other important factors in the antenatal care of the woman with cardiac disease are:

- the prevention or correction of anaemia
- the prevention of infection, by avoiding exposure (visitors, crowds etc.) and by treating even the most minor infections immediately
- the limitation of weight gain, avoiding excessive weight which could add to the strain on the heart; dietary management may include sodium restriction to prevent excessive fluid retention
- the continual and careful observation to identify any worsening of the heart condition or to detect any other complication.

Labour
Labour and delivery increase the stress on both the mother and the fetus. Continuous and exact observation (monitoring) is of the greatest importance. Intervention (such as forceps) is indicated when maternal or fetal response to contractions indicate the beginning of oxygen deprivation. Analgesics are usually prescribed by an anaesthetist; epidural analgesia is often used.

Following delivery
After the placenta has separated and the uterus has contracted, the blood which had been supplying the placenta is redirected into the normal maternal circulation. This adds suddenly about 500 ml to the circulation and the patient must be carefully observed for the development of cardiac failure. After 24 hours this danger should have passed because of the physiological diuresis following the withdrawal of the oestrogen-producing placenta.

The remaining postnatal period is usually normal and uncomplicated. If the woman has severe heart disease, she would be advised against breast feeding.

DIABETES

Pre-existing frank or clinical diabetes can become unstable during pregnancy. As the pregnant woman is usually in the younger age group, her diabetes is more likely to be the juvenile-onset (rather than the milder, mature-onset) type of diabetes.

Gestational diabetes is a temporary diabetic condition which arises because of the changed carbohydrate metabolism during pregnancy. Its effects can be as severe as those of pre-existing diabetes.

All pregnant women have routine urine tests for glycosuria at every visit. A positive test is an indication for a glucose tolerance test (GTT) to be performed. GTT is now becoming a routine investigation in many centres at 32 weeks.

Effects upon the mother
The pregnant diabetic woman is more likely to succumb to infection, particularly vaginal, urinary tract and puerperal infection. Wound healing is

often delayed, and pre-eclampsia occurs in about 25% of diabetic pregnancies. Pre-existing diabetes which was formerly stabilised can become unstable and both pre-existing and gestational diabetes can become severe and difficult to control.

Effects upon the fetus

Glucose crosses the placenta and in poorly controlled maternal diabetes the fetus is exposed to hyperglycaemia. This causes increased secretion of fetal insulin which, in turn, causes the fetus to grow unusually large. Excessive liquor (polyhydramnios) is common, and the incidence of fetal malformations is two to three times higher in diabetic mothers. Induction of labour may be necessary before term to prevent difficulty at delivery, or polyhydramnios which may cause premature labour or rupture of the membranes: in both cases the baby is at risk because of immaturity. After birth the baby is prone to hypoglycaemia and this is most likely to arise 2 to 4 hours after birth.

Management

The pregnant diabetic woman is managed by a specialist team consisting of an obstetrician, a physician, and a dietitian. The delivery is attended by a paediatrician.

During pregnancy

The control of diabetes becomes more difficult as the pregnancy advances. The woman visits every 2 weeks, for diet and insulin adjustment, until 34 weeks when she is usually admitted to hospital for stabilisation of the diabetes and further assessment. An amniocentesis may be performed at 35 to 36 weeks to assess the maturity of the fetal lungs, and labour may need to be induced if pre-eclampsia arises. If possible the pregnancy is allowed to continue to term.

During labour

A vaginal delivery is normal, unless there is some obstetrical complication. Continuous fetal monitoring is usual. Birth trauma associated with an over-large baby is less common as diabetic care improves. Even so, difficulty delivering the shoulders can still be a problem.

A continuous dextrose infusion is maintained throughout labour, with (usually) 2-hourly blood glucose estimations and insulin given accordingly.

During the puerperium

The woman with gestational diabetes, or the mild diabetic, will return to normal over the first postnatal days. Lactation can be successfully established in these patients.

The severe diabetic may have to suppress lactation because it tends to interfere with the control of diabetes. It is important for the woman to be re-established on her insulin and diabetic diet before she is discharged from hospital.

Some very severe diabetics cannot breast feed because of vascular damage within the breast tissue.

Initial care of the baby

In response to maternal hyperglycaemia, the fetal pancreas has been producing excessive quantities of insulin; this persists for a period after birth and so the infant is prone to develop hypoglycaemia.

To prevent hypoglycaemia glucose is administered immediately after birth. For example, IV dextrose 50%, 2 ml per kilogram is given as a statim dose, followed by continuous IV therapy of 10% dextrose solution as well as early, frequent, high calorie, oral feedings.

Blood sugar is monitored, using Dextrostix, hourly for 4 hours and then before each feed.

URINARY TRACT INFECTION

Pre-existing asymptomatic urinary tract infection may flare up because of the pregnant woman's physiological reduction of the normal defence mechanisms of the urinary tract. Infection most often occurs between 20 and 28 weeks.

Severe infections may arise, with symptoms of sudden onset of nausea, vomiting, tachycardia, pyrexia, and loin and abdominal pain. The urine often has an offensive smell and contains protein.

The woman with severe urinary tract infection is at risk of anaemia, pre-eclampsia, chronic pyelonephritis and renal damage. The fetus is at risk of prematurity and growth retardation.

Management
Admission to hospital is necessary to achieve rehydration and correction of fluid balance. Reduction of temperature is urgent. Symptoms are relieved with anti-emetics and effective analgesics. Anaemia is corrected and antibiotic chemotherapy started. Catheterisation is avoided unless absolutely necessary. Careful observation to exclude threatened abortion or premature labour is important. Intravenous pyelogram, cystoscopy and renal biopsy are deferred until several weeks after delivery.

Prevention
The routine collection of a mid-stream specimen of urine from every pregnant woman early in her pregnancy—at the first visit—is now recommended, to screen for asymptomatic bacteriuria.

ANAEMIA

The pregnant woman needs to be fit and healthy and have a competent oxygen-carrying capacity in order for her body to supply the fetus with its oxygen needs. Anaemia during pregnancy makes the mother less able to withstand blood loss and more susceptible to infection. If the anaemia is severe she is prone to the development of cardiac failure. Anaemia can also cause fetal hypoxia and premature labour.

Anaemia is investigated if the woman's haemoglobin level drops to 11 g (75%), or below. It is not always evident by external signs; any symptoms are usually vague (lassitude, fainting, palpitations and so on). For this reason, haemoglobin estimations are done at the first visit, and subsequently as indicated. In most cases adequate nutrition and prophylactic oral iron-therapy are satisfactory measures to compensate for the physiological anaemia (haemodilution) of pregnancy.

Pre-existing anaemia is, however, a problem that needs active attention. There are three main causes:

- iron deficiency
- folic acid deficiency
- thalassaemia minor.

Iron-deficiency anaemia
This may be due to inadequate dietary intake, poor absorption, hyperemesis, heavy menstrual losses, repeated frequent pregnancies. Small continuous blood losses (e.g. as in haemorrhoids) can contribute.

Iron-deficiency anaemia is treated by the administration of iron and by dietary management. If there is no rapid response to iron therapy or if the haemoglobin levels are below 8 g (55%), packed cells are given.

Folic-acid-deficiency anaemia
Folic acid is necessary for tissue growth and the production of red blood cells. The pregnant woman's requirements of folic acid are increased five times above the requirements of the non-pregnant woman. A diet rich in green leafy vegetables and animal protein is usually adequate to cover the increased requirements.

Most at risk are those with a history of antepartum haemorrhage or growth-retarded baby, those with poor socio-economic conditions, a current multiple pregnancy, or four or more previous pregnancies.

Specific management is the daily administration of folic acid in tablet form combined with dietary improvement if necessary. Some doctors prescribe folic acid daily as a preventive measure to all of their patients; others only to those at risk.

Thalassaemia minor
This is an inherited defect, occurring in Mediterranean people. Specifically it occurs in 6% of women born in Greece, and 4% of women born in Italy. There is abnormal haemoglobin synthesis resulting in reduced numbers of red blood cells and early haemolysis.

Normally thalassaemia is symptom free, apart from the woman having a lowered haemoglobin level. During pregnancy there will be further reduction in the haemoglobin and the woman will be unable to cope with any extra physiological stress. For example, a moderately severe infection could precipitate heart failure.

As thalassaemia minor is not an iron-deficiency anaemia, it cannot be treated with iron. Folic acid is given prophylactically to ensure that there is no complicating folic acid deficiency. The woman is observed carefully throughout the antenatal period so that infection and other body stresses can be prevented.

Blood transfusion will raise the haemoglobin, but is usually reserved for a crisis.

ESSENTIAL HYPERTENSION

Pre-existing hypertension may have already been diagnosed and the patient may already be under treatment for the condition. It may, on the other hand, be discovered for the first time during pregnancy.

An elevated blood pressure during the *first 3 months* is suggestive of essential hypertension and so is investigated. Essential hypertension can increase sevenfold the likelihood of pre-eclampsia, and tenfold the likelihood of eclampsia. If pre-eclampsia is superimposed upon essential hypertension the dangers of pre-eclampsia (p. 100) are much more severe, and accidental haemorrhage and fetal death are more likely.

Management

Antenatal care is aimed at the control of blood pressure and the early detection of the first signs of the onset of pre-eclampsia. The woman will be checked at least fortnightly until 28 weeks and then weekly until she delivers. She is encouraged to rest; admission to hospital may be necessary if the conditions at home do not allow satisfactory rest. Sedation, e.g. phenobarbitone 30 mg, *tds*, may be ordered if it is thought necessary.

Antihypertensive drugs such as reserpine and methyldopa may be prescribed to control the hypertension.

The woman is admitted to hospital immediately if *one* of the signs of pre-eclampsia (finger oedema or proteinuria) should appear, and also if there is any further rise of her blood pressure after 28 weeks.

The pregnancy is continued for as long as it is safe. Induction of labour is usual, depending upon the results of urinary oestriol collection (which are done from 34 weeks onwards) or other evidence of placental insufficiency.

SEXUALLY TRANSMITTED DISEASES

Signs or symptoms of syphilis, gonorrhoea and genital herpes simplex arising in the mother during pregnancy require immediate investigation and treatment to prevent the transmission of the disease to the fetus in utero or during delivery.

SYPHILIS

Syphilis may result in infection of the fetus and placenta with the spirochaete *Treponema pallidum*.

Early treatment with large doses of penicillin will be necessary to prevent abortion, stillbirth or the baby being born with congenital syphilis.

Blood is taken routinely from all patients at their first antenatal visit for VDRL or USR testing. The test may be repeated later in suspicious cases.

If the mother is diagnosed as having syphilis and is treated, her baby will still need to be investigated in the early postnatal period, and will possibly need further penicillin therapy. The signs of congenital syphilis are a brownish rash on the buttocks, sores about the mouth and discharge from the nose. Later the classic 'saddle' nose, teeth deformities, deafness and impaired vision may appear.

GONORRHOEA

Gonorrhoea during early pregnancy may cause spontaneous abortion. If the pregnancy continues, and the baby is born vaginally, the gonococcal organisms may enter the baby's eyes (Fig. 10.1). Unless the eye infection is treated promptly it could cause blindness.

The mother may be affected following delivery should the organisms enter even tiny lacerations in the cervix and vagina; puerperal sepsis may result from this.

Any suspicious discharge is examined immediately and if gonorrhoea is diagnosed large doses of antibiotics (the treatment of choice is penicillin) are ordered.

GENITAL HERPES

There are two types of herpes simplex virus (HSV)—type I, which causes common cold sores on the lips, and type II, which causes lesions in the lower genital tract. They can, however, both be found in the opposite sites. Although they are microscopically different, both types produce very similar effects. As with other viruses, HSV are able to remain alive in the body indefinitely after the first infection, travelling along the nerves to a ganglion near the spinal cord where they survive in a dormant state. They may be reactivated at times of physical or emotional stress (or for no obvious reason).

Herpes genitalis is highly infectious and is spread by direct contact with the lesion, i.e. by sexual intercourse and orogenital contact. It has an incubation period of 2 to 7 days, possibly longer, from the time of contact.

Recurrences may occur more frequently and are sometimes a little more severe during pregnancy. Because the herpes virus is a comparatively large virus it does not cross the placental barrier and so the fetus is not affected. But herpes is significant when it is active at the time of delivery; the baby can be infected at any time after the membranes rupture but particularly as he descends through the vagina. Newborn infants are particularly susceptible to serious and sometimes fatal infections with either HSV-I or HSV-II.

Obstetricians are careful to exclude active her-

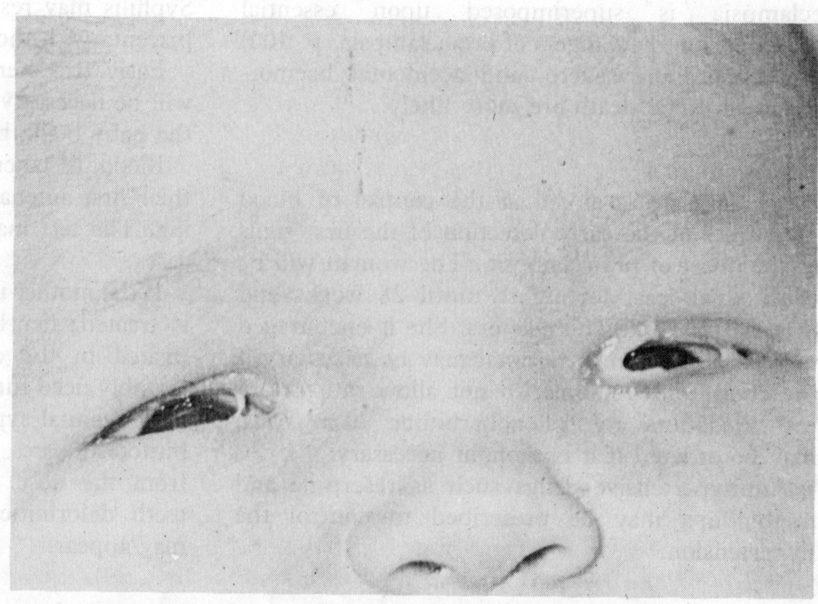

Figure 10.1 Gonococcal *ophthalmia neonatorum*: a profuse purulent discharge develops, and unless treated can lead to blindness; the baby would be nursed in an isolation unit

pes in the 3 to 6 weeks before delivery in a woman who has a history of genital herpes. If viral cultures taken during this period are negative and if there are no active lesions at the time of labour then vaginal delivery is safe, but if there is any doubt the baby would be delivered by caesarean section.

HUMAN IMMUNODEFICIENCY VIRUS (HIV)

Human immunodeficiency virus is the virus responsible for the condition known as AIDS—acquired immune deficiency syndrome. The virus is transmitted mainly in seminal fluid and blood, but also in rectal mucus, vaginal mucus, via the placenta, in breast milk and possibly in saliva. The disease can remain dormant for many years and not progress at all, but when it does it eventually renders the person unable to fight opportunistic infections and there is a high mortality rate in such cases.

AIDS was at first linked almost exclusively to male homosexuals but there are now several cases involving the female partners of bisexual men. It can also occur in heterosexual men who have had sexual contact with prostitutes. Its appearance amongst intravenous drug users is, however, occurring at a rapidly rising rate.

Clinical signs of AIDS may not appear until 3 or 4 years after the disease has been contracted. Antenatal scanning for the presence of antibodies has been recommended, but many years may pass before it becomes routine for all pregnant women. It is certainly indicated in intravenous drug users. As the disease has been in existence for so short a time, there are very few completed studies on its effects upon pregnancy outcome and on the baby. But the baby may contract the virus before, during or after the birth and if so, the outlook is bleak.

The mother with HIV infection is likely to have emotional and social problems associated with the probable low survival prospects for herself and her baby. If she is an intravenous user of a drug of dependency, she and the baby may both be experiencing the effects of withdrawal. Breast feeding is usually contra-indicated, but the mother would be allowed normal contact with her baby unless she has open skin lesions.

RHESUS INCOMPATIBILITY

The Rhesus (Rh) system is a series of antigens present in the red blood cells of approximately 85% of people. Because the Rhesus factor is antigenic, any Rh-positive blood entering the bloodstream of a person with Rh-negative blood will cause the formation of antibodies against the Rh factor.

When Rh-positive cells encounter these antibodies, the antibodies will react with and destroy the red blood cells. This process will lead to anaemia. The breakdown of haemoglobin results in excessive circulating bilirubin which can escape into the tissues, resulting in jaundice.

- If the mother is Rh negative and the father Rh negative, the fetus will be Rh negative, and there will not be any Rh incompatibility.
- If the mother is Rh negative and the father is Rh positive (heterozygous), there is a 50–50 chance of the fetus being Rh positive. Where the father is homozygously Rh positive, the fetus will be Rh positive.

There is normally no communication between the fetal and maternal bloodstreams, but *at the time of abortion or delivery* some fetal cells *may* get into the maternal circulation. It is not completely understood how they enter the maternal bloodstream; it is believed to be due to miniature leaks from the maternal surface of the placenta at the time of its separation.

Fetal cells entering the maternal Rh-negative circulation are not harmful unless they are Rh positive; then the mother will produce antibodies.

It is rare for a first pregnancy to be affected unless the mother has had a previous encounter with the Rh factor, perhaps from a blood transfusion. In a subsequent pregnancy, however, any antibodies present in the mother's circulation will pass through the placental barrier from the mother to the fetus. If *that* fetus is Rh positive, the antibodies will react with the fetal blood cells and destroy them, leading to anaemia and jaundice. So, Rh incompatibility will not usually affect the first fetus, but could affect subsequent pregnancies in progressive degrees of severity.

In recent years, gammaglobulin (anti-D) has been given to the Rh-negative woman within 72 hours of her delivering an Rh-positive baby, to *prevent* the formation of antibodies.

Antenatal management

Blood is tested at the first visit, then later in pregnancy (usually at 28, 32, 34, 36 weeks) for the presence of iso-agglutins. If these tests are positive, and the levels rising, an amniocentesis is performed to examine the liquor and measure the quantity of bilirubin from fetal red cell destruction.

If levels are found to be high, labour is induced, bearing in mind the risks of immaturity. If induction is felt to be unwise, an intrauterine transfusion of Rh-negative blood may be given. The blood is put directly into the fetal peritoneal cavity under ultrasound vision.

Management following birth

The cord is cut quickly at delivery, and a specimen of cord blood collected.

The baby is observed closely for the first 4 days for the development of jaundice. Blood is taken daily, or more often, for serum bilirubin estimations, and treatment is given according to the results.

Phototherapy may bring the bilirubin level low enough to avoid the danger of kernicterus (p. 199), but a severely Rh-affected baby will often need an exchange transfusion to remove the circulating antibodies and correct the anaemia. Rh-negative blood (about 200 ml) is given, usually via the umbilical vein, using a two-way tap, with 10 ml of blood being withdrawn from the baby and discarded for each 10 ml of blood being injected.

ABO incompatibility

A mother with the blood group 'O' may sometimes carry antibodies to 'A', 'B' or 'AB' blood. These antibodies can cross the placenta and cause haemolysis, even in a first pregnancy. It is more common than Rh incompatibility but usually less severe. Very occasionally a baby may be severely affected by ABO incompatibility and will require an exchange transfusion.

PRE-ECLAMPSIA-PREGNANCY-INDUCED HYPERTENSION

Pre-eclampsia (also called Pregnancy-induced Hypertension P.I.H.) is a condition peculiar to pregnancy, and is characterised by oedema, hypertension and proteinuria.

Pre-eclampsia is commonest after 28 weeks gestation. Its cause is unknown, but certain predisposing factors are:

- its peculiarity to pregnancy
- it affects mainly primigravidae
- overdistension of the uterus (as in twins, polyhydramnios, fetal abnormalities)
- complicating medical conditions such as renal disease, essential hypertension, diabetes
- placental dysfunction, e.g. infarction or degeneration
- a higher incidence when the diet is of poor quality.

Pre-eclampsia does not necessarily recur in a subsequent pregnancy. Its main effect is arterial constriction, which causes a rise in blood pressure and reduces the effective blood supply to many of the body organs and tissues including the placenta—thus causing fetal deprivation.

Dangers of pre-eclampsia

Uncontrolled or untreated pre-eclampsia may lead to eclampsia (see p. 102), placenta abruptio (p. 106), renal failure and permanent hypertension. The placenta may become infarcted, limiting the oxygen and nutrients available to the fetus. Intrauterine growth retardation can occur and hypoxia may leave the fetus unable to withstand the normal stresses of labour. In severe cases the fetus dies from anoxia before labour.

Diagnosis
The clinical *signs* usually appear well before the symptoms, and treatment is commenced as soon as two of the three signs are recognised:

- oedema—of the face, legs, hands (tight wedding ring), feet; sudden weight gain
- blood pressure—a steady rise through pregnancy, or a rise of more than 20 mmHg systolic or 10 mmHg diastolic above the early pregnancy reading
- proteinuria—solid protein particles present in the urine after it has been boiled; due to actual kidney damage, it is a sign that the pre-eclampsia is serious.

Symptoms appear late in the disease process and are a danger sign of impending eclampsia:

- gastric—vomiting, epigastric pain
- visual—blurring of vision, specks and flashes of light, loss of sight
- frontal headache
- oliguria.

Management
Antenatal care aims to prevent the development of pre-eclampsia, or at least to recognise it in its very early stages. Particular supervision is given to those women who are in the high-risk groups. The underlying cause is the pregnancy, which is not removed until delivery.

Early diagnosis
The weight, blood pressure and urine of all patients is checked and oedema searched for at every antenatal visit.

Excessive weight gain is a cause for concern, and elevation of blood pressure by more than 20 mmHg systolic or 10 mmHg diastolic is an indication for admission to hospital. If proteinuria is found, the woman is admitted immediately.

General treatment
The woman will need to rest in bed (toilet and bathroom privileges may be allowed). She may find it hard to understand the need for hospitalisation, bed-rest and quiet when she feels well and has no symptoms.

A high protein diet, with no added salt, is usually ordered. She is generally allowed a free fluid intake but should be reminded that her fluid intake and output are being carefully recorded and so to be aware of this. The sudden change to bed-rest, added to her physiological predisposition to constipation, may make the administration of gentle aperients necessary.

Observation
4-hourly recording of vital signs, fetal heart and oedema rate is usual unless there is an indication to check these more frequently. A diastolic reading of 90 mmHg is almost always recorded in red on the patient's chart. These observations should be made with as little disturbance to the woman as possible. She is weighed each day. Urine is tested fully at least once daily, and specifically for protein every 4 hours.

Investigations
Medical investigations may include:

- a mid-stream urine specimen, to exclude urinary infection
- blood examination, especially for blood urea levels (to assess any kidney damage) and haemoglobin
- a retinal examination—for changes in the retinal blood vessels
- urinary or plasma oestriol and human placental lactogen (HPL) levels to assess the functioning of the fetoplacental unit.

Medical treatment
If the pre-eclamptic condition is mild, sedation, such as sodium amytal 50 mg *tds* plus night sedation, is usually sufficient to bring the blood pressure down to safe levels. When the condition is more severe, intramuscular sodium phenobarb (200 mg, every 8 hours), sodium phenytoin (100 mg, every 8 hours) and diazepam (10 mg every 6 to 8 hours) might be ordered, either singly or in combination.

Hypotensive drugs such as propranolol, reserpine and methyldopa are occasionally used. Diuretics are not given as they can be quite dangerous with this condition.

Induction of labour

It may become necessary to terminate the pregnancy to prevent pre-eclampsia from developing into eclampsia. The decision is made considering the relative risks to both mother and baby should the condition worsen, and the risks of immaturity (if the pregnancy is terminated).

Labour is usually induced using both artificial rupture of the membranes and Syntocinon infusion. The labour would be monitored throughout, and the baby most probably would be delivered using forceps to reduce the pushing effort during the second stage. Ergometrine is not given following delivery as it can cause elevation of the blood pressure. Syntocinon is often used as a substitute.

The woman will need continued careful observation for a minimum 24 hours following delivery; sometimes for several days. Eclampsia may still arise in the postnatal period.

In those cases where the cervix is not 'ripe' or the fetal head is not fixed, or where the mother is an 'elderly' primigravida a caesarean section is performed instead of inducing labour. It is also performed immediately if there are signs of fetal distress or if labour fails to progress well.

ECLAMPSIA

Eclampsia is a rare condition which may develop suddenly, with or without preceding pre-eclampsia. It is characterised by fitting which resembles that of a 'grand mal' of epilepsy except that there is usually no loss of sphincter control. Eclampsia is most often seen during or immediately following labour.

Warning signs

A fit may be preceded by:

- a sudden increase in the severity of pre-eclampsia and the appearance of symptoms (see above)
- increased drowsiness
- rolling of the eyes
- twitching
- irregular breathing.

The fits may vary in length, severity and number. If fitting is severe the mother may develop heart failure and pulmonary oedema and become critically ill. Other complications are cerebral oedema, cerebrovascular accident, separation of part of the placenta and disseminated intravascular coagulation (DIC). Fetal deprivation of oxygen can lead to fetal death.

Management

During a fit the first priority is to ensure a clear and satisfactory airway. The woman is protected from physical injury by the usual nursing methods. Magnesium sulphate, a neuromuscular sedative, may be given to prevent further fitting. Diazepam is also sometimes prescribed.

Minimal lighting and absolute quiet are essential when there is any danger of fitting. Occasionally the hospital administration will seek police co-operation to re-route traffic, or will recommend the halting of nearby building works, as even fairly remote outside noises can initiate further fitting.

Eclampsia is fortunately becoming less common as a result of improved antenatal care. It is still, however, responsible for a number of maternal deaths each year, and its effects upon the quality of life of those who survive it may not be good.

HYPEREMESIS

Hyperemesis is defined as excessive vomiting during pregnancy. Its exact cause is not known, but is possibly caused by an over-reaction to chorionic gonadotrophin or the increased levels of oestrogen. It occurs more commonly in first pregnancies and in those with higher than normal levels of HCG, such as multiple pregnancies and hydatidiform mole. Psychiatric and emotional factors (such as a negative response to the pregnancy and poor family relationships) are often, but not always, associated with hyperemesis.

The dangers of hyperemesis include dehydration, fluid and electrolyte imbalance, weight loss, ketosis and, in extreme cases, oligura and jaundice.

Management includes admission to hospital, bed rest, fluid replacement by intravenous therapy and careful recording of fluid intake and output. Small dry meals may be offered frequently (e.g. 6 times a day) and clear fluids 1 hour after the meals. Vitamins, especially B complex, C and K may be given by either the intravenous or intramuscular route, and anti-emetics and mild or moderate sedatives are sometimes prescribed.

The woman is nursed in quiet well-ventilated surroundings, in a single room at first if possible. The condition is explained to her and to her family and their co-operation is sought. This may sometimes involve restriction of visiting until the vomiting has ceased. Referral to a counsellor, chaplain or social worker may be appropriate.

MULTIPLE PREGNANCY

The incidence of twins is about once in every 80 births, and that of triplets is 80 times that again—once in every 6400 births. These figures are fluctuating, however, due to the increasing use of fertility drugs and in vitro fertilisation procedures. As twins are the most common multiple pregnancies and are most likely to be met by the student nurse, this section concentrates on them, rather than on triplets or greater multiple births.

Causes

Multiple births, especially of *fraternal* twins (where two ova are fertilised), tend to run in families. They are passed down through both the father and mother, often skipping a generation. They are more common in mothers over the age of 35.

It is not known why *identical* twins occur, that is, why one ovum or inner cell mass (p. 31) should divide to develop into two babies. Identical twins are more common in younger mothers.

Fertility drugs act upon the hypothalamic-pituitary system, causing the release of follicle stimulating hormone. If FSH is released, it may be in greater quantities than desired although as research and techniques improve more accurate doses are able to be calculated.

High levels of FSH lead to increased ovarian follicular stimulation. In some cases this results in more than one ovum being released and subsequently fertilised.

Table 10.1 compares the features of binovular and uniovular twins.

Where there is doubt as to whether the twins are fraternal or identical, further studies to establish the genotype are done.

Table 10.1 Types of twins

	Binovular (fraternal)	Uniovular (identical)
Origin	Two ova	One ovum
Incidence	75% of twins	25% of twins
Sexes	May be opposite	Always the same
Likeness	As in any brother or sister resemblance	Identical (same genetic make-up) (minor differences, stature, fingerprints)
Chorion	Two separate chorions	One or two chorions
Placenta	Two separate placentae may be fused but the two placental circulations remain separate	One or two placentae depending upon when the division occurred placental circulations may communicate

Diagnosis of twins

Twins are suspected when either weight gain or uterine growth is large for dates. Now that ultrasound techniques are widely available, diagnosis and exclusion of other causes (excessive amniotic fluid, fibroids, hydatidiform mole, wrong dates) is easy, and can be made early. Later, twins may be discovered by excessive fetal movements or parts, palpation of two heads, or simultaneous auscultation of two fetal heart rates by two different examiners who find a variation in rate of at least 10 beats per minute.

With antenatal care now so widely available it has become rare for a twin pregnancy to remain undiagnosed until the time of delivery. (Even so, the fundus is always felt before the administration of intravenous oxytocin to hasten the third stage of labour.)

Effect of twins upon pregnancy

Apart from the emotional, social and financial

aspects (see below) a multiple pregnancy may be complicated by:

- minor disorders being more troublesome
- polyhydramnios (excessive liquor)
- pre-eclampsia (more common)
- anaemia (more likely)
- low placental implantation covering a larger area (antepartum haemorrhage)
- fetal/placental insufficiency
- premature labour, due to increased uterine tension.

Labour

Labour may be complicated by:

- malpresentations, especially of the second twin, often involving breech or transverse lie
- early rupture of the membranes (increased intrauterine tension) before the first fetus is securely engaged in the pelvis—danger of prolapsed cord
- premature separation of the second fetus's placenta, following the delivery of the first baby and the subsequent reduction in the size of the uterus.

Following delivery

There is a predisposition to:

- maternal post-partum haemorrhage—due to considerably stretched uterus and to the large placental site(s)
- prematurity of the babies, and the hazards involved therewith.

Management of multiple pregnancy

Multiple pregnancy does involve more hazards than a single pregnancy, to both the mother and the fetuses. Therefore, extra antenatal supervision is given. Advice and treatment are usually indicated to ensure:

- sufficient rest to improve uterine blood flow (the mother may be hospitalised to prevent premature labour)
- an adequate, well-balanced diet, with iron and folic acid supplements
- prompt relief of minor disorders and discomforts
- early recognition of complications such as pre-eclampsia or low placental implantation.

Labour management involves:

- palpation and perhaps turning of the second fetus after delivery of the first
- prompt and careful clamping and tying of the cord (in case it is a uniovular pregnancy with communicating placental circulation).

The impact of multiple births

The prospect of having two (or more) babies instead of only one may come as a shock to the woman and her husband, especially if there is no family history of multiple births or if the mother has not had infertility treatment.

Although they become very 'special' as future parents, the woman's predisposition to problems with the pregnancy and confinement deserves consideration. The couple should still attend antenatal education and childbirth preparation classes, even though intervention (perhaps by induction, monitoring and assisted delivery) in labour is more likely. They should *anticipate* a normal and natural labour experience, but should understand that intervention may be necessary to achieve the best quality of life for the babies.

The parents should be aware that the babies may be small, and may therefore be separated from the mother to be cared for in a nursery setting. Lactation may need to be established by breast expression; a tiring and tedious business at times. The parents may have to cope with the anxiety of people close to them, or with misunderstanding about their own response to the situation.

Not all twin babies are premature, small, or weak. The average weight of twins born at full term is about 2.7 kg, which is quite a satisfactory weight for normal management in hospital and for going home at the usual time.

There are social, financial and emotional aspects of knowing that a baby is expected, and these aspects are likely to be even more of a problem when there is more than one baby. Where there are already 'too many children' for the parents' emotional or financial resources to cope with, the news could seem to be a disaster. Social workers, especially those employed full time in the maternity area, have access to many avenues of relief; many doctors routinely offer all multiple pregnancy patients the opportunity of discussion with a social worker.

The postnatal midwife or Infant Welfare sister will know details of local support groups for multiple pregnancy parents. These voluntary bodies provide mutual support, guidance and advice, and often run an equipment-lending service. They also participate in research programmes with the aim of providing knowledge for the future management of multiple pregnancies.

ANTEPARTUM HAEMORRHAGE (APH)

Antepartum haemorrhage is defined as any bleeding which occurs from the genital tract after the 20th week of pregnancy and before the onset of labour. It is regarded as placental in origin until proved otherwise. Incidental causes could be vaginitis or cervical polyps or inflammation, but are comparatively rare.

The two main causes of antepartum haemorrhage of placental origin are placenta praevia and abruptio placentae.

Placenta praevia

Placenta praevia is a condition of abnormally low implantation of the placenta in the uterus (the placenta is normally situated high in the upper segment) (Fig. 10.2). Placenta praevia is described in types:

Type I:	the placenta encroaches upon the lower segment
Type II:	the placenta encroaches upon the margin of the cervical os
Type III:	the placenta covers the cervical os when closed
Type IV:	the placenta lies centrally over the cervical os.

Placenta praevia causes antepartum haemorrhage because the placenta, which cannot stretch, lifts away from the lower segment when it stretches in the later weeks of pregnancy. Painless bright bleeding occurs as the blood vessels supplying the separated part of the placenta are exposed. Initial bleeding is scant and often settles, but it will recur so the woman must be admitted to hospital as each succeeding episode will be more severe and the baby could at any stage need to be delivered. With limited activity only allowed, the hospital stay can be tedious and the woman can find it emotionally hard to sit and simply wait until the fetus is sufficiently mature to be born.

Ultrasound is done to confirm the location of the placenta. Vaginal examination is never performed unless in an operating theatre set up for immediate caesarean section because of the danger of uncontrolled and severe bleeding resulting from

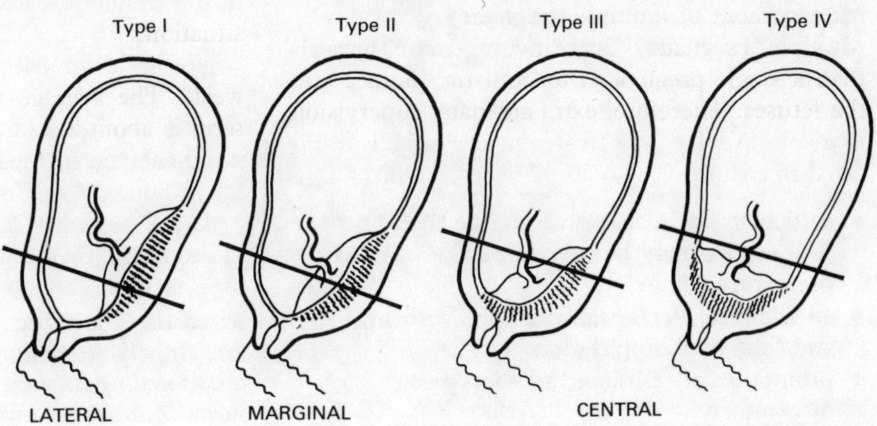

Figure 10.2 Placenta praevia.

digital palpation. Types I and II placenta praevia are sometimes able to be managed by induction of labour and careful monitoring, but Types III and IV will require caesarean delivery.

Abruptio placenta

Abruptio placenta is the premature separation of a normally situated placenta (Fig. 10.3). The resultant bleeding may be revealed, when the blood escapes from the vagina, or concealed, where the bleeding is retained in the uterus. It may be associated with pre-eclampsia or essential hypertension, or it may follow a fall or direct blow to the abdomen. Minimal placental separation may cause little or no pain or alteration in maternal vital signs or fetal heart rate, but moderate to severe abruption can cause severe pain, shock and fetal death unless delivery (by caesarean section) is immediate. It is vital, therefore, that no instance

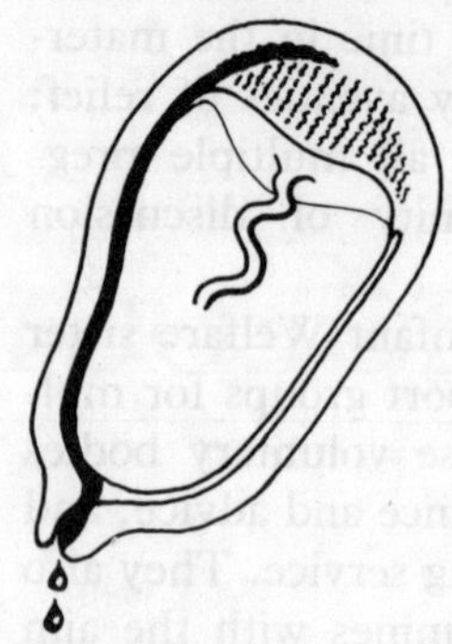
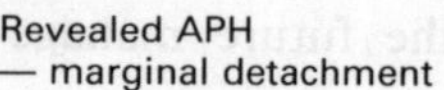

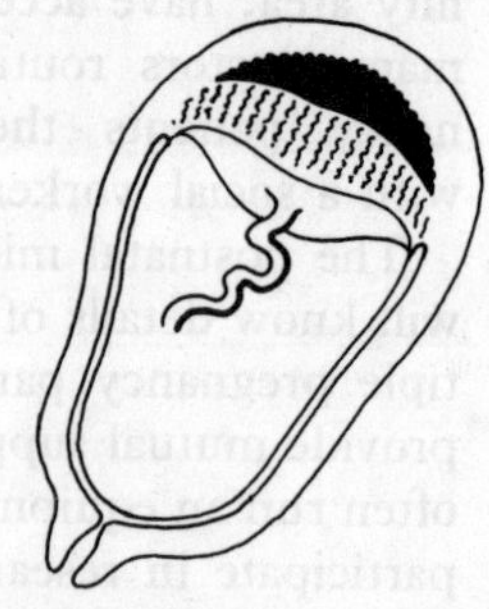

Figure 10.3 Abruptio placenta.

of bleeding at any time during pregnancy be ignored, and also that any abdominal pain is investigated without delay.

11

PHYSIOLOGY OF LABOUR

Chapter outline

Key words

contraction	normal labour
effacement	nullipara
fontanelle	primipara
mechanism of labour	retraction
moulding	'show'
multipara	vertex

Labour is the process by which the products of conception (the viable fetus, placenta and membranes) are expelled from the uterus via the vagina into the external environment. It normally occurs at a time when the uterus can grow no larger, when the fetus is sufficiently mature to survive outside and still small enough to pass through the birth canal.

Normal labour

Normal labour is that which:

- occurs at term (neither premature nor post-mature)
- has a spontaneous onset (not induced)
- is completed after 4 hours, and before 24 hours from the time of its onset (neither precipitate nor prolonged)
- has the (single) fetus presenting by the vertex (top of the head), with the occiput in the anterior part of the pelvis
- is achieved without artificial aids (such as forceps)
- involves no complications (such as excessive haemorrhage)
- involves spontaneous delivery of the placenta.

STAGES OF LABOUR

Labour is divided into three stages:

- The first stage is the stage of dilatation, which lasts from the onset of labour until full dilatation of the cervix.
- The second stage is the stage of expulsion, which lasts from full dilatation of the cervix until the delivery of the baby.
- The third stage is the stage of separation and delivery of the placenta. This lasts from the delivery of the baby until the delivery of the placenta and membranes.

In some centres, the hour or two following the completion of labour is regarded as the 'fourth stage'. This period is one of dramatic change in the woman's body, when complications arising from labour or delivery are likely to occur. The most common complication at this stage is that of bleeding due to the uterus going into a state of relaxation. Other emergencies may arise in the apparently healthy woman, such as a reaction to administered drugs.

The newly delivered woman is kept in the labour ward area or taken to a 'fourth stage' or recovery room where there are suitable facilities to cope with such emergencies, and is observed for at least 1 hour.

THE FACTORS OF LABOUR

The factors involved in labour are:

- the *powers*—contraction and retraction of the uterine muscles plus the voluntary muscular efforts of the mother i.e. contraction of the abdominal muscle and the diaphragm during the 'pushing' or 'bearing-down' phase)
- the *passages*—the bony pelvis, cervix, vagina and pelvic floor (displacement)
- the *passengers*—mainly the fetus (specifically the fetal head), plus the placenta, membranes and liquor.

THE POWERS

The *primary* power of labour is that provided by the contraction and retraction of the uterine muscles.

Contraction

This is the temporary shortening and thickening of the uterine muscles. Contractions are involuntary, are under the control of the sympathetic nervous system, and are probably indirectly influenced by the endocrine system. *Strong* uterine contractions, such as at the end of the first stage of labour, exert an intrauterine pressure of 45 mmHg.

Retraction

Retraction is shortening that persists after a contraction. The muscle fibres do not relax completely at the end of a contraction, but *retain* some of the shortening and thickening (Fig. 11.1).

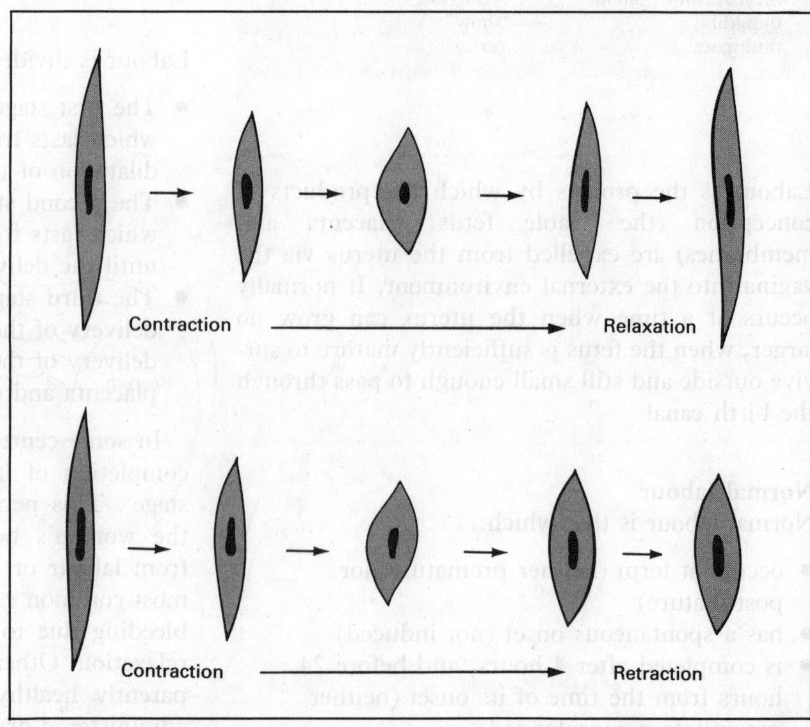

Figure 11.1 Retraction leading to progressive shortening and thickening of the uterine muscle.

Retraction is a special property of uterine muscle.

As a result of retraction, the upper segment of the uterine wall gradually becomes shorter and thicker, and the uterine cavity becomes smaller. Meanwhile, the contracting and retracting muscles of the upper segment cause the specialised fibres of the lower segment and the cervix to be pulled upwards and outwards, to cause *effacement* and *dilatation* of the cervix (see p. 110).

Secondary powers—'bearing down'

The secondary powers (the abdominal muscles and diaphragm) are used in the *second* stage of labour. They are used during 'bearing down' or 'pushing'; they are the mother's voluntary expulsive efforts.

The diaphragm is made rigid by the chest being filled with air and the glottis closed to hold in the pressure. The muscles of the abdominal wall are held in tightly. These actions almost double the pressure on the fetus and reduce the amount of room in the abdominal cavity so that the fetus is pushed down towards that area where there is least resisting pressure, into the escape route, through the pelvis to the vagina.

Pushing is of tremendous assistance in overcoming the resistance of the pelvic floor muscles. Although it involves voluntary muscles, pushing becomes *involuntary* when the pressure of the fetal head on the pelvic floor becomes very strong (just as a loaded rectum brings about an expulsive urge to open the bowels). Sometimes, at 'crowning' (when there is a danger of tearing the perineum), pushing is better controlled and replaced by 'panting', with the mouth and glottis open and the abdominal muscles relaxed.

THE PASSAGES

The fetus must pass through the bony pelvis (Fig. 11.2), the cervix and the vagina to be born. It must also overcome the resistance offered by the pelvic floor and the surrounding structures.

The bony pelvis

The true pelvis is that which lies below the pelvic brim (ileopectineal line), and is the confined space through which the fetus must pass.

Pelvic inlet

The fetus must first enter the pelvic brim. In the

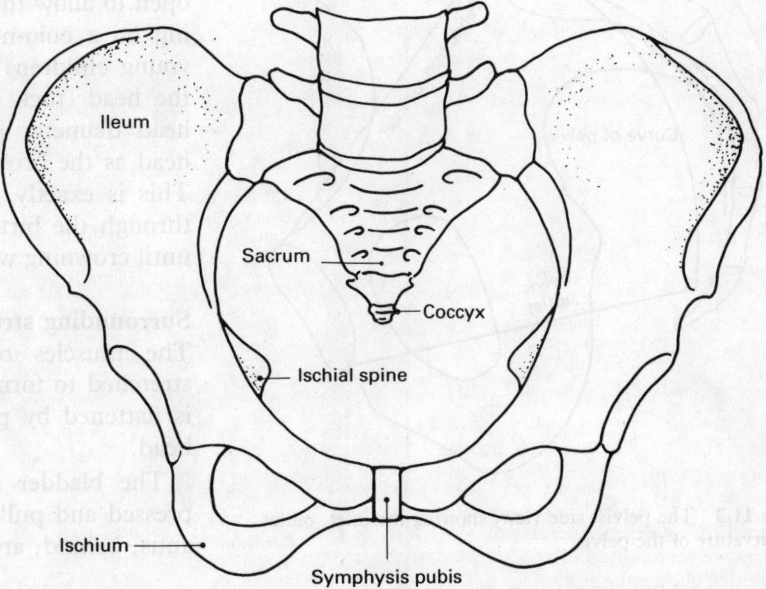

Figure 11.2 The pelvis.

normal female (gynaecoid) pelvis, the brim, which extends from the back of the top of the symphysis pubis to the sacral promontory, measures:

- 11 cm anteroposteriorly (front to back)
- 13.5 cm laterally (side to side).

Pelvic inclination

The pelvis does not sit at right angles to the spine but is inclined or tilted forwards, with the brim at an angle of 60° to the horizontal when erect (Fig. 11.3).

Pelvic cavity

The pelvic cavity (between the inlet and the outlet) is circular in shape and curves forwards. Its average measurement is 12 cm in diameter.

Pelvic outlet

The pelvic (obstetric) outlet is bordered by the two ischial tuberosities (spines), the back of the lowest

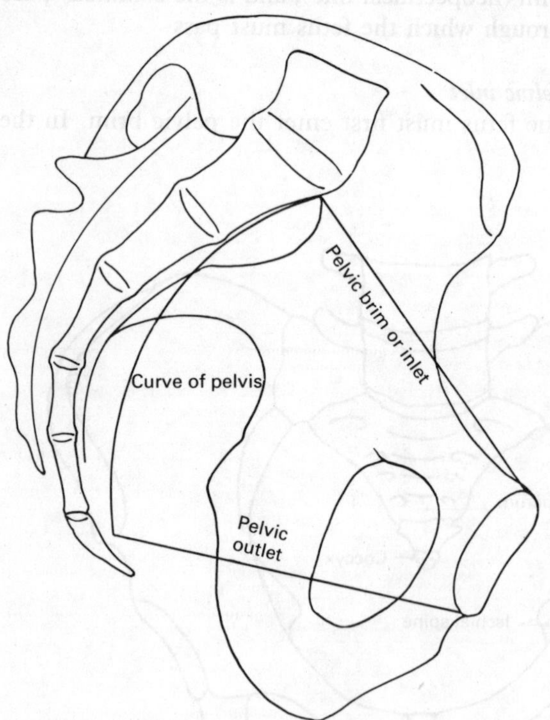

Figure 11.3 The pelvis, side view, showing the inlet, outlet and curvature of the pelvis.

part of the symphysis pubis, and the sacrococcygeal joints. It measures:

- 13.5 cm anteroposteriorly
- 11 cm laterally.

These measurements are a reversal of those of the pelvic inlet.

To negotiate the birth canal, the fetal head must undergo a series of passive movements—the mechanism of labour (Fig. 11.4).

Soft passages

The soft parts of the birth canal are the lower segment of the uterus, the external cervical os, the vagina and the vulva. Once full dilatation of the cervix has occurred, there is a continuous canal with the fetal head dilating the vagina and its vulval orifice.

Effacement and dilatation

The lower segment of the uterus (see p. 57) must be pulled upwards and outwards—*effaced*—and the cervical os must be stretched open—*dilated*—far enough to permit the fetal head to pass through.

This process can be likened to an upside-down version of the process of pulling on a firm-collared polo-neck jumper. The head first stretches out the tube-like neck until it is continuous with the rest of the jumper, then the neck hole itself is forced open to allow the head to go through. When pulling on a polo-necked jumper most people (even young children) instinctively find it easier to flex the head (tuck in the chin) so that the smallest head diameter passes through, then extend the head as the brow and face emerge from the hole. This is exactly what happens to the fetus going through the birth canal. The head is first flexed, until crowning when extension occurs at the vulva.

Surrounding structures

The muscles of the pelvic floor (p. 19) are stretched to form a gutter, and the perineal body is flattened by pressure from the advancing fetal head.

The bladder and urethra, in front, are compressed and pulled upwards, and the rectum and anus, behind, are pushed downwards.

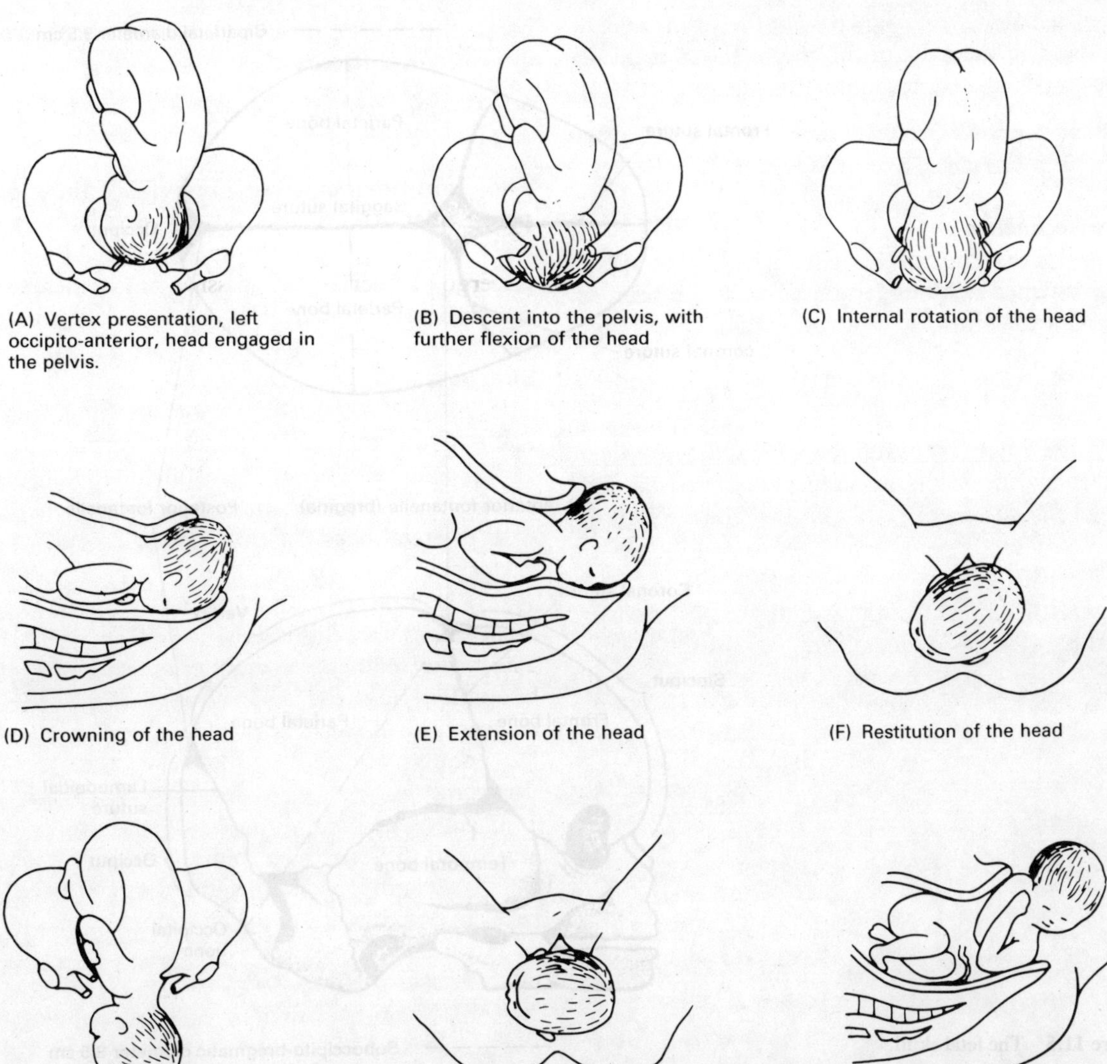

Figure 11.4 The mechanism of normal labour.

THE PASSENGERS

The main passenger through the birth canal is the fetus, and the most significant part of the fetus (because it is the largest) is the fetal head. The head is wider than the shoulders, and makes up approximately one-quarter of the baby's length. 96% of babies are born head first.

The fetal skull
Superior and lateral views of the fetal skull are shown in Figure 11.5.

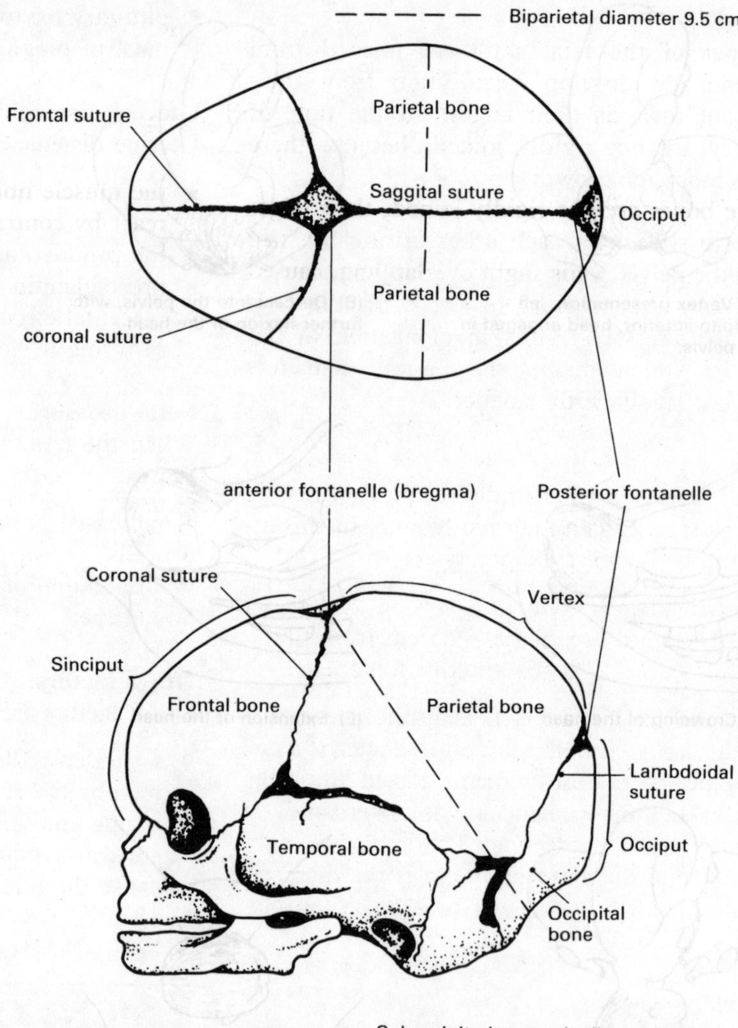

Figure 11.5 The fetal skull.

The vault of the skull is made up of five bones:

- two frontal bones
- two parietal bones
- one occipital bone.

Sutures

The lines of junction between the bones are called sutures. The main ones are:

- frontal—between the two frontal bones
- coronal—between the frontal and parietal bones
- sagittal—between the two parietal bones
- lambdoidal—between the parietal bones and the occiput.

Fontanelles

Fontanelles ('little fountains'—they pulsate) are the areas at which two or more sutures meet.

- The anterior fontanelle (called the *bregma*) is the large diamond-shaped fontanelle (2.5 × 1.25 cm) formed by the junction of the parietal and frontal bones.
- The posterior fontanelle is the smaller, triangular-shaped, junction of the parietal and occipital bones.

Moulding
The bones of the fetal skull are formed from membrane and develop calcification from their centres out towards their edges. At the time of birth they are not rigidly joined, because there must be room for growth.

As the bones are not rigidly joined, their edges are able to slide over each other during the trip through the pelvis. This slight overlapping, caused gradually by the pressure of the birth canal, is called moulding. It results in elongation of the fetal head which makes the largest diameters slightly but significantly smaller.

Attitude
The fetal head is in an attitude (see p. 9) of flexion (chin tucked in) during normal labour. In this attitude, the two largest diameters are

- the biparietal—9.5 cm
- the suboccipito-bregmatic—9.5 cm from the nape of the neck to the anterior fontanelle.

When the fetal head is flexed, the presenting part is the *occiput* and the largest diameter is a circular shape. The head remains flexed until the resistance of the perineum is overcome at 'crowning', when it extends. The extended, sub-occipito-frontal diameter of 10 cm is the diameter which distends the vulva just before the face appears.

CAUSES OF THE ONSET OF LABOUR

The exact causes of the spontaneous onset of labour are still unknown, but there are several interconnected contributing factors.

Changes in hormone levels
Hormone level changes are probably due to placental aging and are as follows:

- progesterone levels fall (muscle relaxation diminishes)
- oestrogen and prostaglandin levels rise
- pituitary oxytocin is released (suppressed for most of pregnancy).

Uterine distension
Uterine distension causes the following to occur:

- the muscle fibres, stretched to their limit, react by contracting
- the production and release of myometrial prostaglandin F
- placental circulation may be interfered with, resulting in hormonal changes (as above).

Fetal pressure
When the fetus has grown to its limit in utero, it causes:

- increased pressure and tension on uterine walls
- stimulation of the distended uterine wall to contract.

Other factors
Other factors are:

- a sudden reduction of pressure when the membranes rupture
- strong emotional disturbances (via the cortical-hypothalamic-pituitary chain) may cause the release of oxytocin.

SIGNS OF THE ONSET OF LABOUR

Early signs of the approach of labour are:

- 'lightening'—the sinking of the fetal head into the pelvic cavity due to it having less room in utero and to the symphysis pubis widening slightly; it often brings relief from respiratory embarrassment and heartburn and may appear at 36 weeks in the primigravida but not until labour in the parous woman whose abdominal muscles are laxer
- frequency (of micturition) due to the pressure of the fetal head upon the bladder
- Braxton-Hicks contractions, felt as the irritable stretched uterus is distending the

abdominal wall, making it thinner and the skin more receptive to sensation.

Contractions

Uterine tightenings or contractions, occurring regularly and producing discomfort and sometimes pain, are a sign of 'true' labour when they continue and increase in frequency. The contractions can be felt by an examiner when the uterus becomes hard and tense. The woman may complain of discomfort beginning at the back and coming around to the lower abdomen.

Show

A 'show' is the appearance of mucus (often blood-stained) from the vagina (Fig. 11.6).

The mucus is thick and difficult to wipe away. It comes from the cervix, where it has been acting as a protective plug (the operculum) during pregnancy. Its appearance is an indication that the cervix is starting to dilate.

A small amount of blood may accompany the mucus (sometimes blood appears on its own). This blood comes from the rupture of tiny capillaries in the cervix (as it begins to open) and from the decidua underlying the chorion (as it lifts from the lower uterine wall as the lower segment starts to stretch).

Dilatation of the cervix

Gradual dilatation of the external cervical os is an indication of the progress of labour when associated with uterine contractions. Dilatation is discovered or verified by vaginal examination.

Engagement of the presenting part

The presenting part (usually the head) of the fetus 'engages' or sinks into the pelvis. In a primigravida this may occur 3–4 weeks before labour starts. The abdominal walls in a multipara are less firm and engagement may not occur until labour has started.

Formation of a bag of forewaters

The formation of a bag of forewaters (liquor trapped in front of the presenting part) can be felt on examination. The bag becomes tense during a contraction, and may rupture. Rupture of the membranes can occur at any time during labour, but it classically occurs at the end of the first stage of labour. It can also occur before labour starts, and so cannot be strictly regarded as a sign of the onset of labour. If liquor is discovered at any stage before or after labour has commenced, and if engagement of the head in the pelvis is not absolutely certain, the vagina should be visually examined by a doctor or midwife to check that cord prolapse has not occurred.

THE FIRST STAGE

The average duration of the first stage of labour is 10–12 hours in a primigravida, and about 4–6 hours in a multipara.

Contraction and retraction of the uterine muscles leads to a reduction in the size of the uterine cavity, with shortening and thickening of the upper uterine segment and lengthening and thinning of the lower uterine segment. Therefore:

- the cervix is taken up—effaced (Fig. 11.7)
- the head begins to descend in the pelvis
- the membranes (which are non-elastic) detach from the stretched lower uterine segment
- a bag of forewaters forms in front of the fetal head

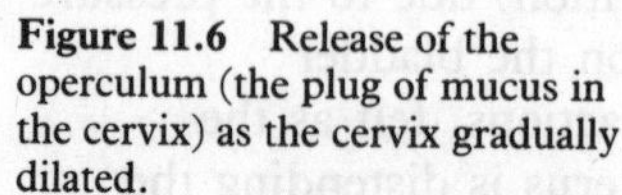

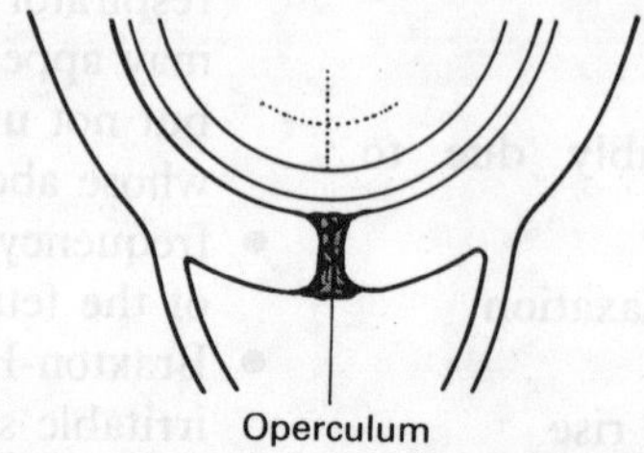

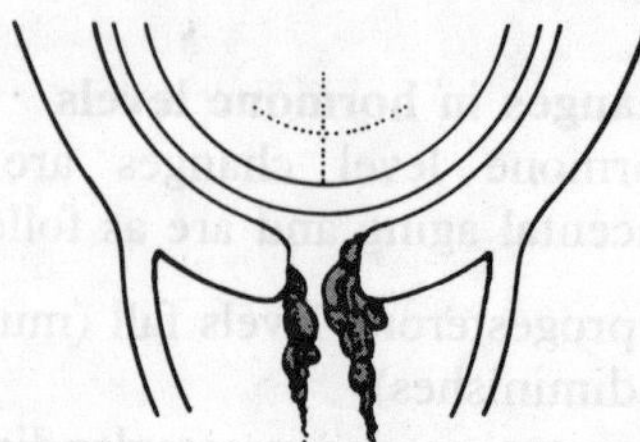

Figure 11.6 Release of the operculum (the plug of mucus in the cervix) as the cervix gradually dilated.

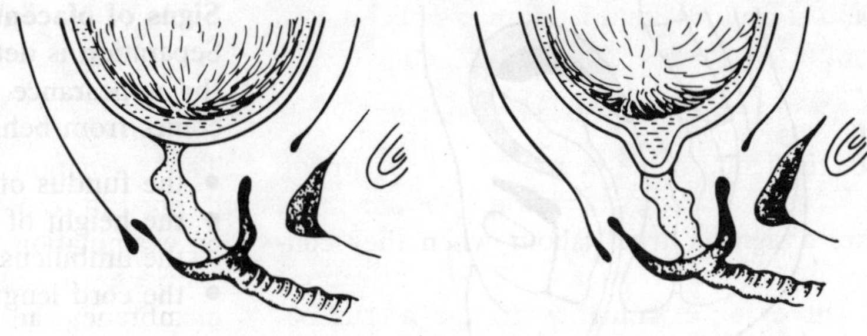

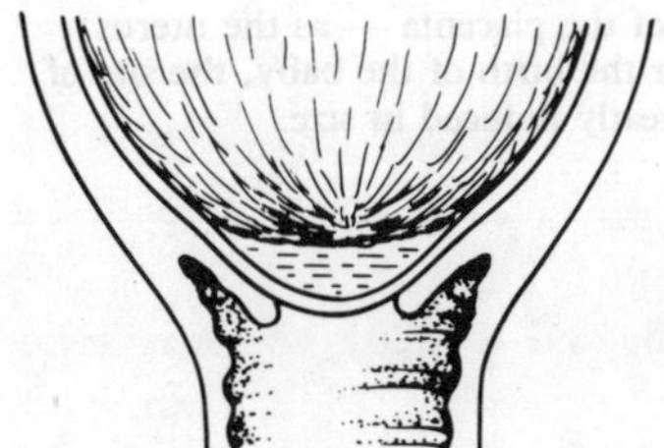

Figure 11.7 Process of 'taking up' of the cervix by which its canal becomes continuous with the lower uterine segment.

- the cervix is gradually dilated (effacement and dilatation occur simultaneously in multiparae), by the pulling up of the lower segment and by the downwards pressure of the forewaters or head.

At the end of the first stage:

- the cervix is fully dilated
- the uterus, cervix and vagina form one continuous canal
- the membranes rupture (if this has not already happened)
- there will be strong uterine contractions usually every 2 to 3 minutes, lasting between 50 and 60 seconds each
- the fetal head will have descended into the pelvis.

THE SECOND STAGE

The second stage of labour is the stage of full descent and expulsion of the fetus. The second stage lasts for an average of $\frac{3}{4}$–1 hour in a primigravida and for about 15–30 minutes in a multipara. The *transition* from first to second stage is often very rapid in a multipara.

The passage of the fetus through the vagina to be born is achieved by:

- strong, long, but perhaps less frequent uterine contraction and retraction
- use of the secondary powers—the abdominal muscles and diaphragm—to assist in pushing the fetus down the birth canal
- displacement of the muscles of the pelvic floor by the advancing fetal head
- considerable dilatation of the vagina (prepared for this by progesterone)
- thinning and lengthening of the perineum (flattened by the advancing fetal head)
- bulging of the vulva and dilatation of its orifice by the emerging head.

All of this culminates in the birth of the baby.

THE THIRD STAGE

Following the delivery of the baby, the uterus is considerably reduced in size. After a brief period,

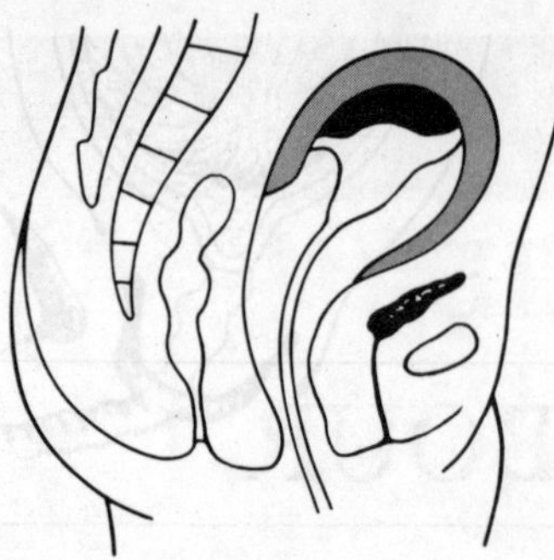

Figure 11.8 Separation of the placenta — as the uterus continues to contract after the birth of the baby, the site of placental attachment is greatly reduced in size.

while it adjusts to the absence of the fetus, the uterus recommences the process of contraction and retraction. Because the placenta is not muscular (and cannot therefore contract with the uterus) it begins to lift away from the uterine wall (Fig. 11.8). When this happens the large blood vessels in the uterine wall behind the placenta bleed and fill the retroplacental space with blood. When this space is filled with blood, the bleeding stops and the blood will clot.

Further uterine contraction causes further placental separation and retroplacental bleeding until the entire placenta has separated and descended, and has been expelled with some assistance from the voluntary powers (bearing down by the mother).

This process can take from 5 minutes to half an hour, with contractions recurring every 2 to 3 minutes. Oxytocic drugs are often prescribed to speed the placental separation. There is usually no difference in the duration of the third stage between multiparae and primiparae.

During placental descent, the membranes are stripped from the uterine walls by the weight of the placenta.

Signs of placental separation and descent

Separation is detected by observing the vagina for the appearance of a small rush of blood which comes from behind the placenta. At descent:

- the fundus of the uterus is firmly contracted
- the height of the fundus drops to the level of the umbilicus
- the cord lengthens at the vulva.

Control of bleeding

After the placenta has separated and delivered, the uterus is left with a large raw area—the placental site. This area has been supplied with enough blood to provide every physical need of the fetus, and so it contains large, open-ended, blood vessels, which could pour out enough blood to cause the woman to bleed to death rapidly if there were no way of stopping the flow.

Bleeding from the placental site is controlled naturally, and excessive bleeding is prevented, by:

- continued strong contraction and retraction of the uterus, reducing the size of the placental site; the criss-cross muscle fibres act as 'living ligatures', closing the blood sinuses at, and reducing the blood flow to, the placental site
- clot formation in the sinuses of the placental site.

The 'fourth stage'

The 'fourth stage' of labour is the name sometimes given to the hour or two following labour; at this time the most important physiological task is the maintenance of strong uterine contraction and retraction. This can be aided by giving oxytocic drugs such as ergometrine maleate, syntocinon or Syntometrine prophylactically or therapeutically. These drugs are often given at the end of the second stage of labour, after the presence of a previously undiagnosed twin has been excluded. Oxytocic drugs may make the *signs* of separation less obvious because of the speed and firmness of the subsequent uterine contraction.

12

CARE OF THE WOMAN IN LABOUR

Chapter outline
Admission to hospital
- Husbands and labour companions
- History and examination
- Preparation procedures

The first stage
- General care
- Prevention and relief of pain and fatigue
- Assessment of progress
- Observing the fetal condition
- Observing the mother's condition

The second stage
- Care and observation

Birth of the baby
- Positions for delivery
- Conduct of the delivery

The third stage
- Examination of the placenta and membranes

Documentation
Witnessing the birth of a baby
- Helping with labour care

Key words

accoucheur	paracervical
Brandt-Andrews method	partogram
cardiotocograph	pudendal
caudal	transition
epidural	Wharton's jelly

Hospital care for labour is the most usual practice in this country and so the nursing student's experience will, with rare exceptions, be limited to observing childbirth in a hospital setting.

The givers of care during labour, the midwives and doctors, hold a wide range of attitudes and have many different approaches to childbirth. Practices vary from one hospital to another, sometimes even from one delivery suite or labour ward to another within the same hospital. A book such as this can cover only that which the student might see during her period of clinical experience in the maternity unit. Some of the procedures and patterns of management which are described here are no longer carried out in some hospitals. They have been included because they are routine in other places. It would be fair to say, however, that in almost every instance, the right of the woman to choose her options in labour care is respected. She, in turn, is expected to be responsible in considering both the welfare of her baby and her own physical condition as she makes those choices.

Childbirth in our technological age is a very different experience from the childbirth of even one generation ago. It is very easy to understand why there is a swing back to nature. Technology has been developed to meet almost every need of the pregnant and labouring woman: as a baby machine she will be kept in good working order. Technological advances have both saved lives and improved quality of life. Yet, as these valuable aids become less restricted to the specific purposes for which they were designed, and become more routine, problems arise. There are emotional needs at every phase of labour, brought on by anxiety, fear, loneliness, pain, excitement and joy. Even in normal labour these needs exist, and if they are not met at least as well as the physical needs, the woman's whole outlook on childbirth and perhaps her subsequent sexual enjoyment could be affected adversely.

ADMISSION TO HOSPITAL

When her booking is accepted the mother-to-be is

most usually given printed information telling her what to expect during her hospital stay. Prominent in this information is a statement reminding her to telephone the hospital when she thinks that she might be in labour. This has a double purpose. The midwife who speaks with the woman will, by careful questioning, be able to assess approximately what the woman's body, in particular her cervix, is doing. If the midwife estimates that labour is in the very early phase of first stage she may recommend that the woman remain at home for a while longer, perhaps taking two paracetamol tablets to take the edge off early contractions and allow the woman to sleep. It can be very disheartening to arrive in hospital too early, and the possibility of good rest and sleep is undoubtedly lessened in strange surroundings. The other purpose of a pre-admission telephone call is so that the labour ward can be made ready and, if necessary, extra staff allocated to the department.

When the woman arrives at the labour ward she and her husband or companion are welcomed by the midwife who will take responsibility for her care. Ideally the couple will have visited the department as part of an antenatal class tour (or by private arrangement) and so the set-up will not be totally strange to them. In most cases labour is established, but still in first stage, when they arrive. The couple are shown into an admission/preparation room, or directly into their labour room. Everything is unpredictable in midwifery, including the time available for interview, history-taking and admission/preparation procedures.

It is not uncommon for contractions to diminish in strength and frequency for a short period after admission to hospital. This may be due to an adrenalin surge which occurs as a result of the excitement of coming in, or it may be due to a (perhaps unconscious) fear of the unfamiliar place, unknown people, pain or labour itself. The increased adrenalin can act upon the uterus to inhibit contractions. If the woman is in true labour, however, the strength and pattern of contractions is soon re-established as she overcomes her first nervousness and relaxes.

HUSBANDS AND LABOUR COMPANIONS

Husbands are made welcome in the delivery suite. As well as his presence usually being a great comfort to his wife, the husband can take an active part in providing physical comfort and giving encouragement. The husband who has participated in antenatal education and childbirth preparation classes can usually regard the whole of labour (not just the delivery) very positively; it is right for him to be there.

Now that the presence of husbands in labour wards is accepted and has become the norm, it must be remembered that there are some who do not want to be there and some whose wives do not want them present. About 10 or 15 years ago husbands were suspected of being rather strange if they wanted to be there; now they may be criticised if they do not have that desire. As long as they are made comfortable in their choice the couple will usually be happy. The state of mind of her husband can be very important to the woman in labour.

Most hospitals expect the couple to plan together about this during pregnancy and to resolve their feelings before coming into hospital. Sometimes the mother may prefer to have the company of a close friend instead of her husband. Whatever the situation, it is usually understood that the husband or friend will accept the discipline of the institution, will be responsible about his or her own state of health at the time, and will be willing to leave if requested by the doctor or midwife.

HISTORY AND EXAMINATION

The first important facts to be ascertained concern the progress of the labour:

- when the contractions started, and when they became regular

- the frequency, duration and strength of contractions now
- the state of the hormones, and the colour of the liquor if they have ruptured

While these facts are being sought, the midwife will be observing the mother, noting her general appearance and her response to contractions, and gauging her overall approach to labour. Some women are excited and challenged by labour, others are fearful—most are a little of both.

The midwife will then examine the woman and record:

- temperature, pulse, respirations, blood pressure
- abdomen—appearance, old scars, palpation
- vaginal loss (including description of liquor)
- evidence of oedema
- contractions—felt for strength and timed for frequency and duration
- results of rectal or vaginal examination if done (these are not routine in most places)
- fetal heart rate, rhythm and response to contractions

Urine is tested as soon as it is available and a fluid balance record is started. The woman's doctor is notified of her admission and is told the results of the initial examination. He will then give instructions as necessary.

Other history taking

Many centres keep their patients' medical notes in the delivery suite or in a place easily accessible to the delivery staff, and so the essential medical and obstetric information needs only to be revised and checked. The important points are:

- *Blood group and Rh factor*: most women are asked to carry their blood group card with them at all times during pregnancy and to bring it into hospital when in labour. Verbal information is not satisfactory, the official card must be seen and a signed notation made on the patient's records.
- *All previous pregnancies, labours and their outcomes*: birth weights, whether the children are still alive and well, whether they were breast fed, when and where the babies were born, whether there were any complications or problems, and any previous experiences that the woman wants to discuss.
- *General medical information*: any previous illnesses, operations, drug or other sensitivities, and the woman's general health during this pregnancy.
- *Medications or treatment*: all current medication or treatment.

PREPARATION PROCEDURES

Shaving

Shaving of the pubic, vulval and perineal area is no longer routine in many centres. Some doctors issue standing instructions, others leave the matter to the discretion of the midwife who acts according to the desires of the woman.

Shaving of the perineal area removes any hairs which might, in the event of a perineal tear or episiotomy, be caught up in the wound or be a source of infective organisms. Clipping, rather than shaving, is becoming more common as it involves less risk of skin injury.

Enema

Like shaving, enemas are no longer routine, and after a full explanation of the procedure the midwife allows the woman to decide whether or not she wishes to have one. Enemas are not given in strongly-established labour or when the presenting part is not engaged in the pelvis if the membranes have ruptured.

The purpose of giving an enema to a woman in labour is to empty the lower bowel. This, in effect:

- allows more room in the pelvis for the descent of the fetal head
- may stimulate contractions (in a reflex way)
- prevents contamination by faeces at the time of delivery
- proves more comfortable during the early puerperium.

It can also, as a bonus, increase the woman's co-operation at the pushing stage. The desire to push is interpreted in a way which resembles closely the overwhelming urge to open the bowels. (We never take a strongly-labouring woman to the toilet when she desperately wants to go—we look for the fetal head.) If the woman can be reminded that the lower bowel has been emptied by the enema and she is therefore not likely to soil the bed, she will not be inhibited from pushing when she should be pushing.

The enema will be either plain water, soap and water, or one of the disposable types. If the woman is having contractions, the experience may not be a pleasant one, particularly during the time between the enema's administration and its return. The woman will not want to be left alone at this time and she probably will not want to make intelligent conversation either.

General hygiene
Although the final thing that many women do before leaving home is to have a bath or shower, after an enema most will appreciate another wash.

At this time any necessary or advisable aspects of hygiene are attended to. Hair is washed perhaps, or brushed into a suitable and comfortable style for labour. Nails may need attention—long fingernails especially can be a hazard both to the mother and to others, during labour and the postnatal period. Any skin or mouth lesions observed are recorded and brought to the attention of the doctor if they are significant.

The woman is then transferred to her room. Some hospitals have 'first-stage rooms, where there are curtains, bedspreads, sitting rooms, and a general atmosphere of relaxation. If she desires it she is given a sedative or analgesic, according to her progress in labour.

THE FIRST STAGE

A healthy woman who has undergone a programme of good antenatal care and education, enters hospital in the most favourable condition to undergo the stresses of labour.

During the first stage of labour, the care is aimed at maintaining the mother's condition at its best, relieving symptoms without harming the mother or the fetus, and observing the progress of labour and its effect on the mother and the fetus.

GENERAL CARE

Ideally, the first stage of labour is passed in quiet surroundings, with the midwives and the woman establishing a good relationship. If it is a first labour, the woman will have some feelings of apprehension and perhaps worries about how she will behave, no matter how well she has been prepared. Even for a woman who has been through the labouring experience several times, each labour has probably been different; she will also almost certainly encounter at least some new midwives and doctors.

No matter what the labouring woman's previous experience, whether as a patient, a midwife or a doctor, the midwives will still make sure that she understands what is going on in this labour.

Comfort
The bed is kept dry—liquor may be draining continuously. Mouth care is important, especially if oral fluid intake is limited. Frequent hand and face washes are appreciated, and vulval washdowns are performed every 4 hours.

Backache is common; it can be eased by slow firm massage to the base of the spine. The use of a large bean-bag (instead of pillows) is becoming popular as an effective means of back support during labour.

Activity
The woman is normally encouraged to ambulate until labour advances to the stage where it is safer or more comfortable for her to stay in bed. Some form of activity or distraction is advised, perhaps reading or knitting, or revision of relaxation and breathing techniques.

Fluids
A record of fluid intake and output is kept during labour. The frequent intake of small amounts of non-aerated, clear fluids, e.g. water, glucose

drinks, fruit juices—about 75 ml per hour—is encouraged. Intravenous fluids are usually only necessary when the woman has a poor intake, is vomiting or has a poor urinary output.

Voiding

Urinary output is observed. The woman is encouraged to empty her bladder at least every 2 hours, because a full bladder can inhibit uterine action and can occupy pelvic space. The bladder is catheterised only if the woman is unable to void after some time and then only after the usual nursing measures have been tried.

All urine passed during labour is tested for acetone and protein. If a trace of protein shows on the stick test, the urine is boiled. Pre-eclampsia can still emerge for the first time when the woman is in labour.

Food

It used to be taught that 'when labour starts, peristalsis stops'. That is *almost* true; the absorption of food from the stomach and intestine is slowed down considerably. Because of this, and because of the possibility of general anaesthesia becoming necessary, solid food is usually withheld during labour; custards, jellies and pureed food are recommended. The mother's appetite is usually only for light foods in any case.

With a relatively empty stomach, there is the risk of a build-up of highly acid gastric secretions. If these are vomited and inhaled, they can cause a rapidly-spreading and serious chemical pneumonitis (Mendelson's syndrome). An alkaline mixture such as magnesium trisilicate (15 ml) or one of the proprietary antacids is given regularly (2- to 4-hourly) in many centres to reduce the gastric acidity.

PREVENTION AND RELIEF OF PAIN AND FATIGUE

The pain of labour is caused by the combination of:

- the stretching of the lower segment (and subsequently the cervix)
- ischaemia (hypoxia) of the uterine muscles.

As the contractions increase in strength, they pull harder on the cervix; these stronger contractions also restrict the flow of oxygen to the uterine muscles thus leading to ischaemic pain.

Fatigue is caused by the enormous amount of energy used by the body. It is worsened by anxiety, which in turn causes tension, preventing relaxation of the rest of the body and possibly leading to exhaustion.

Pain relief in labour has three basic aims:

- to minimise the experience of pain and tension, while allowing the woman to be as alert as she wants to be
- to keep both the woman and the fetus as free from any depressive effects of medication as possible
- to achieve these ends without interfering with uterine contractions.

Pain has three components:

- stimulus—the cause of pain
- threshold—the level at which pain intensity registers
- reaction—how the individual interprets pain and reacts to it.

The *stimulus* of pain in labour cannot be eliminated, short of doing a caesarean section and thus stopping the labour. Some abnormalities, such as malpresentation, can increase or prolong the stimulus and so increase the potential pain.

The *threshold* of pain in labour can be lowered by fear, lack of understanding, and by physical problems—fever, tiredness, dehydration acidosis, tension. The pain threshold can be raised by the use of drugs, physical and psychological well-being, relaxation, and distraction.

Reaction to pain in labour is a very individual response. It depends upon the woman's personality, emotional state and level of understanding, her cultural, family and educational background and her previous experiences.

The woman who undergoes a normal labour with good antenatal preparation and education, careful preventive care, the support and companionship of a competent midwife and with well-timed suitable analgesia when indicated, is likely to have a 'good' labour experience.

Timing of pain-relief

Pain intensity is normally related to the amount of cervical dilatation, and so the various ways of lowering the pain threshold can be employed in relation to dilatation (Fig. 12.1).

Relaxation

Relaxation is revised and practised from the beginning of labour and continued throughout, as well as encouragement, companionship and distraction. Distraction, in the form of concentrating upon breathing patterns, is employed more intensely as the first stage reaches its climax.

Sedatives and hypnotics

These drugs are restricted to *early* labour. They are useful then, when they can help to produce a good sleep from which the woman wakes with restored energy and often with some progress of labour achieved.

They are not given after the pain intensity rises because they do not relieve pain, and sedation can produce an inability to co-operate readily.

Narcotic analgesics and tranquillisers

These can be given, either singly or together, from the time contractions or back pain become distressing. They can be administered until it is no longer wise to given them because of the danger of the baby being born while still under their effects. These drugs cross the placenta, and can cause neonatal respiratory depression. Pethidine is currently the most common narcotic analgesic used in midwifery, and promethazine and diazepam are the most common tranquillisers.

Inhalation analgesia

Gas and air (most commonly nitrous oxide and oxygen) administered through a mask by the mother herself, is commonly used once labour is established and the contractions are causing some distress. It can be used in conjunction with learned relaxation techniques or with narcotic analgesia.

Nitrous oxide acts within 5 seconds, does not accumulate in the system, and allows rapid recovery. Modern inhalational apparatuses have a built-in maximum cut-off mechanism so that they

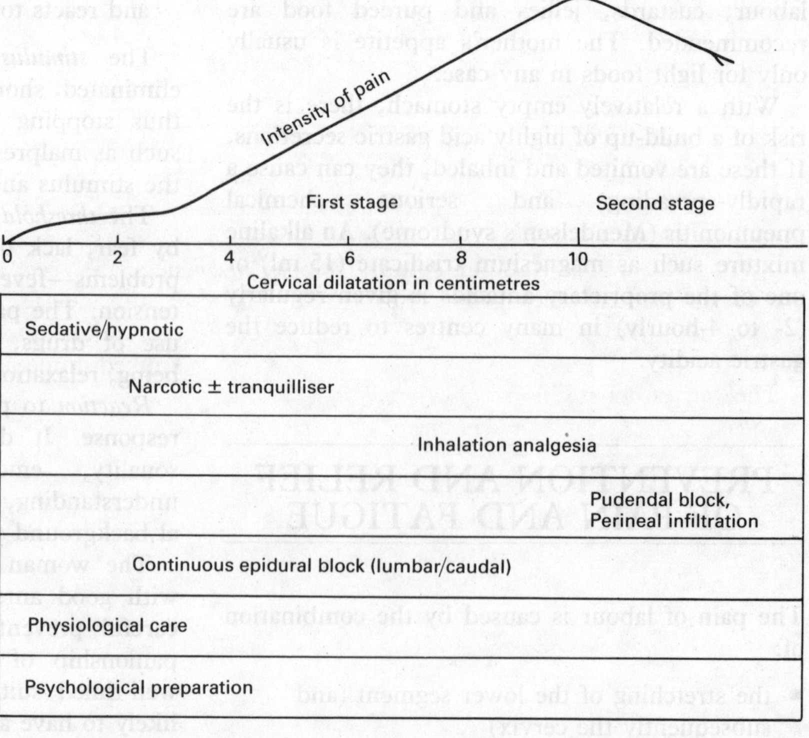

Figure 12.1 Timing of various methods of analgesia in relation to pain and to cervical dilation (Source: Moir D D, 1986 Pain relief in labour, 5th edn. Churchill Livingstone, Edinburgh, p 40)

deliver no more than 70% nitrous oxide and no less than 30% oxygen. If there is any indication of fetal distress such as fetal tachycardia or bradycardia, the machine can be set deliver to 100% oxygen immediately.

The woman applies the mask as soon as she feels the contraction begin. If a midwife or nurse is sitting with her and feeling for contractions (which can be felt from the outside a few seconds beforehand) she can apply the mask when she is told that a contraction is starting. She breathes steadily on the mask throughout the contraction until it begins to fade. The gas proportion is adjusted according to its effect upon the pain sensation or the mother's response. In some it causes weepiness; in others, laughter. It is usually begun at 30% nitrous oxide and increased to about 60% by the end of the first stage of labour. Other inhalation agents, trichlorethylene and methoxyflurane, are occasionally used, but are less favoured because they accumulate in the body.

The equipment used for inhalational anaesthesia is always maintained in perfect working condition because damaged or perished tubing, connections or face masks will cause leakage of the gases, thus reducing the desired effect. At the start of labour the midwife ensures that the woman knows how to hold the face mask in the correct position so that it is close-fitting and effective.

Epidural block

Epidural block involves the administration of local anaesthetic solution into the extradural space surrounding the spinal cord from which the nerves supplying the uterus (lumbar epidural block) or the cervix (caudal block) arise (Fig. 12.2). The solution is spread by gravity. It is a sterile procedure.

The anaesthetist inserts a needle into the epidural space. A catheter may be threaded through the space, and a local anaesthetic solution is injected through the catheter which is taped carefully in position. Bupivacaine or Lignocaine is usually chosen, using the minimum effective dose for the shortest possible time. The woman lies on her left side for the duration of the procedure.

Epidural block enables the mother to cope with, and cooperate during a difficult and potentially very painful labour. Unless prolonged, this form of analgesia in itself has no effect upon the fetus. It is indicated when maternal physical stress could be dangerous. (e.g. in pre-eclampsia, essential hypertension, or cardiac disease). It is commonly used for caesarean section, and is part of the 'active management of labour'.

Because sensation to the area is absent, the woman will feel neither contractions nor the overwhelming urge to push during the second stage of labour. This means that she must have her contractions felt by an observer(the midwife) who can tell her when each contraction is beginning and ending, in order to make full use of the secondary powers at the right time. Forceps delivery is more common with epidural analgesia is used, because of the patient's reduced ability to push effectively and because there is a degree of pelvic floor relaxation which interferes with internal rotation of the fetal head as it descends.

Epidural analgesia is not used in the presence of infection, bleeding disorders or haemorrhage, or where the patient is opposed to its use. There are sometimes complications, usually minor ones such as headache, backache and bladder disturbances. Sometimes the headache persists for days and can be a most unpleasant experience. The anaesthetic agent can cause preganglionic interruption which can cause vasodilation and thus hypotension. This is a more serious complication, and is constantly watched for during the procedure. Most anaesthetists routinely begin an intravenous infusion of fluid (e.g. Hartmann's solution) and many run in 500 ml before beginning the epidural. The mother's vital signs and her state of mental alertness are recorded frequently. Signs of systemic (toxic) shock reaction to the local anaesthetic agent are watched for, and resuscitation measures are applied immediately.

Because of the potential danger associated with the administration of epidural analgesia, it is always done by an experienced anaesthetist in a hospital properly equipped to deal with emergencies.

Pudendal and paracervical blocks

A pudendal block involves the injection of local anaesthetic solution into the area close to the pudendal nerve. A paracervical block is injected into the tissues of the external cervical as (Fig.

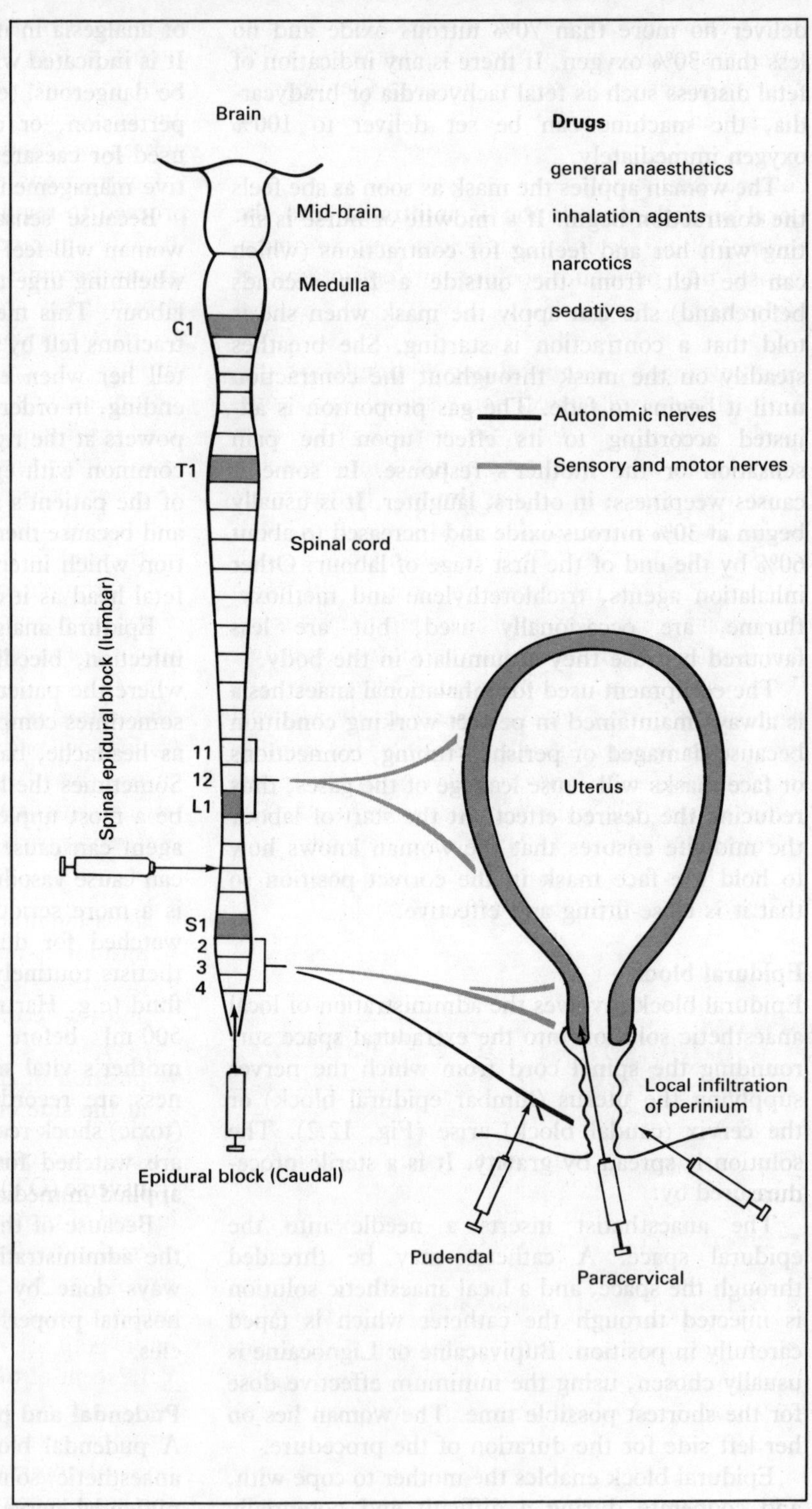

Figure 12.2 Sites of action of analgesics (Source: Holdcroft A 1975 Analgesia and anaesthesia. Nursing Mirror 3 July: p 60).

12.2). These blocks provide analgesia for the end of the first stage and for the second stage of a difficult labour or when a forceps delivery is anticipated.

Perineal infiltration
Local anaesthetic solution is infiltrated into the perineal skin, ideally in sufficient time to anaesthetise the perineum before an episiotomy is performed.

Transcutaneous electrical nerve stimulation
Transcutaneous electrical nerve stimulation, commonly known as TENS, is a method of pain control used in several areas of medicine, especially with chronic pain. It has limited, but at times useful, application to the management of pain relief in labour. The TENS device involves a small pad attached to the mother's skin in the lumbar/sacral region. This pad is connected by wires to a hand-held control which the mother operates. When she feels a contraction beginning she depresses a button which causes a small electrical impulse to be sent though the skin. This impulse interferes with the sensory nerve pathway to the brain so that the pain stimulus is reduced. The effectiveness of the TENS device depends, to a large extent, upon the mother's understanding of its functions and attitude to pain relief.

ASSESSMENT OF PROGRESS

The progress of the first stage of labour is measured by:

- observation of contractions
- abdominal examination
- vaginal (or rectal) palpation.

Many hospitals and birth centres use a partogram to record both progress and vital signs. Figure 12.3 shows a partogram recording a typical normal labour.

Contractions
The pattern of contractions should show a gradual increase in frequency, strength and duration. Frequency is timed from the start of one contraction until the start of the next, and duration is from the beginning of abdominal tightening until the tightening (contraction) disappears.

Contractions often begin as 'niggles' and then proceed to regular mild, short contractions 15–30 seconds long, occurring every 10–15 minutes. As labour becomes established they gradually build up until they are strong, long contractions lasting to 50–60 seconds, and recurring every 2–3 minutes.

Contractions are felt by the midwife with her hand resting lightly on the uterine fundus, and are timed over at least three consecutive contractions. They are observed hourly during early labour, half-hourly as labour advances, and quarter-hourly by the end of the first stage.

In primiparae, the change of character of the contractions is gradual; in multiparae it occurs much more rapidly.

Abdominal palpation
Abdominal palpation (Fig. 12.4) is performed to ensure that the fetus is positioned correctly for a normal labour, and to assess the descent of the presenting part.

Correct positioning of the fetus is when the:

- lie is longitudinal
- attitude is one of flexion (of the whole fetus)
- presenting part is the top of the head (vertex) and the leading part of the vertex is the occiput
- position of the occiput in the pelvic cavity is at the side or the front (transverse or anterior)

Thus, occipito-anterior (OA) or occipito-transverse (OT) (sometimes the term lateral is used instead of transverse—occipito-lateral (OL) are the normal positions for labour, and comprise about 85% of vertex presentations. Left-sided occipital presentations are more common than right-sided ones; both are normal.

Descent of the presenting part is followed in the first stage by abdominal palpation, in the second stage by perineal observation and post-anal palpation. Abdominal palpation assesses whether or not the head is engaged, and when it is it assesses the relationship of its widest part (the biparietal

MRS S Grey
(Identification details)

PARTOGRAM

BOOKING: ROOM No. PATIENT I.D.

ADMISSION DATE: 23/1/1990 Time: 23.20 Doctor Notified: ✓ Time: 23.40

REASON FOR ADMISSION: Regular contractions with backache LABOUR COMMENCED: 22.00

CONTRACTIONS: None Irregular (Regular) Frequency 5-6/60 mins Show mucoid

MEMBRANES: (Intact) Ruptured Date / / Time: liquor

Height of fundus 2 finger-breadths ↓ Xiphisternum Presentation Vertex Position Left occipito anterior

Presenting part, Station head 2-3 fingers above brim Foetal Heart Rate 144 regular

Temp 36.6 Pulse 92 B.P. 130/80 Weight 70 Kg Oedema slight fingers only

URINE: Colour Straw S.G. 1010 Reaction pH 6 Albumen trace on boiling

Sugar neg Acetone neg Bile neg Blood small

Prep none Enema none Shower yes

PATIENT PROGRESS REPORT

Date

Date and Time	
23.1.90	Admitted to labour ward. In early established labour.
23.40	Ambulating. Comfortable with contractions. Backache less after shower. Analgesia and delivery options discussed
01.30	Showered again. Contractions more painful. Would like to try half dose of Pethidine
01.40	Doctor given progress report. Ordered IM Pethidine 50mgms now and repeat in 30 minutes if required
01.45	IM Pethidine 50mgms given
02.15	More relaxed and comfortable. No backache
03.20	Rectal pressure with contractions. Bright mucoid show.
03.23	Spontaneous rupture of membranes. Clear liquor. Urge to push.
*	Dr notified of progress - will come for delivery.
03.30	Head on view with contractions. Spontaneous pushing
03.35	Perineum distended - stretching well
03.40	Normal spontaneous delivery of a living girl, baby
03.41	Abdomen palpated to exclude multiple pregnancy. IV Ergometrine 0.25 mgm given
03.44	Placenta and membranes delivered (Brandt's Andrews method)
03.45	Perineum, vagina and cervix examined. Very small posterior vaginal laceration involving mucosa only. Not sutured
03.50	Fundus palpated - firm central, 2cm below umbilicus. PV loss minimal
04.00	Baby to breast. Attached and sucked well.

Figure 12.3 Partogram, charting a normal labour.

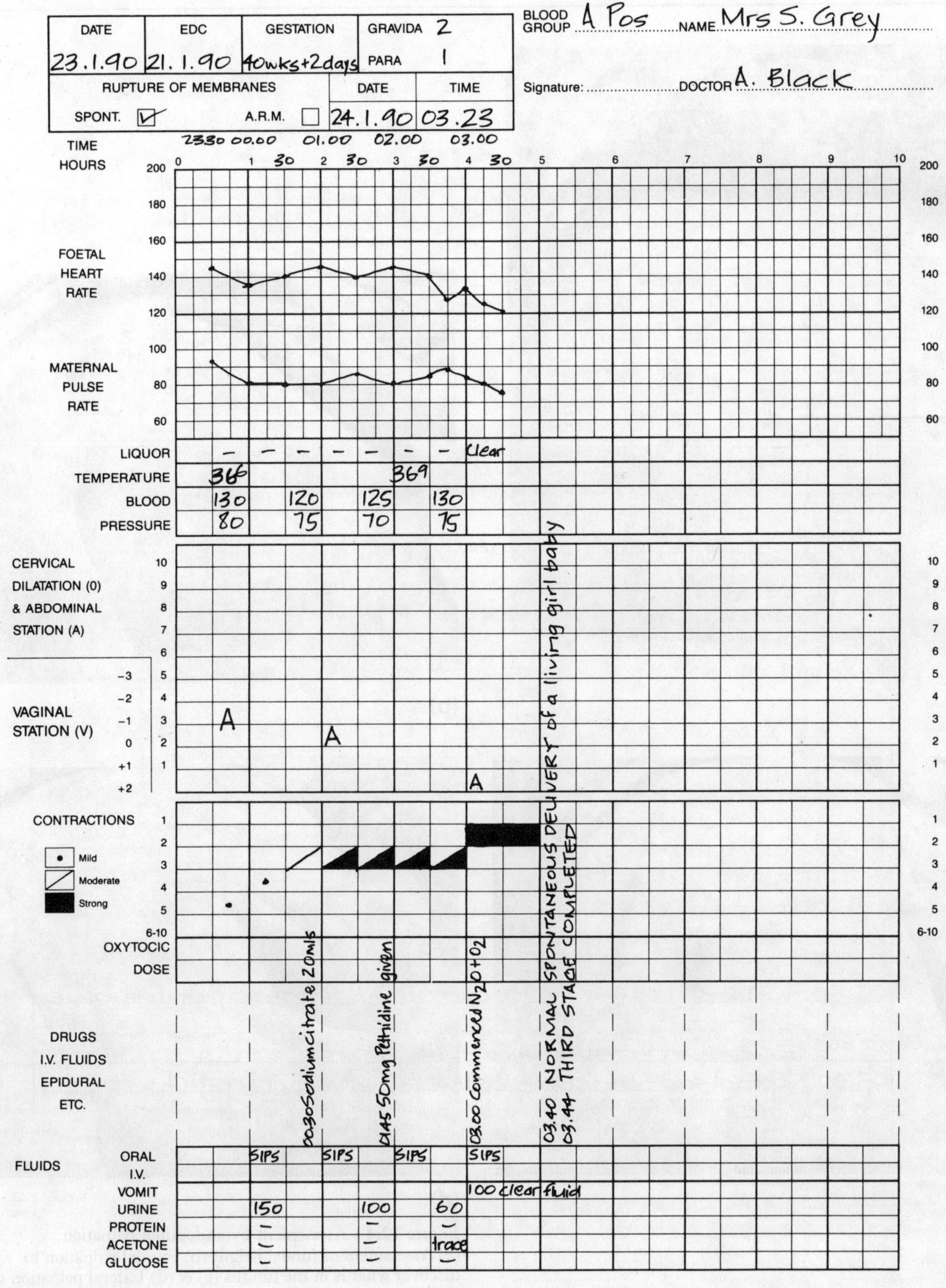

DATE	EDC	GESTATION	GRAVIDA 2
23.1.90	21.1.90	40wks+2days	PARA 1

RUPTURE OF MEMBRANES		DATE	TIME
SPONT. ☑	A.R.M. ☐	24.1.90	03.23

BLOOD GROUP A Pos NAME Mrs S. Grey

Signature: .... DOCTOR A. Black

TIME 2330 00.00 01.00 02.00 03.00

HOURS 0 1 30 2 30 3 30 4 30 5 6 7 8 9 10

FOETAL HEART RATE 200 180 160 140 120

MATERNAL PULSE RATE 100 80 60

	0	0.5	1	1.5	2	2.5	3	3.5	4
LIQUOR		–	–	–	–	–	–	–	Clear
TEMPERATURE	366						369		
BLOOD PRESSURE	130/80			120/75		125/70		130/75	

CERVICAL DILATATION (0) & ABDOMINAL STATION (A) 10 9 8 7 6 5 4 3 2 1

VAGINAL STATION (V) −3 −2 −1 0 +1 +2

A A A

CONTRACTIONS 1 2 3 4 5 6-10

• Mild
Moderate
Strong

OXYTOCIC DOSE

DRUGS I.V. FLUIDS EPIDURAL ETC.

0030 Sodium citrate 20mls

0145 50mg Pethidine given

03.00 Commenced $N_2O + O_2$

03.40 NORMAL SPONTANEOUS DELIVERY of a living girl baby

03.44 THIRD STAGE COMPLETED

FLUIDS	1	2	3	4
ORAL	SIPS	SIPS	SIPS	SIPS
I.V.				
VOMIT				100 clear fluid
URINE	150	100	60	
PROTEIN	–	–	–	
ACETONE	–	–	trace	
GLUCOSE	–	–	–	

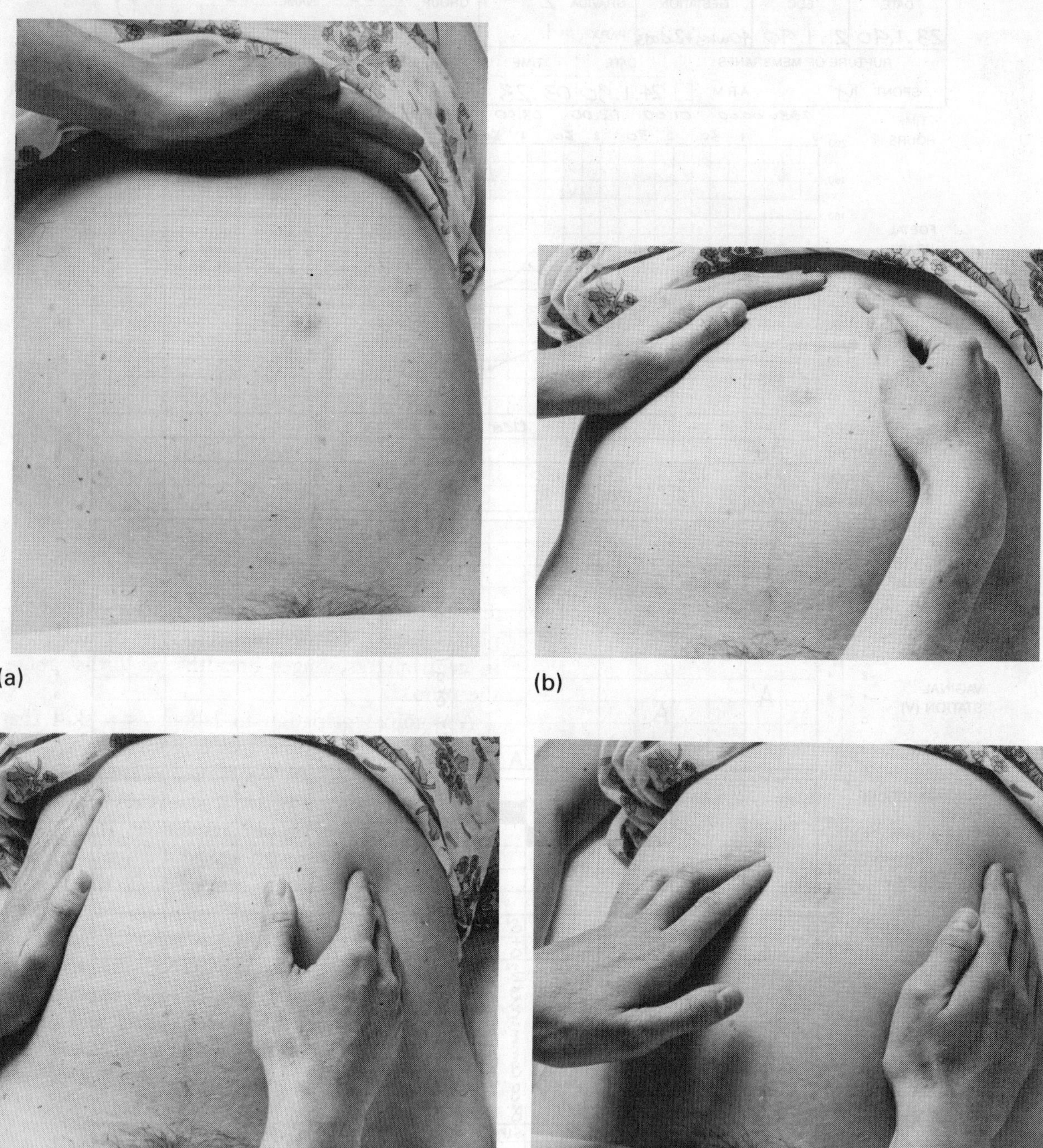

Figure 12.4 Assessment by abdominal palpation
(a) Assessment of fundal height (b) Fundal palpation to discover what is in the fundus (c) & (d) Lateral palpation to identify the fetal back (e) Pawlik's palpation to assess engagement of the head (f) Pelvic palpation — two-handed technique to identify the relationship of the fetal head to the pelvic brim and degree of flexion of the head (g) Auscultation: listening to the fetal heart.

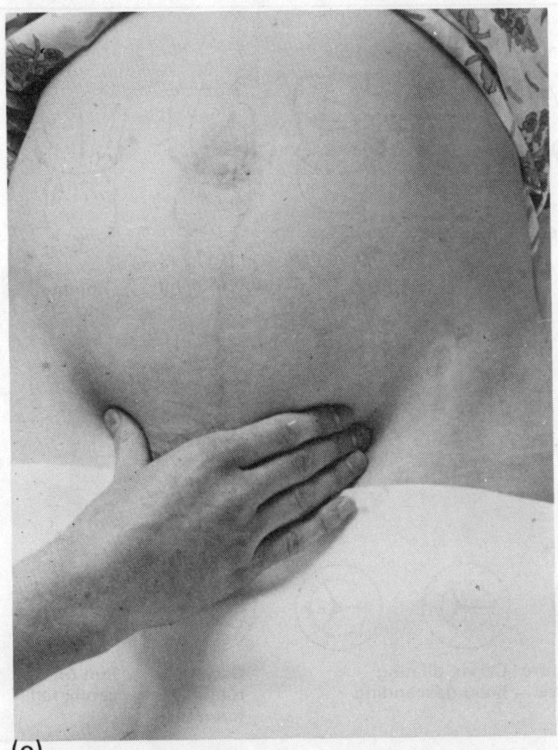

(e)

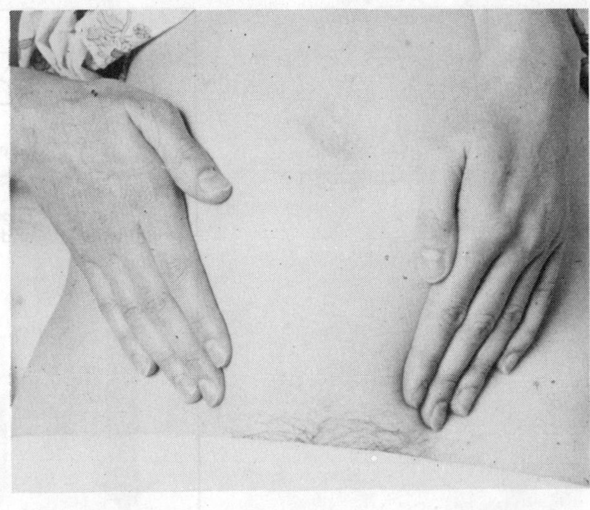

(f)

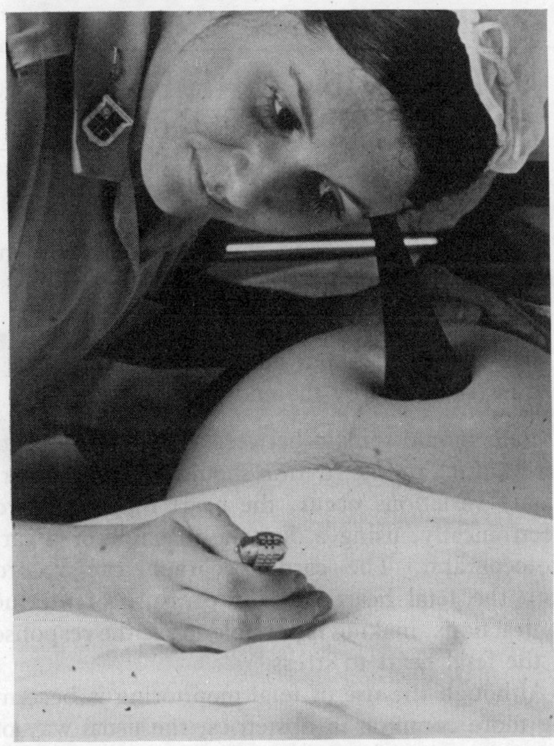

(g)

diameter) to the pelvic brim (in front, the symphysis pubis). This relationship may be described in centrimetres, finger breadths or 'fifths' above the brim.

Abdominal palpation in labour is a skill that takes quite some time to develop. The student nurse will most likely observe palpation performed by the doctor or midwife. If she is invited to palpate herself, she should remember that she is feeling not only through the abdominal wall and possibly a layer of fat, but through the uterine muscle and perhaps a fair quantity of amniotic fluid. Therefore, it is not a disaster if her initial palpation is not particularly successful. Even so, she should attend carefully to the explanations given on how to identify the fetal parts, and should be careful to stand on the patient's righthand side, have warm hands, and not attempt to palpate during a uterine contraction.

Vaginal examination

The progress of labour can be estimated more accurately by vaginal examinations than by abdominal palpation, but as few vaginal examinations are performed as possible because of the danger of introducing infection, especially after the membranes have ruptured. When a vaginal examination is performed, it is as a 'sterile'

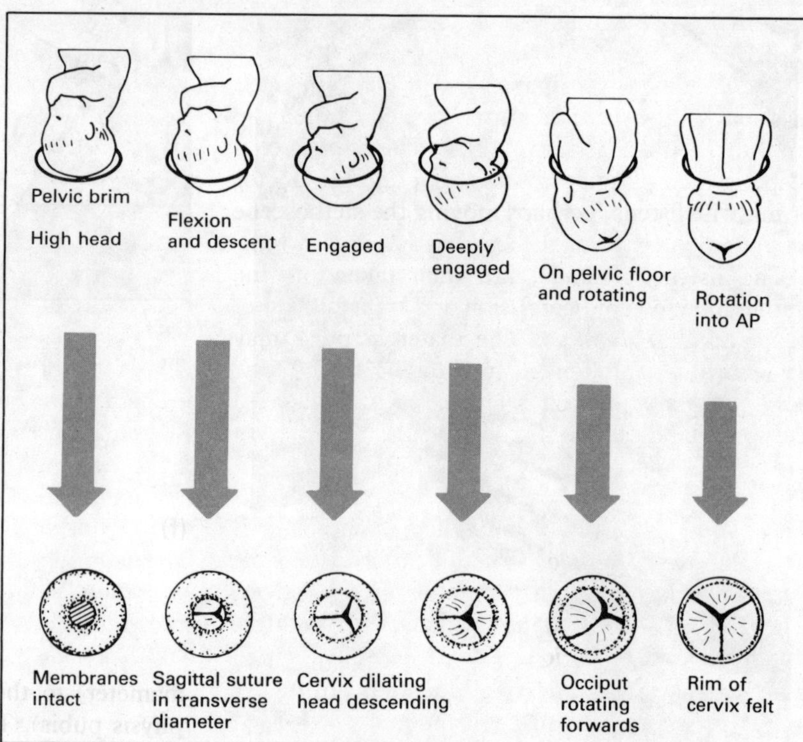

Figure 12.5 Diagrammatic representation of head descending through the pelvic brim and findings per vaginam.

procedure, with the examiner scrubbed and wearing sterile gloves.

Vaginal examination will show:

- the state of the membranes (whether ruptured or not—if unruptured, the presence or otherwise of a bag of forewaters)
- the degree of descent of the fetal head, recorded in centimetres above or below the ischial spines
- the attitude of the fetal head and the position of the presenting part
- the degree of effacement, thinning and dilatation of the cervix (Fig. 12.5).

Rectal examination

Rectal examination is an aid to assessing cervical dilatation and the station of the presenting part of the fetus. These can be felt through the thin anterior rectal wall. The rectal examination is unlikely to introduce infection and is not as time-consuming or disturbing to the woman as a vaginal examination, but can be painful. It is no longer done routinely.

OBSERVING THE FETAL CONDITION

Fetal heart

The fetal heart rate and rhythm is the main indicator of the fetal condition. It is observed:

- hourly in early labour
- half-hourly as labour advances
- quarter-hourly by the end of the first stage.

Its rate should remain between 120 and 160 beats per minute, and its rhythm should remain regular. If any variations occur, the heart may be heard electronically, using a doptone machine or a cardiotocograph. The cardiotocograph can record both the fetal heart and the pressure of uterine contractions, making it possible to see the response of the fetal heart to stress.

Although the use of fetal monitoring is becoming more common in obstetrics, the usual way of intermittently recording the fetal heart is aurally, using a special trumpet-shaped metal or plastic stethoscope (Pinaud's fetal stethoscope, Fig. 12.4G).

The abdomen is palpated and the approximate position of the fetal heart is located, using the anterior shoulder as a landmark. The fetal stethoscope is then placed over this spot and the doctor or midwife listens, perhaps moving the stethoscope around slightly, until the heart is heard clearly.

The listener's hands, are then taken off the stethoscope to avoid confusion and transmission of finger arterial impulses. The maternal pulse may be felt while simultaneously listening to the fetal heart; this avoids confusion with the maternal uterine arterial pulses.

Liquor

Clear liquor is an indication of fetal well-being. It if is meconium-stained, it could indicate that the fetus is, or has been, in a state of physical stress. The passage of meconium while still in utero usually follows a period of fetal oxygen deprivation, leading to vagal nerve stimulation and thence to gut peristalsis and anal relaxation.

During labour, the amount and description of draining liquor is recorded every time the fetal heart is checked.

OBSERVING THE MOTHER'S CONDITION

The woman's response to labour is noted and recorded throughout. Often fetal distress will arise as a result of maternal physical distress. Signs of particular importance are:

- pulse rate above 96 beats per minute
- temperature above 38° C
- blood pressure more than 20 mm systolic or 10 mm diastalic above the patient's pre-labour recording (also, any diastolic reading above 90 mmHg)
- urinalysis showing protein or acetone
- low urinary output, dehydration
- anxiety, distress, fatigue
- nausea or vomiting
- abnormal reaction to pain or to analgesics administered.

The woman's condition in the first stage of labour should remain good. If there is any departure from this ideal, she is always carefully assessed by her doctor.

THE SECOND STAGE

The second stage of labour is found by many women to be much more bearable than the first stage, because they finally have something positive to do: it is the stage of pushing and delivery.

Just before second stage, when the cervix is almost, but not quite, fully dilated, the signs of *transition* may appear. Transition is usually brief, generally lasting for only a few minutes, but it can be frightening because its onset is quick. It is at transition that many a mother has said 'I want to go home!', and as many husbands have said to the midwife 'Why can't you do something?' The mother feel nauseated or suddenly vomit, she may start to shake all over, and she often feels that she is losing control of herself, which can be especially distressing when remaining in control is of great importance to her. An experienced midwife will constantly and positively reassure the mother through this stage, encouraging her and her companion through the few contractions until the signs of the second stage occur.

Signs of the second stage

Signs of the second stage are:

- the cervix is found to be fully dilated on vaginal examination
- the membranes usually rupture, if this has not happened already, as there is no longer a cervical 'shelf' to support them
- contractions are long (50–60 seconds), strong, and perhaps slightly less frequent (occurring every 3–5 rather than 2–3 minutes)
- there may be a trickle of blood from the vagina
- the woman will normally have an overwhelming desire to push
- the anal sphincter may dilate ('pout')
- the perineum may bulge

When any of these signs appear, the others are quickly looked for. The mother is never left without the constant presence of a midwife or a doctor at this stage.

CARE AND OBSERVATION DURING THE SECOND STAGE

The basic pattern of care for the second stage of labour is the same as the first stage, except that now:

- the mother is helped into a position which is both comfortable for her and suitable for the midwife to observe progress
- the mother's pulse is recorded quarter-hourly and her blood pressure, as indicated
- the fetal heart is recorded between each contraction
- sips of water or small chips of ice are offered after each contraction, and the mother's face and neck are wiped with a cold cloth if she wishes
- the bladder may be emptied by catheter, but only if it appears to be obstructing or delaying the descent of the baby's head
- analgesia is restricted to non-depressing types only: nitrous oxide by mask, or caudal or pudendal block, or perineal infiltration
- progress is observed visually, looking for bulging of the anus and then the perineum until the head is seen. Post-anal palpation is done gently and only if necessary
- relaxation between contractions rarely needs to be encouraged at this stage. It will occur naturally, with the mother almost asleep between contractions.
- breathing patterns are done with the mother by her husband or labour companion, or by the midwife: with a natural stimulus to push she will do as her body tells her, but occasionally it is important for her to overcome the pushing urge in order to steady the speed with which the baby's head is born.

When a doctor is to be present at delivery he is summoned according to individual circumstances. As a general rule, he is called when the baby's head is first on view in a primigravida, and as soon as the second stage of labour is recognised when the woman has had a previous vaginal delivery. These guidelines apply only when it is known that the doctor is not far away and is free to come as soon as called. Such details are sorted out earlier in the labour. Some doctors prefer to arrive some time before the actual delivery is imminent.

The second stage proceeds, with the fetus descending through the birth canal under the power of the strong uterine contractions and the bearing down efforts of the mother.

The presenting part distends the anus, the perineum and then the vulva. It progresses until 'crowning'—when the biparietal and suboccipto-bregmatic diameters have escaped under the pubic arch—the head then extends and the brow, face and chin are born.

BIRTH OF THE BABY

POSITIONS FOR DELIVERY

Ideally, the baby will be born with the mother adopting the position in which she feels most comfortable. Much has been written and taught in recent years on the subject of birth positions, and most midwives and doctors are now flexible in this matter. *Squatting* would seem to be the most natural position to adopt, with gravity aiding the downwards pressure of pushing and the pelvic floor muscles relaxed, making it easier for the head to displace. There can, however, be some problems with squatting. It does not allow a good view of the perineum to *predict* possible tearing, nor does it allow perineal support and massage or control of the extended head to *prevent* possible tearing.

Controlled delivery, therefore, necessitates compromise. Becoming more common, and acceptable to most women and their attendants, is the 'supported dorsal' position, where the woman reclines, with her back and head well supported by pillows, and draws up her knees so that she can pull against her legs while pushing down. She pushes her chin down onto her chest and in this curled-up position (Fig. 12.6), gets the maximum benefit of gravity while her attendants can still control the delivery. This 'supported dorsal' position is becoming more and more common.

Other delivery positions (left lateral and lithotomy) are used when indicated. The left lateral position, with the upper (right) leg supported, and the woman lying on her side, is useful when it is important to avoid supine hypotension. This can occur because of the heavy uterus pressing on the inferior vena cava and therefore indirectly jeopardising the fetal oxygenation at this time. The left lateral position also gives a very good view of the perineum. Many women who find this position comfortable during their labour are reluctant to turn over onto the back and are happy to give birth this way.

The lithotomy position is used when closer access to the vagina or vulva is necessary, perhaps for obstetrical intervention such as the application of forceps or when skilled manoeuvres (such as in assisted breech delivery) must be performed. Most doctors and midwives are sensitive to the general dislike of the lithotomy position and if the woman asks them not to use it few would insist upon it unless it was necessary.

Whichever position is used, the woman is exposed as little as possible in order to keep her warm and save her from embarrassment.

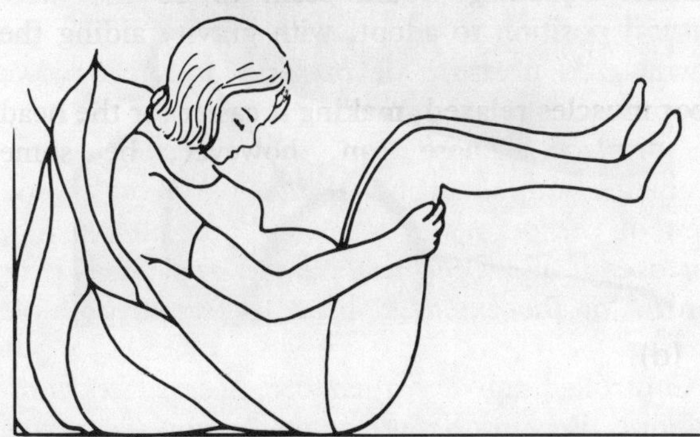

Figure 12.6 'Supported dorsal' position for pushing during the second stage of labour. This position aids gravity, and the back supports help to reduce backache.

CONDUCT OF THE DELIVERY

Figure 12.7 shows a normal delivery. The accoucheur (the person who delivers the baby), wearing a mask, undergoes the surgical scrub procedure and may put on a sterile surgical gown. Sterile gloves are always worn. After swabbing the lower abdomen, thighs, the pubic area and perineum, the (right-handed) accoucheur then:

- places the left hand on the occiput—to maintain flexion and to gently restrain the speed with which the head emerges
- uses the right hand (protected by a towel or combine pad of suitable size) to support or 'guard' the perineum
- while supporting the perineum, feels for the chin and may press very slightly on the chin to maintain flexion of the head
- controls the emergence of the head so that it is born slowly, between contractions
- draws back the perineum with the right hand during the extension of the head and the emergence of the face
- swabs the baby's eyes, and clears away mucus and fluid from the nose and mouth (perhaps using suction for the pharynx)
- waits for the head to restitute, then feels around the baby's neck for the cord
- draws the head down slightly, to see whether the cord is around the neck: if it is and is loose, it can be slipped over the head or pushed back beyond the anterior shoulder; if it is tight it is clamped and cut
- delivers the shoulders during the next contraction, using gentle downward traction until the anterior shoulder has emerged, then lifts the baby upwards to deliver the posterior shoulder and the rest of the baby's body
- places the baby prone on the mother's abdomen (without pulling on the cord) so that the head is lower than the body, to drain the mouth and pharynx (at this stage the time of delivery is noted)
- may aspirate the baby's mouth (to prevent

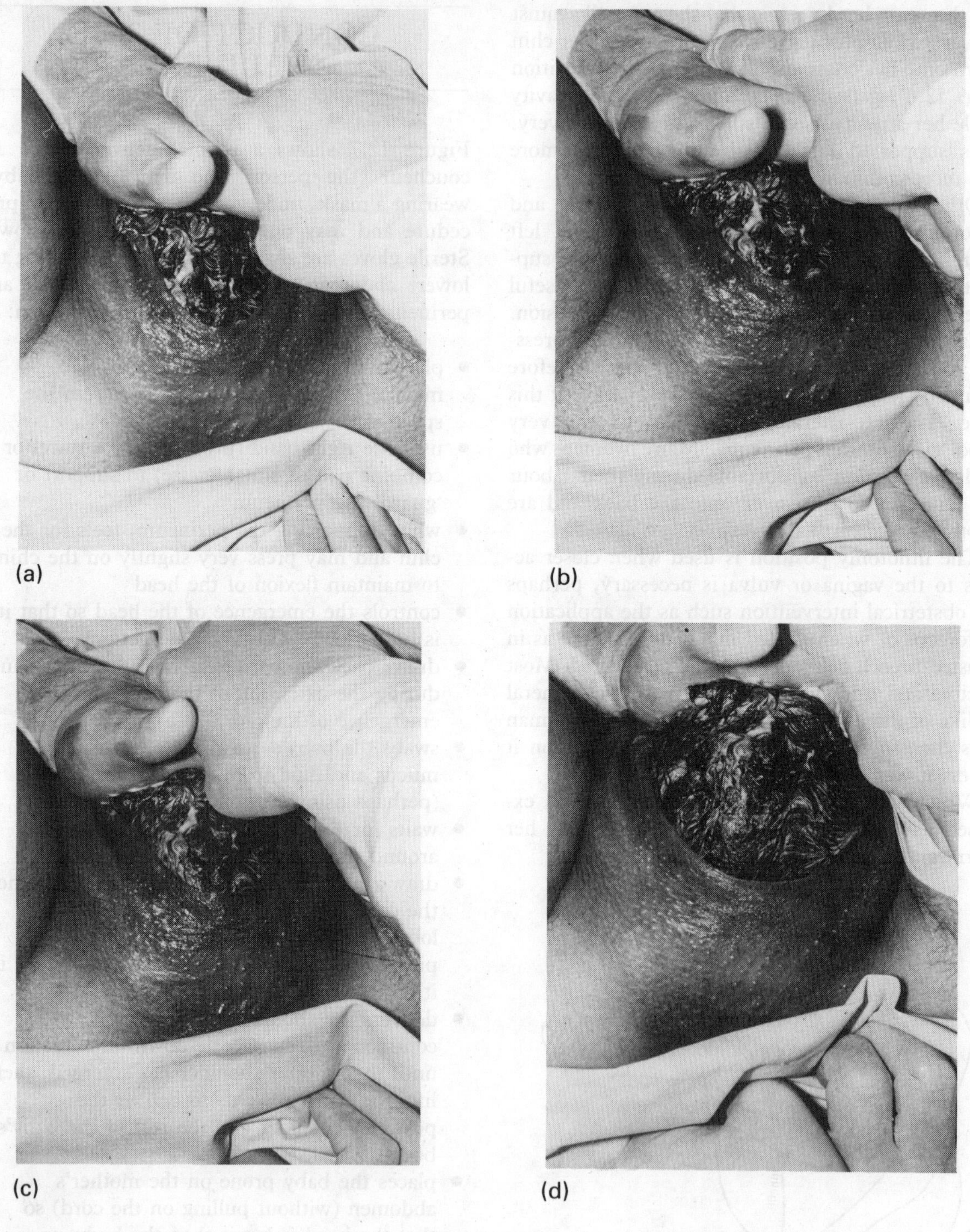

Figure 12.7 Delivery of the baby (a), (b), (c) and (d) gradually increasing distension of the vulva and perineum by the advancing head. Gentle pressure is placed on the occiput to maintain flexion of the head

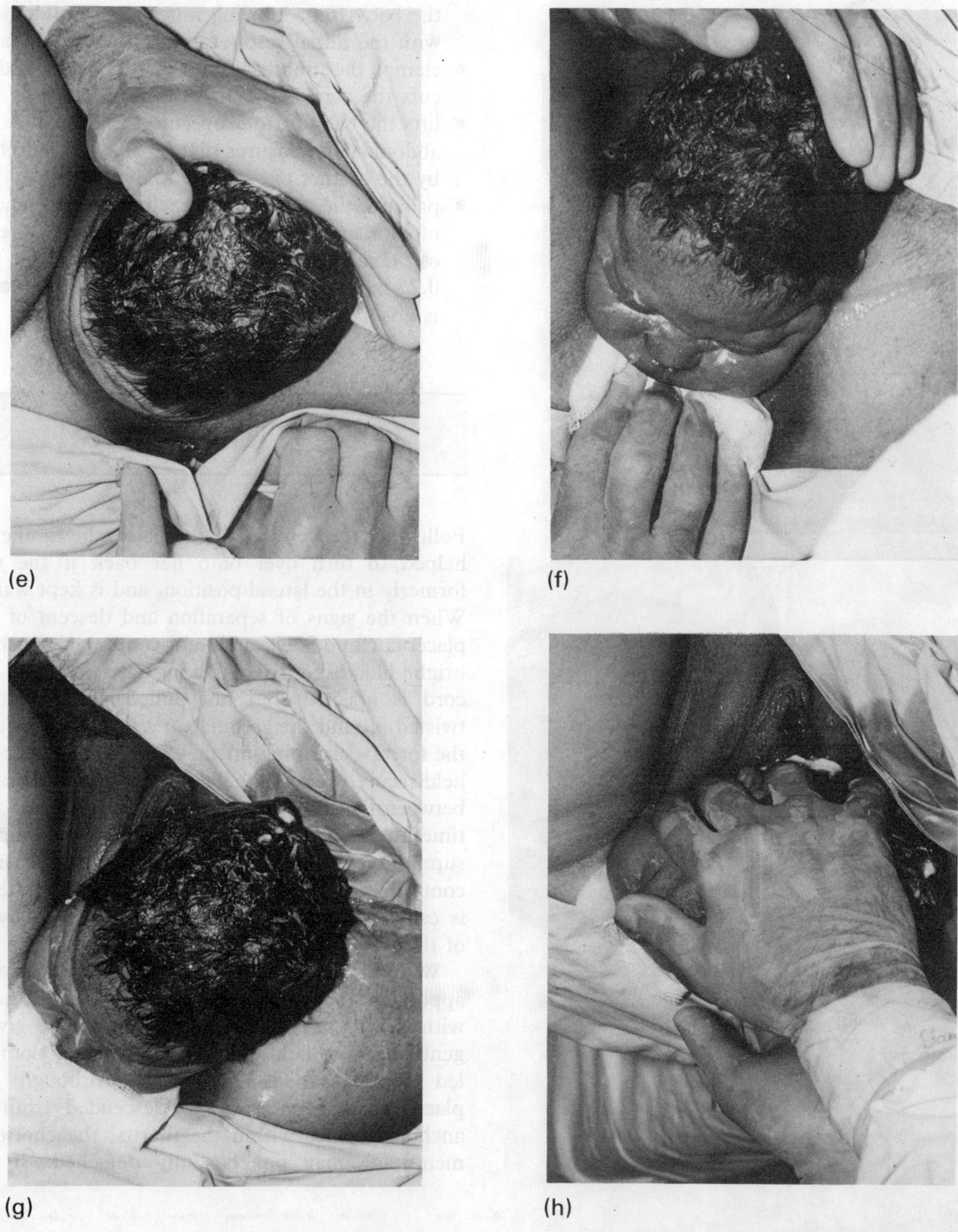

(e) (f) (g) (h)

Figure 12.7 (*contd*) (e) extension of the head and emergence of the brow (f) further extension, with the emergence of the face. The perineum is being drawn back (g) restitution of the head so that it is in line with the rest of the body (h) gentle downwards traction applied to the head to free the anterior shoulder

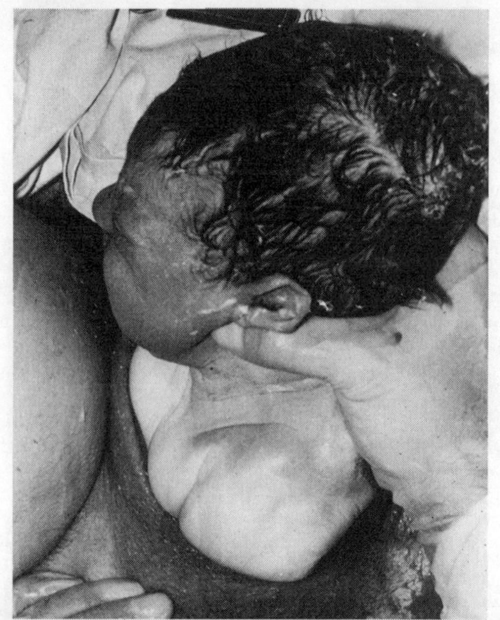

(i)

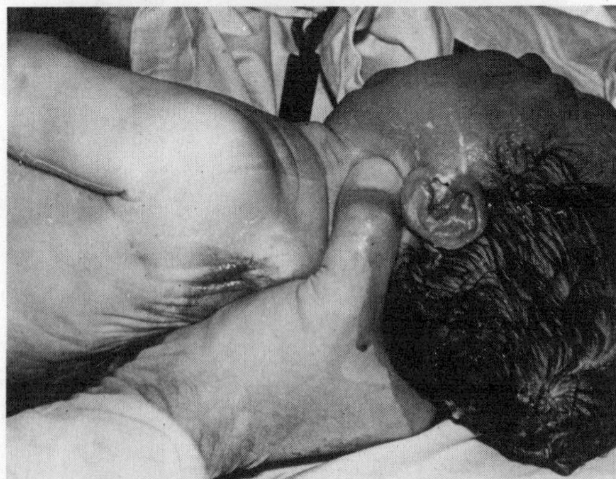

(j)

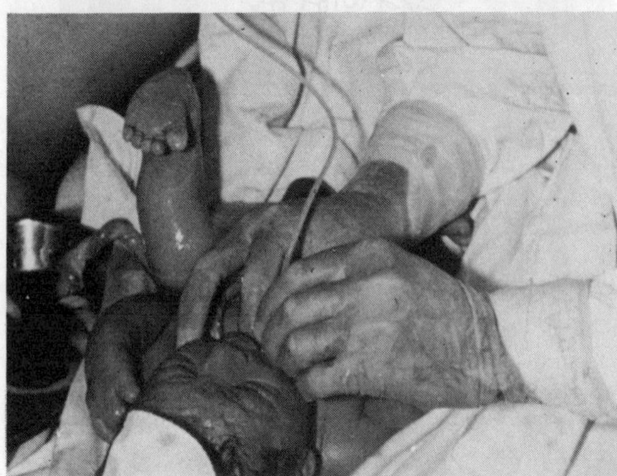

(k)

the baby from inhaling mucus and liquor with the initial respiratory effort)

- clamps the umbilical cord in two places and cuts the cord between the clamps
- lifts the baby further up onto the baby's abdomen and ensures that he is held securely by the mother or assisting midwife
- palpates the abdomen to exclude the presence of another fetus, and if nothing is found the oxytocic injection (usually ergometrine 0.25 mg, or Syntocinon 10 units intravenously) is given (on the doctor's instruction only).

THE THIRD STAGE

Following the delivery of the baby, the mother is helped to turn over onto her back if she was formerly in the lateral position, and is kept warm. When the signs of separation and descent of the placenta (fundus elevated and contracted, gush of bright blood, cord lengthening) are detected, the cord is grasped (but not pulled) and is either twisted around the accoucheur's fingers or around the forceps clamping off the cord. The forceps are held securely across the hand with the cord passing between the third and fourth fingers. During this time, the body of the uterus is supported by gentle suprapubic upwards pressure. This combination of controlled cord traction and support of the uterus is called the Brandt-Andrews method of delivery of the placenta (Fig. 12.8).

With the next contraction the placenta should appear at the vulva, and is slowly but steadily withdrawn. The mother may be asked to give a gentle push to help deliver the placenta. Controlled withdrawal is important. Although the placenta has separated and descended from its anchoring place within the uterus, the chorionic membrane may not be fully detached. If the

Figure 12.7 (*contd*) (i) delivery of the shoulders completed (j) delivery of the rest of the baby's body (k) aspiration of the baby's mouth.

DELIVERY/NEONATAL SUMMARY

DUE DATE: 21/1/1990

Mother's Blood Group: A Pos **Antibodies:** —

GESTATION AT DELIVERY: 40 wks, plus 3 days

Gravida: 2 **Para:** 2

Mrs S. Grey (Identification derails)

PATIENT I.D.

ANTE-NATAL COMPLICATIONS:

MOTHER: DELIVERED 24/1/90 AT 03.40

ACCOUCHEUR: A. Black

Assistant: G. Green

METHOD OF DELIVERY: Spontaneous vaginal delivery

INDICATIONS: (Other than Spontaneous)

MEMBRANES RUPTURED: 24/1/1990 AT 03.23

SPONTANEOUS ☑ A.R.M. (Induction) ☐ A.R.M. (Labour) ☐

INDUCTION INDICATION:

LIQUOR: Clear, copious

OXYTOCICS: (If labour induced)

DURATION OF LABOUR:	**Date**	**Time**	**Duration**
Onset of 1st Stage	23/1/90	22.00	5hr 20min
Onset of 2nd Stage	24/1/90	03.20	20 mins
Completion of 3rd Stage	24/1/90	03.44	4 mins
TOTAL			5hr 44 mins

DRUGS USED IN 3rd STAGE:

I.V. Ergometrine 0.25 mgm at 03.41

Placenta: Delivery: Controlled cord traction

Delivery Time: 03.44 **WT.** 550 g.

Placenta: (Complete) / Incomplete Membranes: (Complete) / Incomplete

Cord: 3 vessels

Remarks: appears normal. Minimal calcification

BLOOD LOSS: COMMENTS:

Before 3rd Stage 50 ml

With 3rd Stage 100 ml

After 3rd Stage 50 ml

Total 200 ml TRANSFUSION: YES ☐ NO ☐

EPISIOTOMY (None) Small Large

LACERATION None Other — Describe

Very small posterior vaginal laceration

Suture Material: not sutured

MEDICATION/ANALGESIC DURING LABOUR:

I.M. Pethidine 50 mgm at 01.45

Nitrous Oxide + Oxygen from 0300 until 0325

DELIVERY ANAESTHETIC:

ANAESTHETIST:

SHARPS/SPLASH INJURY: YES ☐ NO ☐

PAEDIATRICIAN:

INFANT: Sex GIRL BAPTISED / /

(Alive) S.B. Fresh/Macerated N.N.D.

WEIGHT 3420 g. Length 55 cm.

Cord Blood Taken YES ☑ NO ☐ Head Circumference 35 cm.

Infants Blood Group Rh. Pos. Neg.

Direct Coombs

Breast Feeding ☑ Artifical Feeding ☐

Congenital Malformations: None apparent

APGAR SCORE	1 Min.	5 Min.
Heart Rate	2	2
Respiratory Effort	2	2
Muscle Tone	1	2
Reflex Response	2	2
Colour	1	2
TOTAL:	8	10

First breath < 1 min. Respirations established 1 min.

RESUSCITATION:

First breath < 1 mins. Resp. Established 1 mins.

Resuscitation Measures: None necessary

Konakion: 1 Mg. given Cord Round Neck: once loosely

Meconium: not seen Urine: ✓ at birth

IDENTIFICATION: Identification wristlet bearing

Name of Baby of Susan GREY

attached to infant prior to transfer to post-natal ward with mother

Signature: G. Green

TRANSFER TO NURSERY: Baby checked by nursery midwife

DATE: 24/1/90 TIME: 05.00

RELEVANT COMMENTS:

Previous child developed jaundice (ABO incompatibility) at 4 days - needed phototherapy. Please observe this baby

SIGNED G Green

P4

DELIVERY / NEONATAL SUMMARY

Figure 12.8 Typical summary of normal delivery.

placenta is pulled out too quickly, the membrane may tear and some may remain adherent to the decidual wall, providing a potential site for the establishment of infection.

As soon as the placenta has emerged sufficiently to be grasped in both hands, it is twisted gently in one direction to withdraw the membranes. When the placenta and membranes have been expelled, the uterine fundus is felt, and massaged if necessary to ensure a state of contraction. A sample of cord blood may be obtained.

The vulva and vagina are swabbed clean and inspected for tears. Any such tear or an episiotomy is repaired at this stage. The mother's vital signs (temperature, pulse, respirations and blood pressure) are recorded. She is then made clean, dry and comfortable, and she is offered a warm drink.

EXAMINATION OF THE PLACENTA AND MEMBRANES

The placenta and membranes are checked to make sure that they are complete and normal. If they are incomplete, there may be fragments retained in the uterus, preventing efficient uterine contraction and providing a focus for infection to establish. If the placenta or membranes are abnormal the discovery will alert those responsible to check and observe either the infant or the mother (depending on the abnormality) especially carefully.

Gloves are always worn during the examination of the placenta because of the danger of blood-borne infections.

Membranes

The membranes are examined first because they could get torn or ragged and this would make estimation of their completeness difficult. The chorion or outer membrane is continuous with the margin of the placenta. It is checked to see if it is big enough to have contained both the fetus and the amniotic fluid. The amnion or inner membrane is peeled away from the chorion, right up to the insertion of the cord. It is usually always complete.

The membranes are examined for the presence of blood vessels, as occasionally there is an extra, separate, placental lobe, and blood vessels must lead somewhere.

Placenta

Maternal surface

Excess blood is stripped from the placenta. This is maternal blood (see below).

The placenta is weighed and its diameter is measured. It usually weighs about one-sixth of the weight of the baby.

The placenta is then laid flat and its colour, consistency and any abnormalities (areas of infarction, calcification, old bleeds) are noted. It is then held slightly cupped, so that all the cotyledons fit together, to check that it is complete.

Fetal surface

The placenta is turned over so that the white glistening fetal surface is uppermost. The position of cord insertion and radiation of the surface vessels is noted.

Cord

The cord should arise from near the centre of the placenta. The cord is examined for true knots, which are very rare, or false knots (outgrowths of Wharton's jelly).

The cut end of the cord is wiped with a swab and then the blood vessels are noted. There should be two arteries and one vein. They should be surrounded by sufficient Wharton's jelly to have protected them.

The cord is measured. Taking into account the part still attached to the baby, the total cord length should be about 55–60 cm.

Charting the findings

All of the findings of the placental examination, along with the estimation of the maternal blood loss during delivery, are recorded on the patient's labour record or summary. Normal findings will read something like this:

Placenta weight: 600 g

	diameter: 20 cm
	complete: appears complete
	calcification: slightly gritty
	any other abnormalities: nil
	cord insertion: central
Membranes	complete: appear complete
	carrying vessels: no vessels seen
Cord	vessels: two arteries, one vein
	thickness: moderate, normal thickness
	knots: nil
	total length: 55 cm
Maternal blood loss	approximately 200 ml

DOCUMENTATION

After the birth of a baby, there are various documents that must be completed in order to have accurate records of the birth in case they are ever needed. The birth details are recorded in the permanent hospital birth register. A delivery summary (such as the one shown in Fig. 12.8) is written up. A copy of the delivery summary is made to go with the baby's records, and the midwife who attached the identification bands or tape to the baby will sign that she has done so. All other documents are completed, including signing for any drugs given to the mother or baby, and signing that all needles and packs used have been accounted for following delivery (and episiotomy or laceration repair).

A claim form for Family Allowance is certified by the doctor or midwife in charge of the conduct of the delivery, and given to the mother. A birth registration form is also given to the mother and she is reminded that she must complete and send it to the Government Registrar as stated on the form within the period set down.

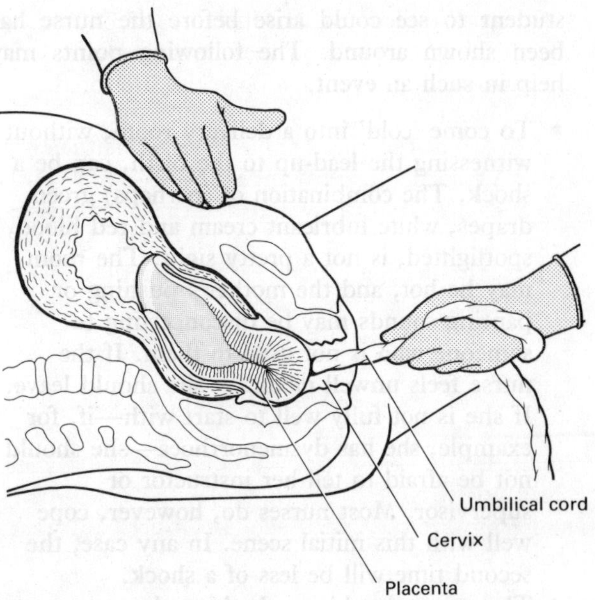

Figure 12.9 Brandt-Andrew's method of delivering the placenta: using controlled gentle cord traction while elevating the uterus.

'WITNESSING' THE BIRTH OF A BABY

One of the reasons for including maternity nursing in the curriculum for the basic education programme for nurses is so that the nurse will be able to cope with the delivery of a baby in an emergency and in the absence of a doctor or midwife. Therefore, the required clinical experience includes the witnessing of a normal delivery.

If the student has not yet had operating room experience, she might find some labour wards intimidating with their overhead lamps, scrub-sinks and sterile trolleys. In most cases she will have an opportunity to see the layout of a delivery room and to ask questions about the equipment that she sees there before she is called to witness a delivery. But midwifery does not always allow for a clinical instructor's orientation programme to be completed, and a normal delivery very suitable for a student to see could arise before the nurse has been shown around. The following points may help in such an event.

- To come 'cold' into a delivery room, without witnessing the lead-up to the birth, can be a shock. The combination of (perhaps) green drapes, white lubricant cream and red blood, spotlighted, is not a pretty sight. The room may be hot, and the mother's pushing or panting sounds may be disconcerting to someone who is not used to them. If the nurse feels unwell or dizzy, she should leave. If she is not fully well to start with—if, for example, she has dysmenorrhoea—she should not be afraid to tell her instructor or supervisor. Most nurses do, however, cope well with this initial scene. In any case, the second time will be less of a shock.
- The nurse should stand where she can see, but where she will not impede the movements of the working staff. She should be ready to move out of the way if necessary. Most likely, she will be told to come closer, but she should not presume to get too close or she may be regarded as an intruder.
- She should remember the basic rules about sterility, and should not touch any sterile surface or item, nor walk between two sterile fields such as a sterile trolley and a 'scrubbed' person.
- She should wear the prescribed dress for the labour room correctly.
- She should remember that she is witnessing a very important and potentially emotional event.
- Although the mother may not be aware of who witnesses the delivery, the father can be very conscious of such things; the behaviour of the nurse is to be beyond reproach. She must be quiet, unobstrusive and must never stare. Afterwards, if an opportunity arises, she can thank the couple for allowing her the privilege of being there (their permission would have been asked beforehand).
- Following the delivery of the infant, the nurse should observe the way he is handled and what procedures are performed. At the same time, she should be alert to observe the delivery of the placenta and the way it is withdrawn from the vagina.
- After this, she does not stand staring at the vulva while an episiotomy or tear is being repaired. Instead, she continues to observe what is happening to the baby, or she goes with the midwife to observe the examination of the placenta and membranes.
- Witnessing a delivery is *not* an everyday event. Even though the nurse will be experiencing many differing emotions, she should remember her usual common courtesy; she will not arrive chewing gum, exclaiming, commenting, or asking questions loudly in the delivery room. Questions *are* encouraged, but later, away from the new parents who might misinterpret the student's lack of knowledge or experience or be frightened by the answers given.
- As most midwives love to teach, they are quite likely to ask questions of the student. They will want to ensure that the student reacted well to the witnessing experience, and that she fully understood what happened and the reasons behind it.

A sound theoretical understanding of the subject is a good base for any clinical experience; this is especially so in midwifery, particularly in the labour ward where events can happen very quickly.

HELPING WITH LABOUR CARE

Nursing students may be given the opportunity to spend some days in the labour ward as part of their clinical experience in maternity nursing. Such an arrangement is, of course, much better than simply being called to witness a birth as an isolated incident.

The midwife responsible for the conduct of the labour will be aware of the legal restrictions of any nursing intervention or care given by a student, so students assigned to labour ward for clinical experience must work within the limits set by that midwife and the clinical teachers. There are, however, a number of positive contributions which a student can make to the care of a labouring woman and her husband or companion, and so enrich her clinical experience.

Some ways of helping could include:

- simply being company in the early stages of labour, when the midwife's constant presence is not necessary. Company is really appreciated in circumstances where the husband or labour companion is not able to be present or when they need a break or change of scene, perhaps to go out for a meal or a walk;
- distracting the couple with quiet conversation if it seems that they would like to talk, and if the atmosphere is right. Their pregnancy experiences and preparations and plans for the baby are usually safe topics and ones which most couples are eager to talk about. It is important that the couple be aware of the student's limitations in knowledge and experience. Sometimes the student will be told of worries or concerns which, with the couple's permission, she should report to the midwife;
- giving basic nursing attention and care both when the woman is ambulating and when she is in bed. Assistance with showering or bed sponging, teeth cleaning or mouth rinses, back massage, hair brushing—all of these will be appreciated. Tidying the labour room, emptying bins and hanging up dressing gowns can also help. Some people hate to be in a mess, and a woman in labour often cannot do much about her surroundings herself;
- provision of ice both in the woman's water jug and in a bowl for her 'cold' face washer, and renewing the ice supply when necessary. Encouraging the woman to keep up an adequate intake of fluids (unless there is any reason to restrict intake) and recording all fluids taken;
- providing a separate supply of iced water for the husband or companion—a small but useful task;
- attending to bladder care by offering bedpans or assisting the woman to the toilet as as appropriate, and recording and reporting results of urine testing;
- caring for the husband—by encouraging him to look after himself by taking occasional breaks from the labour ward and by having meals and drinks to keep his own blood sugar and hydration at satisfactory levels. The student nurse can also observe the husband's response at the time of delivery, when all other eyes may be on the mother.

Other opportunities to participate will be given by the midwives when they recognise a student who is keen to take an active part in maternity care.

13

ASSISTED LABOUR

Chapter outline
Induction of labour
Episiotomy
Instrumental delivery
Vacuum extraction
Caesarean section
Active management

Key words

artificial rupture of membranes—ARM	oxytocin
elective caesarean	prostaglandins
emergency caesarean	Syntocinon

The nursing student will almost certainly encounter patients whose labours have been assisted by one or more intervening procedures. Induction, episiotomy, instrumental (forceps) delivery, vacuum extraction and caesarean section are outlined here.

INDUCTION OF LABOUR

Labour is induced or brought on artificially in those cases where the life or the quality of life of either the mother or the fetus would be endangered if the pregnancy were to continue.

Indications

Fetal

Fetal indications for induction are:

- prolonged gestation—usually if over 41 weeks, over 40 weeks if the mother is 'elderly'
- evidence of placental dysfunction or intrauterine growth retardation
- Rh-affected fetus
- rupture of the membranes near term.

Maternal

Maternal indications for induction are:

- pre-eclampsia
- antepartum haemorrhage
- hypertension
- diabetes
- poor obstetric history.

Methods of induction

Oxytocin infusion

Oxytocic drugs are used to cause contractions of the uterus. Usually a synthetic form of ergometrine called Syntocinon is used, and it is given as an intravenous infusion. The drip rate is carefully controlled, usually by an infusion pump, and the rate is gradually increased until labour is established. The fetal and maternal responses to contractions are constantly and carefully observed.

Prostaglandin administration

Prostaglandins may be used in a similar manner to Syntocinon, i.e. via intravenous infusion, and the same precautions apply.

Prostaglandins, in a gel form or pessary, can be used as a local application to the ripe cervix and upper vagina. It acts especially to 'ripen' the cervix, and in some cases induces labour. Its effect can sometimes be rapid and the woman is usually kept in the delivery suite rather than in a ward bed because of this. Intrauterine administration of prostaglandins is sometimes also employed to induce labour.

Surgical
The amniotic sac is ruptured (artificial rupture of the membranes-ARM). By reducing the tension within the uterus, artificial rupture of the membranes is believed to help to initiate contractions. Usually it is the forewaters that are ruptured. This gives access to the fetal scalp for the application of fetal scalp electrodes, which are connected to a cardiotocograph for continuous or intermittent heart-rate assessment if indicated. If the baby is not delivered within 24 hours, antibiotic therapy may be commenced. A common practice now is to combine both medical and surgical induction, with the oxytocic infusion begun after the artificial rupture of the membranes.

EPISIOTOMY

An episiotomy is an incision into the perineum, to enlarge the vulval orifice during the delivery of an infant.

Indications
Indications for an episiotomy are:

- rigidity of the perineum—where a thick or scarred perineum is causing slow progress of the second stage
- overdistension—where there is a large baby, a breech or other abnormal presentation, or where more room is necessary, such as when forceps are used.
- to hasten delivery—is cases of fetal distress, haemorrhage, cord prolapse, where the baby is premature
- to prevent tearing—a tear will naturally go from the fourchette towards the anus.

A mediolateral incision (Fig. 13.1) is most commonly done, and it is made when the head is stretching the perineum. The area is infiltrated with local anaesthetic prior to making the incision. Following delivery, the episiotomy is repaired as soon as possible to reduce the amount of blood lost. Self-dissolving catgut or synthetic sutures are used for the repair.

INSTRUMENTAL DELIVERY

An instrumental delivery is one in which obstetric forceps are applied to the fetal head in order to assist its delivery (Figure 13.2). Some forceps, such as Keilland's, are designed so that they can rotate the fetal head from an unsuitable position (such as occipito-posterior) to one with a smaller presenting diameter (occipito-anterior). Neville Barnes' forceps are used where the occiput is anterior but where there is delay in delivery, and Wrigley's forceps, which are shorter and lighter in weight, are used for 'life-out' deliveries.

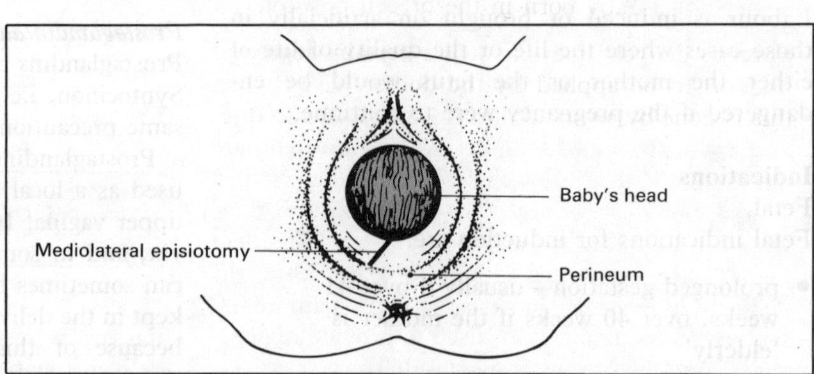

Figure 13.1 Mediolateral episiotomy inicision, directed away from the anus in order to avoid central tearing.

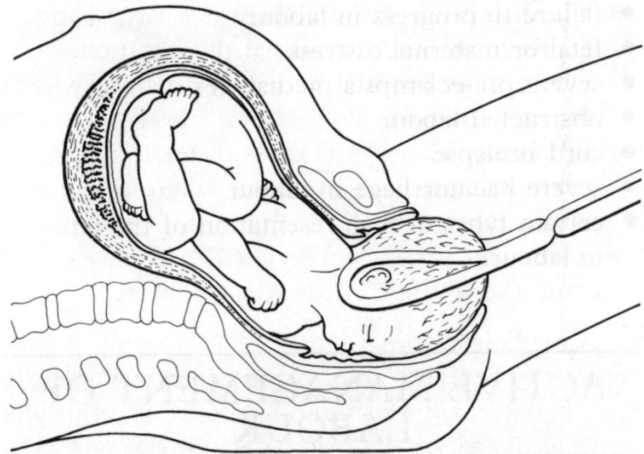

Figure 13.2 Instrumental (forceps) delivery.

Indications

Instrumental delivery is indicated in the following circumstances:

- delay in the second stage of labour; forceps are applied when there has been poor progress after one hour of second stage or after thirty minutes of the head reaching the perineum
- to shorten the second stage when necessary for the welfare of the fetus or the mother, in such conditions as fetal distress, maternal distress and cord prolapse
- where pushing could be dangerous because of the exertion involved, such as in pre-eclampsia, hypertension, and cardiac patients
- to control the delivery of the head, e.g. in the premature baby, or for the aftercoming head of a baby born in the breech position.

Forceps delivery may involve a certain degree of traction to be applied by the doctor. Even when this is done by a very skilled doctor, the procedure may be somewhat disconcerting to those who are unfamiliar with it. For this reason, unless it is a simple low-forceps or 'lift-out' delivery, the woman's husband and any others (such as student nurses) are sometimes asked to leave until the delivery is over. In most cases extra pain relief, such as pudendal block, is used to provide regional anaesthesia before instrumental delivery.

VACUUM EXTRACTION

Another aid to delivery is the use of a vacuum extractor (Fig. 13.3). A cup is attached to the baby's head by creating a vacuum, and the vacuum is maintained throughout the procedure. A chain is attached to the cup and the cup is gently pulled intermittently, at the same time as the mother's uterus contracts.

Vacuum extraction is a useful alternative to low forceps delivery when the mother is tired and unable to push effectively. As well, it is sometimes employed to help rotate a transverse or posterior occipital presentation into the anterior position.

Using vacuum extraction, there is less likelihood of laceration occurring or an episiotomy being needed than with a forceps delivery. Vacuum extraction is, however, comparatively slow, and so would not be used where there is fetal distress.

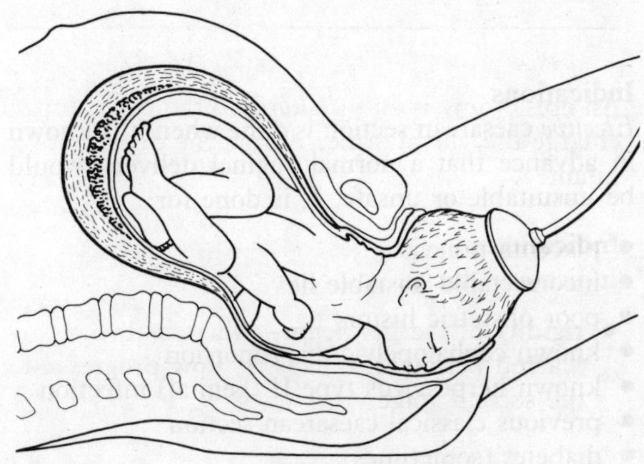

Figure 13.3 Vacuum extraction.

CAESAREAN SECTION

Caesarean section is an obstetrical operation to deliver a viable fetus via the abdominal route.

Types of caesarean section

Lower segment caesarean section (LUSCS)
A transverse incision is made over the lower uterine segment. The lower uterine segment is less vascular than the upper segment, therefore there is less risk of haemorrhage occurring. Also, because the lower segment is outside the peritoneal cavity there is less likelihood of post-operative infection. There is, as well, less risk of uterine rupture in a subsequent pregnancy and labour when the scar is confined to the lower segment of the uterus. Wound healing is usually good because the lower segment is the less active part of the involuting uterus.

Classical caesarean section
The classical incision is used only very occasionally. It is performed when the lower segment is inaccessible because of adhesions or placental obstruction, when there are varicose veins of the lower segment, sometimes for a fetus lying in the transverse position, and for a caesarean hysterectomy.

Indications

Elective caesarean section is done when it is known in advance that a normal vaginal delivery would be unsuitable or unsafe. It is done for:

- placenta praevia
- incorrectable unstable lie
- poor obstetric history
- known cephalopelvic disproportion
- known herpesvirus type II (genital) infection
- previous classical caesarean section
- diabetes (sometimes)
- breech presentation (sometimes)
- severe fetal disease or deprivation, such as erythroblastosis or marked intrauterine growth retardation.

Urgent caesarean section is done for:

- failed induction of labour
- failure to progress in labour
- fetal or maternal distress
- severe pre-eclampsia or diabetes
- obstructed labour
- cord prolapse
- severe haemorrhage in labour
- certain types of malpresentation of the fetus in labour.

ACTIVE MANAGEMENT OF LABOUR

Active management is indicated when there is a need to control and supervise the labour, in anticipation of either fetal or maternal complications. Active management of labour usually involves:

- induction by artificial rupture of membranes
- intravenous oxytocic infusion (Syntocinon) to establish or accelerate contractions
- assessment of progress by regular, e.g. 4-hourly vaginal examinations
- recording the rate of cervical dilatation on a specific chart (partograph, cervicograph)
- adequate pain relief—oxytocin-induced contractions are often abnormally painful, epidural analgesia is preferred
- fetal monitoring (cardiotocograph) as indicated to assess fetal response to contractions
- assisted delivery (low forceps) is common (because of epidural analgesia)
- intervention (if progress slower than satisfactory) by caesarean section

Active management of labour will probably not be the 'beautiful experience' that the parents may have hoped labour to be. It does, however, avoid the hazards of prolonged labour, and in cases of high risk it ensures that labour or delivery does not adversely affect the mother or the baby physically. That is a very important consideration.

14

IMMEDIATE POSTNATAL CARE OF THE MOTHER AND BABY

Chapter outline
'Nature' versus 'modern medical management'
Immediate care of the baby
Immediate care of the mother

Key words
Apgar score
Leboyer-type births
meconium

The basic initial care of the mother (observation, prevention of bleeding, and provision of warmth and comfort) has been mentioned briefly (p. 138), as has the cutting of the cord, clearing the baby's mouth and pharynx, and handing him to either his mother or the midwife.

This is the point at which practices favoured by the hospital, doctor, midwives, mothers and husbands can really differ, and these differences can give rise to misunderstanding and disappointment if they have not been openly discussed beforehand.

Much depends on the condition of the baby, the mother's condition, how alert she is, the expectations of the couple, and the past experiences of her attendants. It would be foolish to give an exhausted or sedated mother her new baby and expect her to 'bond' with him, or even to be safe with him.

It is strongly recommended that the nurse re-read the section 'Adaptation to extrauterine life' on page 43 so that she will understand the principles behind medical or nursing intervention at this stage.

Following an uncomplicated delivery, the baby who breathes readily and has a good Apgar score is given immediately to his mother. He will be dried to prevent heat loss by evaporation, and then wrapped or covered in some way unless there is some provision made for warming the environment to compensate for the often dramatic drop in his external temperature.

The mother and father can then *really* have their baby; they can establish eye contact, stroke him, examine him. This moment, as well as being profoundly moving for the couple and perhaps for any person who witnesses it, is also the time during which they must begin their adjustment to the *real* baby as distinct from the one they have imagined.

'NATURE' VERSUS 'MODERN MEDICAL MANAGEMENT'

The baby's entry into the world is, for him, a time of phenomenal change and shock. Although the medical and nursing professions have always been aware of this, developments in their understanding of physical complications and their efforts to prevent problems such as perineal tearing and heat loss gradually led to a situation in which the natural aspects of the baby's birth became overshadowed by unnatural interventions and procedures.

Leboyer-type births

A French obstetrician, Professor Frederick Leboyer, studied the problem of birth shock for several years, and in 1967 published his theory of 'birth without violence'. It was, in many respects, the direct opposite of the way most hospitals were managing the newborn baby at the time of birth. For the purposes of this book, the main points of the Leboyer-type method are best summarised and

Table 14.1 Comparison of routine hospital and the Leboyer-type methods of management of the newly delivered baby

'Hospital routine' and usual rationale	'Leboyer-type method' and his rationale
Comparatively cool room—for the comfort of the labouring mother	Room warmed—to lessen heat loss, and so that the baby can stay naked
The room may be well lit, perhaps with spotlights—to observe the thinning perineum and to observe the baby's colour	Dim lighting—to lessen the shock for the baby
There may be activity and noise (suction + O_2 machines, verbal encouragement 'push', 'pant', 'look at the baby, it's coming')	Atmosphere of quiet, calm and peace, talking kept to an absolute minimum—to lessen the shock for the baby
Cord usually cut immediately—the baby can be removed to a resuscitation unit for further sucking-out, administration of oxygen, initial examination; also immediate cutting of the cord will prevent any more red cells from entering the baby's circulation	Cord not cut until pulsation has ceased—the baby has, for a short time, two potential sources of oxygen
Onset of respiration may be assisted with suction, oxygen, stimulation (flicking feet)—because of the known dangers of hypoxia	Respiration onset is not assisted routinely—spontaneous respiration is anticipated, drainage of airways achieved by prone position, does not hurt like suction may
The baby may be placed in the dorsal position (on his back) with his body extended, while being attended, for ease of access and observation	The baby lies prone (on his stomach)—resuming his natural attitude of flexion
The baby may be wrapped and attended to before being given to his parents—to prevent heat loss and to make sure that everything is normal	The mother holds the baby as soon as he is lifted on to her bare abdomen (she may, in fact, draw his body from the vagina herself); she strokes him slowly and allows him to remain on his stomach until spontaneous respirations occur
The baby may be taken to the ward or nursery for observation and further management, and is weighed, bathed and checked by nursing staff	The baby remains with the parents and, when ready, is placed in a warm bath—to allow free limb movement and to simulate the intrauterine fluid environment

compared with the standard 'hospital routine', in chart form (Table 14.1).

The compromise

Both Leboyer and 'intervention' have extremely good points. A compromise in the form of 'modified Leboyer births' is now popular in Australian hospitals, as doctors, midwives and potential parents learn to appreciate both sides of the question.

Local warmth (radiant heat-lamps), reduction of light (with good lighting immediately available), parental involvement in the birth with skilled intervention available if necessary, allowing the parents to hold their baby from the start with staff there to guide them and observe the baby; these are the ideals of 'safe-nature' in maternity care.

IMMEDIATE CARE OF THE BABY

Apgar score estimation

The Apgar scoring system gives an index of a new baby's condition at birth, determining his need for help through five easily observed signs:

- colour
- heart rate
- respiratory effort
- muscle tone
- reflex response.

At 1 minute after delivery, and again at 5 minutes, the baby is given a score of 0 or 1 or 2 out of a maximum of 2, for each sign (Fig. 14.1). A total score of 10 indicates that the infant is in optimum condition. If the score is 7 or more, the baby rarely needs special resuscitation. A total score of 6 or less demands immediate attention.

Suction and oxygen

Suction and oxygen equipment is checked before all deliveries. Oropharyngeal suction is no longer routine except where the liquor has been meconium-stained. In such cases it is important that the baby's airway be cleared with gentle but

APGAR SCORING	2	1	0
Heart rate	over 100	less than 100	impalpable or invisible
Respiration	established and almost regular	intermittent, gasping in character	no breaths have been seen
Colour	pink all over	centrally pink but with blue extremities	cyanosed or pale
Muscle tone	good—usually kicking	fair—some movement	none—completely floppy
Response to stimulation (flicking the feet)	vigorous withdrawal	minimal withdrawal	none

Figure 14.1 The Apgar score chart.

thorough aspiration of the mouth and pharynx before the first breath is taken. Inhaled meconium can cause lung irritation and severe respiratory distress. Oxygen via an intranasal catheter is not routine, but is indicated when colour is not satisfactory by 3 minutes after birth.

Cutting of the cord

The baby's cord is clamped approximately 1 centimetre from the abdominal wall, and cut at least 1 centimetre beyond the clamp. In some centres, it is tied with tape before the cut.

Identification

Hospitals vary in their baby identification procedures, but all must observe the state laws. Two identification bands are prepared, one secured around the wrist and one around the ankle. In some countries identification beads are worn around the baby's neck, or an ink imprint of the baby's foot is made as well.

Identification bands should be put on before the baby leaves the delivery bed. If that is not possible they are applied as soon as the opportunity arises. The baby never leaves his mother's presence without his identification bands. The bands are shown to the mother and she is asked to read them aloud and agree that the name is correct before they are applied.

Vitamin K injection

An intramuscular injection of Vitamin K (Konakion) may be given to normal newborn babies as a preventive measure against bleeding tendencies (neonatal haemorrhagic disease). Its natural source, synthesis in the large bowel, is not available until the activity of the digestive system is established following the intake of food. It can take up to 8 days before the baby has satisfactory blood-clotting ability.

The usual dose of vitamin K is 1 mg depending on the size of the baby.

A number of paediatricians are currently questioning the value and necessity of routine administration of vitamin K (especially via the intramuscular route) for a normal mature infant who has had an uncomplicated, unassisted birth.

Initial examination

An initial examination is performed quickly and as soon as possible, so that any findings can be acted upon immediately. The examination looks for:

- satisfactory colour, respiration, and muscle tone
- presence of the reflexes, especially the Moro reflex (p. 160)
- presence and normality of the fontanelles, eyes, hard and soft palates
- obvious abnormalities in the external genitalia
- normal movements in the limbs and digits.

A description of the subsequent, full examination of the newborn baby appears on page 157.

Urine and meconium

Urine and meconium may be passed at birth or soon after. The midwives are alert for this; they make a note if either are passed for the information of those who take over the care of the baby.

Temperature maintenance

The midwife is aware that heat loss can occur rapidly in the newborn baby, especially during procedures which entail exposure of the skin.

He is kept warm by wrapping (not forgetting the large surface of the head), heat lamps or room conditioning. If wrapped, a sheet of insulating material of some sort such as aluminium foil or 'bubble' plastic may be incorporated into or placed outside the rugs. Baby wrapping cloths are usually pre-warmed. It must not be forgotten that the warmest place for a baby is, almost always, in his mother's arms!

Other procedures

The baby may be weighed, measured and washed before being transferred to postnatal or nursery care. Weight may be significant in the calculation of drug dosage or in decisions regarding the management of the baby, therefore it is the most likely of these procedures to be done at this stage. Washing and measuring may be left until the baby has recovered and rested, and are always left until his temperature is stable and at least 36.5°C.

The first 'cuddle' and feed

Unless the baby has urgent need of resuscitation or immediate medical care he is handed to his mother as soon as he is born. The instinctive response of many new mothers is to want to put the baby to the breast quite soon after birth.

This is in accordance with nature; as well as the cord being exactly the right length (from the uterus to the breast), suckling stimulates further uterine contractions and so aids in the expulsion of the placenta. It also aids in the process of 'bonding' between the baby and the mother, and should never be discouraged unless there are absolute contraindications.

Some new mothers may still have to resolve their feelings about breast feeding, or about the baby; the opportunity to feed the baby at this stage should be given, but the matter should not be pushed.

Ideally, the baby will stay with his mother until she is ready to be moved to her postnatal bed. The baby is always transferred in a safe cot, never carried in his mother's, or anyone else's arms.

IMMEDIATE CARE OF THE MOTHER

The mother remains in the delivery suite for at least 1 hour, preferably longer, following delivery. The first hour is sometimes called the 'fourth stage' of labour. Her body is undergoing a great adjustment, and there is the danger of postpartum haemorrhage. The delivery area has facilities for coping with such an emergency.

She is kept warm, helped to achieve a comfortable position, given a sponge bath and perineal wash-down or assisted to shower, the bed linen is changed, and she is offered a cup of tea or other drink.

Observations made and recorded half-hourly at this stage are:

- temperature, pulse, respirations, blood pressure
- fundus—should be firm, central and at or below the level of the umbilicus

- loss—should be minimal (pads should not be soaked in less than 1 hour)
- voiding—a full bladder can prevent proper uterine contraction. As well, there may be oedema of the internal urethral sphincter, causing difficulty in voiding; sitting out of bed in a commode-type chair often helps
- pain—pain should not be excessive, discomfort should be relieved by oral analgesia such as codeine or paracetamol tablets; if not, it is reported.

Visitors

The newly-delivered mother is usually both weary and excited. As she and her husband recover from the work of labour it is important that they spend time quietly enjoying and discovering the baby by themselves. Midwives are careful to leave the couple on their own at this time, apart from doing the necessary checks on the mother's and baby's condition. Appreciation of cultural factors is, however, important here—in some cultures there is a strict order in which family members should greet the new baby and congratulate the parents. Midwives in most labour wards are flexible in this, while endeavouring to protect the newly-delivered mother from becoming overwhelmed and exhausted from visitors.

Transfer to the postnatal area

When the mother's vital signs are proved to be stable and satisfactory, vaginal loss is minimal, her uterus is well contracted, and she has voided, she is transferred to the postnatal ward.

The woman and her husband have just been through a very significant experience; they may be reluctant to leave the labour ward midwives who have shared this with them, for the unknown personnel of the postnatal floor.

It is important, therefore, that their reception when they get there is good. The student nurse often spends a fair proportion of her maternity clinical experience in the postnatal area and so contributes to the couple's impression of the maternity care they receive.

15

EMERGENCY DELIVERY

Nurses are expected to be able to cope with all sorts of emergencies: 'She's a nurse, she'll know what to do'. In an emergency associated with labour, people are probably *not* going to stop to consider whether the nurse that they are calling upon has done specialised midwifery training.

An emergency delivery can occur in a busy, crowded, perhaps dirty place where there may be very few facilities. Or it could occur in a person's home, where conditions are better, but where improvisations will still need to be thought about with some speed. Or it could happen in a *general* hospital (the woman may already be a patient for some other reason), or a mother in strong labour might go to the nearest medical facility because she feels that she will not have time to reach a maternity hospital. Even in a hospital, unless it is *specifically* equipped and staffed for maternity patients, adaptations will have to be made. Wherever the emergency occurs, it *will* be an emergency; it will be upsetting for the woman and her husband, and their anticipated birth experience will be somewhat of a frightening ordeal unless it is handled very well.

The nurse might become involved when the labour is still in its early stages. Alternatively, she may not come upon the scene until labour is too far advanced for her to even turn her back on the woman, let alone consider going to a telephone to send for extra assistance.

The emergency may arise in a 'near' situation; near to other more experienced people, near to transport, a doctor, a hospital. Or it may arise in a very distant situation (e.g. trapped in the outback by flood-waters), where there is no option but to help the woman right through her labour, assist her with the baby's birth and ensure the best possible care of both the mother and the baby afterwards.

Because of the many variations that can arise, the management of an emergency delivery can only be based upon the application of principles. These principles, with her knowledge of the details described in the preceding four chapters, and serious attention and careful observation during maternity clinical experience, will enable the nurse to 'cope' as she is expected to be able to, because she is a nurse.

The first task that the nurse must undertake is that of establishing that the woman *is* in labour. She must know well and be able to recognise the signs of the onset of labour. After this, she must be able to assess, approximately at least, how far the labour has progressed. She must realise that there are differences between the usual progress of the labours of a primigravida and a multipara, and she must remember this when planning her actions, adapting her management of the situation to enable the best possible outcome in the available time. Table 15.1 outlines the principles of the management of an emergency delivery.

There is a lot more to think about than just putting on the kettle—although that could well be useful when the emergency is over!. Some other points worth remembering follow.

- The safest and warmest place for the baby is usually in his mother's arms.
- Suckling causes the uterus to contract and so is nature's way of preventing postpartum haemorrhage.
- Identification labelling is very important, as the baby could well be separated from the mother.

Table 15.1 Management of an emergency delivery

Principle	Actions	Details of actions
Labour can be:		
frightening	reassurance	calm assessment and action; the woman is never left alone; husband also considered and given some positive role.
complicated	summon assistance	sensible message including where to come, description of signs, parity, state of membranes, any known obstetric or medical problems
painful	assist relaxation, promote physical comfort, distract from pain	relaxation encouraged, attention to bladder, bed, warmth, back massage, revise (or teach basic) breathing patterns, other mental exercises
embarrassing	provide privacy	close doors, improvise screens, minimise exposure use people's backs to make a 'wall'
long or exhausting (distant situation)	relieve symptoms, continually reassure, prevent exhaustion	all of the above actions, plus: fluids and light foods as desired, relaxation techniques taught, encourage to void 2-hourly; lying on side
Delivery can be:		
sudden	find a safe place	lie woman down, don't allow her to 'go to the toilet' when she feels bowel pressure, check for the head (visual check only) when woman feels the urge to push
damaging (both to the baby's head and to the mother's perineum)	prevent sudden expulsion of the head	encourage 'panting' (do it with her) for the delivery of the head; gentle restraint to flex baby's head while supporting the perineum; adequate lighting to see properly.
the cause of later infection	ensure best possible cleanliness	clean hands of helpers*, clean place for the woman to lie on (insides of unread newspapes, clean towel or sheet), wipe away or cover any faeces that escape *hands off' policy in any case
The newborn baby can be:		
slow to breathe	after ensuring clear airway, stimulate respirations	clear mouth with soft cloth, 'strip' nose of mucus and fluid. Allow 1 minute for baby to recover from shock of birth then stroke baby's back, flick feet, mouth-to-mouth resuscitation if indicated
(is) prone to infection	minimise contact with potentially infecting materials	ensure cleanest possible surroundings, clean hands of helpers, clean wrappings.
(is) prone to heat loss	minimise exposure, provide warmth	light fires or heaters (must be safe), pre-warm towels and wraps in oven if possible; warm room, dry and wrap baby immediately (remembering large area of head), give baby immediately to mother
(later) separated from his mother	allow opportunity for bonding	allow mother time to cuddle, examine, breast feed, her baby; make sure that the father has an opportunity to hold his baby before they are taken off to hospital
	label both baby and mother for identification	details of name, the delivery, time and place of birth, should be written on cloth or strong card; this should be tied to the wrist or ankle before the mother and baby are separated

Table 15.1 (*contd*)

Principle	Action	Details of actions
The placenta and membranes can be		
slow to deliver	maintain uterine contractions	put baby to breast—suckling stimulates contractions; massage fundus gently, observe fundus and blood loss, encourage voiding
torn during extraction	control to allow spontaneous placental delivery	never pull on cord; wait until signs of separation appear before asking mother to give a push, then gently extracting, twist placenta to ease membranes out
The newly-delivered mother can be:		
prone to blood loss	maintain uterine contractions exclude non-uterine causes of bleeding	massage fundus, put baby to breast; if really severe, aortic compression may be attempted examine vagina and vulva for fresh bleeding; apply local pressure if necessary
upset, cold and exhausted	provided physical and emotional comfort	give praise and encouragement, reassure; keep warm, provide nourishment, prevent further blood loss, allow to rest

- Aid should be summoned as soon as possible, but the strongly-labouring (pushing) woman should not be left alone, even to summon aid.
- It does not really matter whether or not the cord is cut, but it should be tied, in two places, perhaps with cotton tape or a piece of cloth. Bleeding should not occur from the placenta, because placental circulation ceases with the onset of the baby's respirations.
- The placenta can be wrapped up with the baby, perhaps first being placed in a clean plastic bag if it is especially messy. It must accompany the baby to hospital in every circumstance. If the cord is cut, it should be cut no less than 5 cm from the baby's umbilicus after ensuring that it is tied securely.
- It *does* matter if the cord is cut with any object which has not been sterilised. The umbilical vein leads directly into the liver, and infection can be dangerous.
- The mother and baby and placenta are sent off to hospital, or a doctor is summoned, as soon as possible. Both the mother and the baby will need to be fully examined to ensure that everything is normal, and they will both need to recover from the experience of emergency delivery.

Legal aspects

In emergency situations, the nurse has no different status from any other member of the public. She will, however, be expected to have some knowledge and competence, and so if she does render assistance in an emergency what she does will be judged by what one would expect of the reasonable nurse.

She should make every attempt to summon the aid of a medical practitioner or a registered midwife. She must also endeavour to transfer the mother and the baby to hospital or to a medical practitioner as soon as it is safe and possible.

Concealing a birth

Concealing the birth of a baby is a criminal offence for which there is, in many places, a penalty of imprisonment. A person who became involved in the concealment of the birth could be prosecuted as being an accessory. It is irrelevant whether the child was born alive or was stillborn.

16

THE NORMAL NEWBORN BABY

Chapter outline

Full examination of the newborn baby
Subsequent care of the baby
- Rooming-in
- Nursery-based care
- Daily examination
- Temperature control
- Hygiene and skin care
- Weight recording
- Nutrition and elimination
- Cord care
- Phenylketonuria screening
- Fingernails
- Visitors
- Clothes

Minor problems
- Thrush
- Sore buttocks
- Neonatal breast engorgement
- Skin rashes
- Common birth marks
- The 'unsettled' baby

Circumcision
Mild (physiological) jaundice
- Phototherapy

Key words

caput
cephalhaematoma
fontanelles
Guthrie test
milia
mongolian spots
moulding
'relaxation bath'
rooming-in

FULL EXAMINATION OF THE NEWBORN BABY

When the baby has rested and recovered from his experiences of birth and adaptation to extrauterine life, and when his temperature is stable he will be carefully, thoroughly and systematically examined.

The midwife who conducts this examination will have reviewed the mother's antenatal history, giving special attention to the results of the mother's previous labours and any problems then or with the just-completed pregnancy. She will also have studied the mother's labour summary and noted the findings of the baby's initial examination, the Apgar scores, and any treatment or medication given to the baby.

Before being examined, the baby is fully undressed. Many hospitals provide overhead warming lamps to help to prevent heat loss. In any case, the examination is done in a warm place, with good lighting, and the baby is placed upon a safe, flat surface. Most midwives try to do the examination at a time when the baby is awake but quiet; crying, although giving good vision of the mouth, may affect the accuracy of the other findings.

Table 16.1 shows the usual methods of examining the various body parts, the expected initial findings, and possible developments which may arise in the first 7–10 days. Findings are recorded clearly on a fill-in card or sheet and are kept with the baby's records: they provide information for planning the baby's individual care.

Weight

The baby is weighed without clothes; this first weighing always checked by a second midwife, then recorded on the baby's chart and cot card. The average weight of a normal full-term infant is about 3.5 kg. It is normal for up to 10% of the birth weight to be lost in the first 2–4 days, and for birth weight to be regained by the 10th–14th day.

Table 16.1 Characteristics of the normal newborn baby

Body part	How examined	Initial fiindings	Later developments (first 7–10 days)
Head			
Size	Measured around occipito frontal circumference	Average circumference 35 cm	There should be no increase in size in the first week
Fontanelles and sutures	Gently palpated	Anterior fontanelle no tension or depression; posterior fontanelle and sutures palpable; there may be some overriding of the sutures	Posterior fontanelle may close, overriding of sutures disappears
Shape	Inspected and palpated	Elongated (moulding–Fig. 16.3)	Moulding reduces most in first 48 hours, 'normal' shaped head by 7–10 days
		Soft spongy area (caput–Fig. 16.4A)	Reduces by 48 hours
		Unilateral or bilateral soft swelling (cephalhaematoma–Fig. 16.4B)	Reduced by 3–4 days; baby observed for jaundice
Face			
Colour	Inspected	Pink to red	
Appearance	Inspected and palpated	symmetrical at rest and when moving (e.g. crying); sucking pads present in cheeks; small petechiae may be present	
Eyes			
Appearance	Inspected; lids may need to be opened gently	Eyes dark blue, sclerae white; placed symmetrically; small subconjunctival haemorrhages common	Sclerae may become yellow if baby becomes jaundiced.
Eyelids	Inspected	Lids able to be opened; close properly when baby at rest; blink reflex present; slightly oedematous; 'stork marks' (dilated capillaries on upper lids) are common; lids moist	Oedema disappears within 24 hours; moist eyes should not become 'sticky'
Pupils	Inspected; tested with torch	Round in shape, equal in size; react to light	
Lenses	Inspected	Clear	
Ears			
Shape	Inspected and palpated	Well-formed, correctly positioned, cartilage present	
Hearing	Baby subjected to sudden noise	Moro response (Fig. 16.2)	
Nose			
Appearance	Inspected	Symmetrical; often flattened; milia (blocked sebaceous glands) common–Fig. 16.5	Flattening disappears after 24 hours
Nostrils	Inspected	Symmetrical and patent; breathes without difficulty–no flaring; mucus often present for a short time after birth	
Mouth			
Lips	Inspected, touched gently	Lips pink; occasionally temporary slight cyanosis; touching elicits sucking reflex response	
Tongue	Inspected	able to protrude (no tongue tie), but normally rests inside the mouth; clean and pink	
Palate	Inspected and palpated	Hard and soft palate fused	
Gums	Inspected and palpated	Clean and pink; very occasionally one or two teeth may be present	

Table 16.1 (*contd*)

Body part	How examined	Initial findings	Later developments (first 7–10 days)
Neck			
Appearance	Inspected and palpated	Short and straight; no webbing, oedema or masses	
Movement	Head put through range of normal movements	Moves freely from side to side and from flexion to extension	
Chest			
Size	Measured at level of nipples	Circumference average 34 cm	
Movement	Inspected	Expands symmetrically with respirations; no sternal retraction	Breast may swell (at 3–4 days) in response to withdrawal of placental hormones, and may secrete a fluid ('witch's milk'–Fig. 16.6)
Breast	Inspected and palpated	Breast tissue palpable in both male and female infants	
Nipples	Inspected from axilla to groin, both sides	Symmetrical; no axillary nipples	
Heart rate	Ausculated	120–160 beats per minute; clear and regular	
Abdomen			
Shape	Inspected and palpated	No masses felt; slightly prominent but not distended	
Movement	Inspected	Moves up and down with respirations	
Umbilicus	Inspected and palpated	Cord blue/white; three vessels in stump; clamp secure, no bleeding	Cord dries and necroses; separates at about the 7th day, leaving umbilicus clean and dry
Genitalia			
Female	Inspted and palpated, gently separating labia	Labia and clitoris often prominent (Fig. 17.7); vernix present in folds; vaginal introitus visible; mucoid 'show' sometimes present	May have slight vaginal blood loss ('spotting') for the first few days, due to withdrawal of placental hormones
Male	Inspected and palpated	Large in relation to body; scrotum contains both descended testicles (or testes can be drawn down easily); foreskin is adherent to glans; urethral meatus is central on tip of penis	
Limbs			
Appearances	Inspected and palpated, hands brought together at the umbilicus	Limbs should be symmetrical, rounded, and feel warm; arms are long enough for hands to meet at the level of the umbilicus; legs are in proportion to length; limbs usually flexed when baby is sleeping	
Movement	Taken through full range of movements	Limbs and extremities able to withstand full range of passive movements	
Extremities	Inspected and palpated	May be slightly cyanosed; 10 fingers and 10 toes (no extra digits–Fig. 16.8); nails are often long; no webbing; grasp reflex present in fingers and toes; feet may turn inwards, but this can be passively corrected	Cyanosis usually disappears after 4–6 hours
Hips			
Movement	Ortolani's test (Fig. 16.9) for congenital dislocation of the hip	Hips able to be abducted to 90° (with the baby supine and the hips and knees flexed) without feeling any 'click'	

Table 16.1 *(contd)*

Body part	How examined	Initial findings	Later developments (first 7–10 days)
Back			
Appearance	Inspected and palpated with the baby supported in the prone position; examiner runs a finger right down the spine from the nape of the neck to the anus	Spine intact, no gaps or growths of hair; spine straight, easily flexed; occasionally a small dimple is present at the base of the spine; fine hair may cover shoulders and upper back	
Anus	Inspected by separating buttocks; in some centres a rectal thermometer is inserted	Anus patent; thermometer inserted easily, showing meconium on removal	

Measurements

The baby is measured bare as part of the full examination. There are, of course, variations in measurement according to the height and build of the parents, but average measurements are:

- crown to heel (legs extended) 50 cm
- head circumference 35 cm
- chest circumference 34 cm

Measuring is repeated as indicated. In some hospitals the head circumference is routinely re-measured 2–3 days after birth, looking for increase in size, to exclude hydrocephalus.

Colour

The baby should be a clear pink colour. There may be some cyanosis of the feet and hands for the first 24-hours.

Respirations

The respiratory pattern is slightly erratic for the first few hours after birth, with a rate of between 40 and 60 breaths per minute. After 2 hours it should have settled to around 40 breaths per minute, with the baby at rest. Respirations are counted by observing the rise and fall of the abdomen.

Posture

The normal baby (Fig. 16.1) will adopt an attitude of flexion naturally, similar to his curled-up attitude in utero. Where there has been an abnormal presentation such as a breech or face, the baby may continue to lie with his legs or head extended for a few days.

Movements

When undressed and awake the baby should be able to move his limbs vigorously and freely. His neck should be able to move from side to side and from flexion to extension. Muscle tone should be firm.

Reflexes

The reflexes present in the normal newborn are:

- Moro
- grasp
- sucking
- seeking ('rooting')
- stepping.

Moro or 'startle' reflex

This is a sign of satisfactory neuromuscular co-ordination. Its absence is suggestive of cerebral damage. The Moro reflex is present for a few weeks after birth. It consists of the baby throwing out his arms (Fig. 16.2) and then bringing them together in an 'embracing' movement. The thighs and legs may also respond in this manner.

The baby will demonstrate the Moro reflex in response to sudden external stimuli. It can be demonstrated by lowering the baby's head a few inches, quickly, with the baby on his back. Loud noises and sudden touching, especially with cold hands will also prompt the reflex.

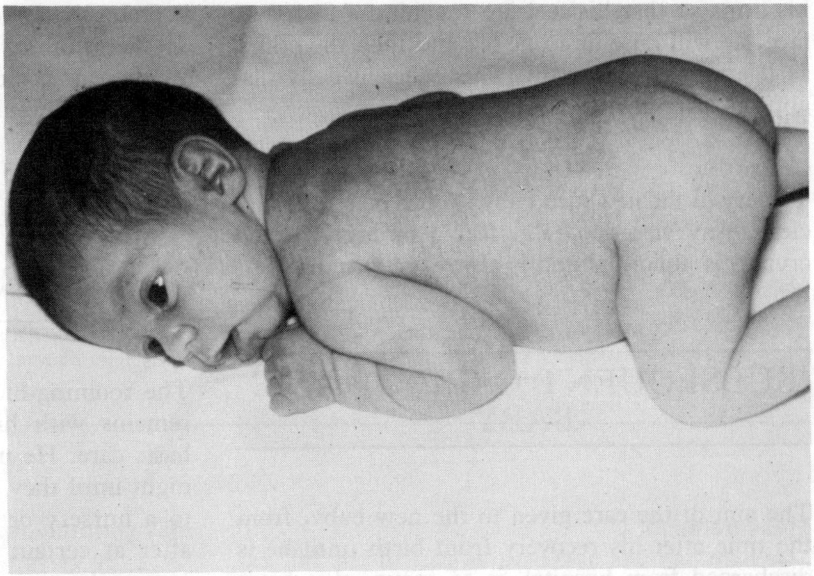

Figure 16.1 The newborn baby adopts an attitude of flexion.

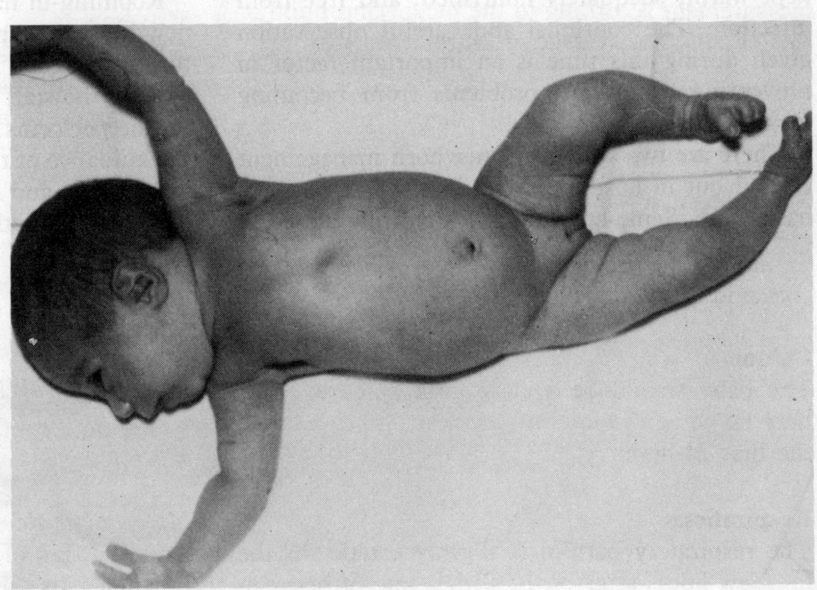

Figure 16.2 The arms are thrown out as part of the Moro or 'startle' reflex.

Grasp reflex
The grasp reflex can be very strong and the baby can sometimes be lifted clear of the surface upon which he was lying when he is grasping on to an attendant's finger.

Sucking reflex
A mature normal baby will attempt to suck at any object which touches his lips. The swallowing reflex is also present.

Seeking or 'rooting' reflex
When the baby's cheek is touched he will turn his head to that side, seeking or searching for a nipple.

Stepping reflex
If the baby is held upright and supported under

his arms so that his feet are touching a firm surface, he will raise first one leg and then the other, as if attempting to walk. This reflex usually disappears after about 48 hours.

Crying
The cry of the newborn baby should be strong and clear. Any variation (e.g. feeble or high-pitched crying) is abnormal and is always reported.

SUBSEQUENT CARE OF THE BABY

The aim of the care given to the new baby, from the time after his recovery from birth until he is discharged from hospital, is to ensure that he is kept warm, adequately nourished, and free from infection. The continual and careful observation given during this time is an important factor in preventing any minor problems from becoming major.

There are two systems of newborn management carried out in hospitals: rooming-in and nursery-based care. Some hospitals work entirely upon the rooming-in system for all normal babies of well mothers; others are flexible in that they offer the mothers a choice, or 'partly room-in'. Very few hospitals now use a totally nursery-based system.

ROOMING-IN

The rooming-in system is one in which the baby remains with his mother and she performs his basic care. He may stay with his mother day and night until they are both discharged or he may go to a nursery or an observation bay to be looked after at certain times, such as overnight and at visiting hours.

Rooming-in has many advantages. It allows the new mother, especially the primipara, the opportunity to really learn to care for her baby, and enables the staff to answer questions as they arise. As she performs all of the basic care herself, under the guidance of the midwives, she gains confidence in handling and feeding her baby. Because no two babies are exactly alike, she is going to discover

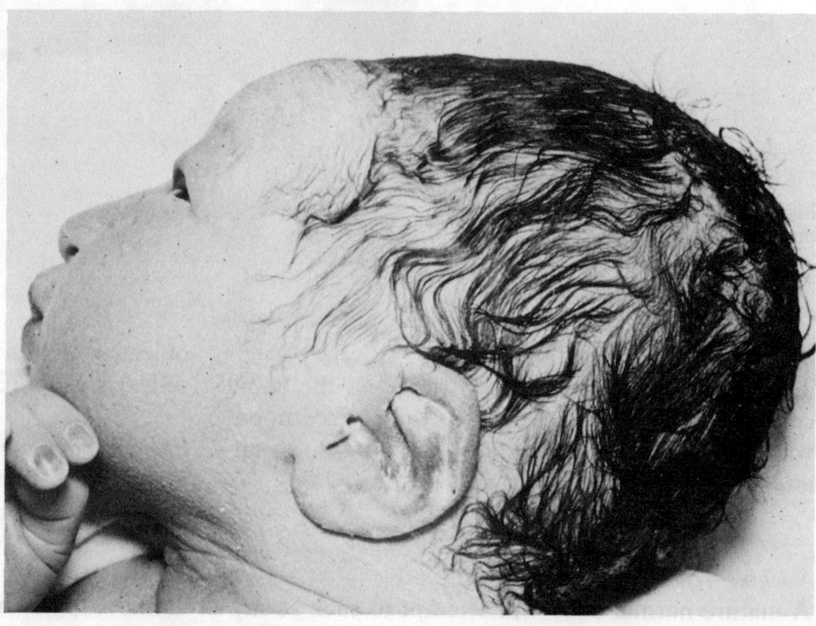

Figure 16.3 Moulding.

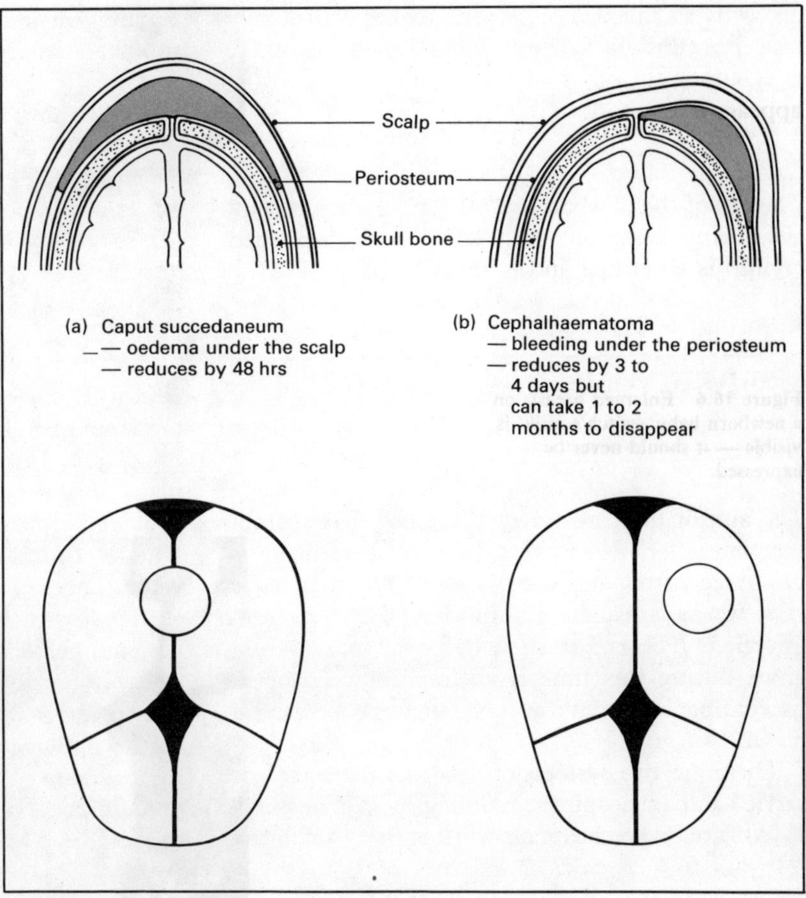

Figure 16.4 Caput, cephalhaematoma.

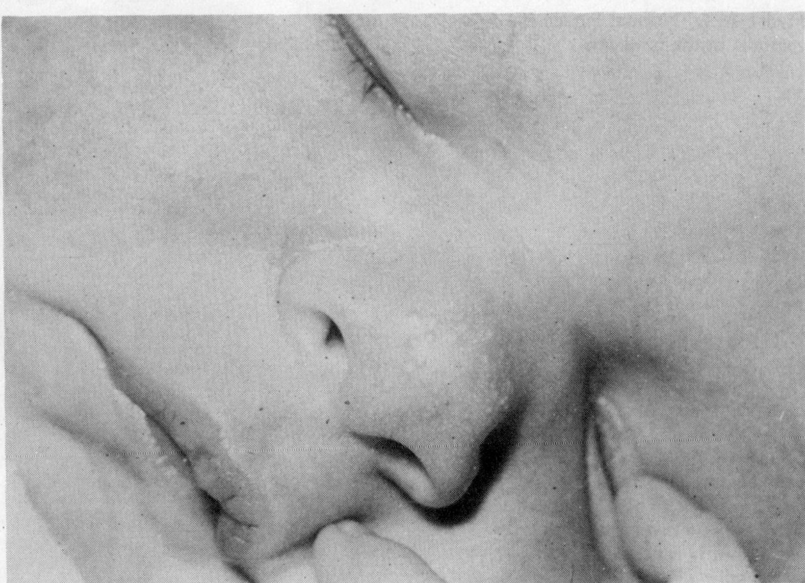

Figure 16.5 Milia — these spots should never be squeezed

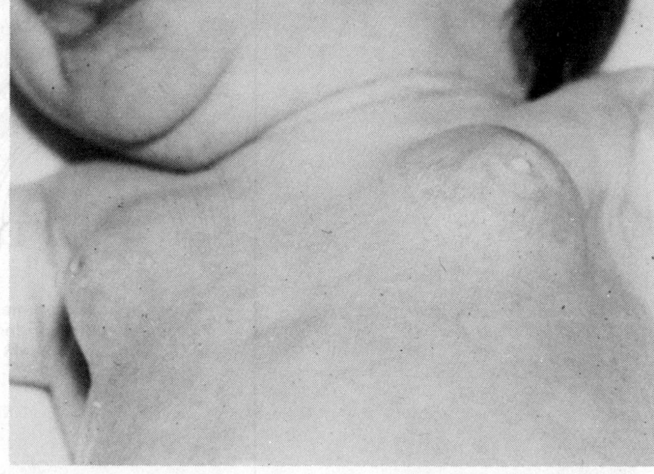

Figure 16.6 Enlarged breasts on a newborn baby; 'witch's milk' is visible — it should never be expressed.

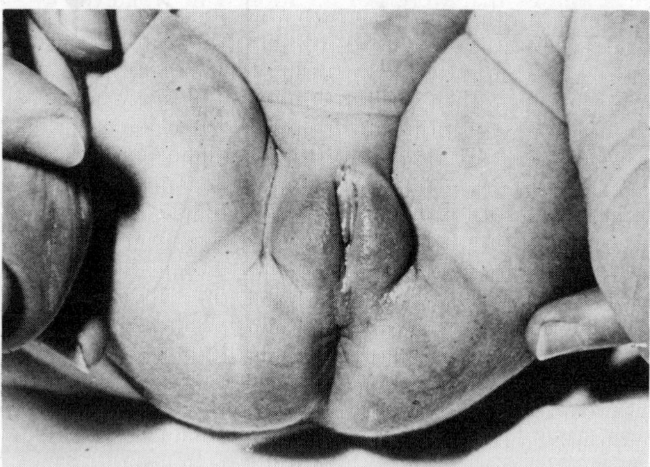

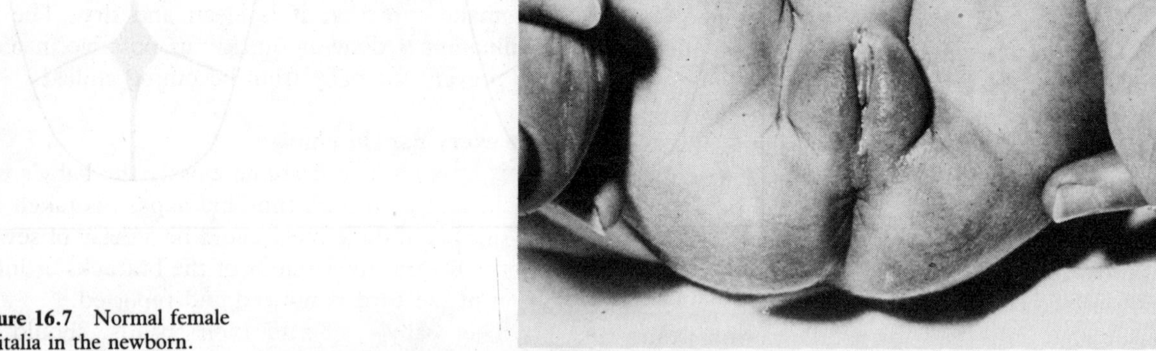

Figure 16.7 Normal female genitalia in the newborn.

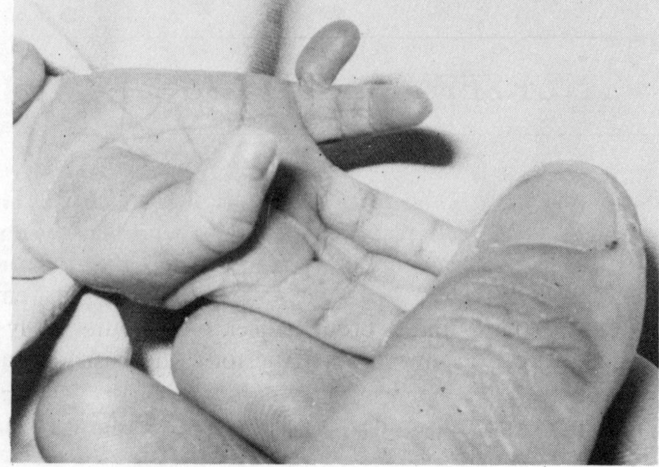

Figure 16.8 Accessory digit; this would be treated by tying with fine cord such as black silk; where there is bony involvement the extra digit is usually left untreated.

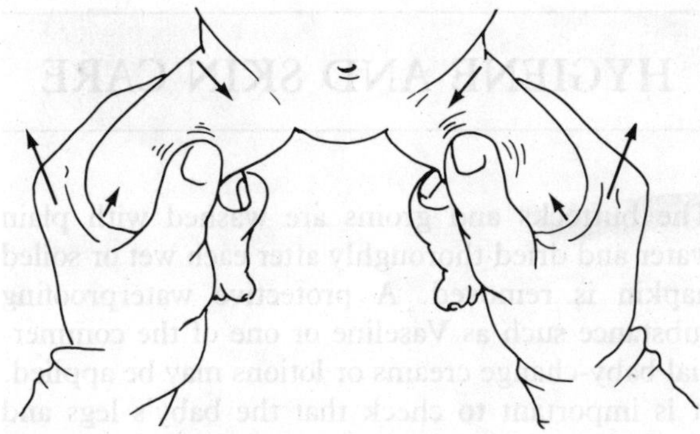

Figure 16.9 Ortoloni's test for congenital dislocation of the hip.

little things that were not mentioned in whatever books she has read or that not happen to other babies that she had anything to do with. Rooming-in also considerably reduces the risks of cross-infection.

There is one possible (but preventable) disadvantage to rooming-in. Unless the mother is well-disciplined with herself about using every opportunity for rest, she could waste a lot of rest time and become very tired. If the staff are alert to this, and help her to organise her day well this problem should not occur.

All mothers who room-in their babies are reminded that should a complication such as jaundice arise, rooming-in may possibly have to be suspended until the baby is fully normal again and does not need special observation or care.

NURSERY-BASED CARE

With this system the infant spends much of his hospital stay in a nursery, cared for by a nursery staff as distinct from the postnatal staff that cares for the mother. The baby is taken out to his mother for feeds and is brought back to the nursery to settle. The nursery staff perform the basic care of the baby, but in most hospitals the baby's parents are free to wander in and out of the nursery at any time.

Nursery-based care, to be successful, depends very much upon good co-operation and liaison between the separate staffs of the nursery and the postnatal ward.

DAILY EXAMINATION

In most hospitals the baby's clothing is completely removed each day in order to wash and perhaps bare-weigh him, but also to observe any departures from normal. The baby's skin is observed for rashes, blotchiness, unusual spots or dryness, and the skin colour for evidence of the onset or deepening of jaundice. Previously discovered problems will be re-checked. The eyes, nose, mouth and fingers are examined in good lighting for any signs of infection, and the cord is examined to make sure that it is clean and dry. The examination is done as quickly as possible in order to prevent the baby from becoming chilled.

At every napkin change

It is important to examine closely the baby's buttocks and cord each time his napkin is taken off. If this is not done there could be a delay of several hours before any soreness of the buttocks or infection of the cord is noticed and reported.

The baby's identification bands should be deliberately checked at every napkin change.

TEMPERATURE CONTROL

The new baby's temperature regulating centre is not yet fully functioning and so cannot cope well with extremes or sudden changes in his external environment. Most hospitals nowadays are centrally-heated or air-conditioned, but even so the baby's temperature needs to be checked regularly and his blankets and wrappings adjusted accordingly.

The usual method of checking the temperature

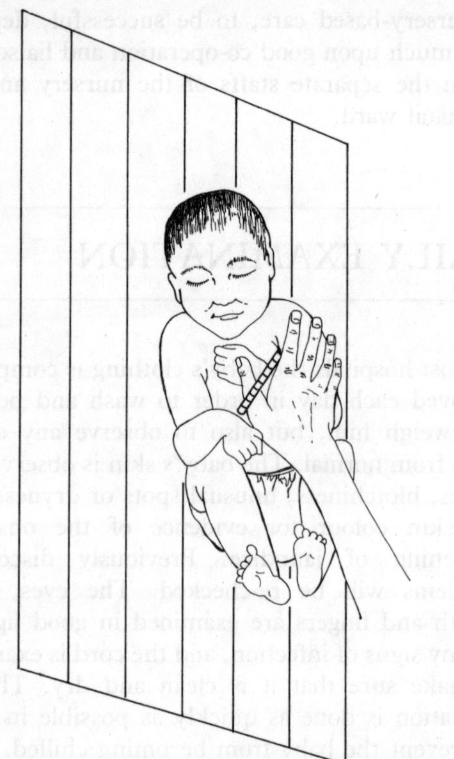

Figure 16.10 The axilliary temperature should be maintained at 36.5° C.

is by placing a thermometer under the axilla and holding it in place (Fig. 16.10) for 1 minute. Rectal temperatures are taken in some centres. The aim is to keep the axillary temperature, which is 0.5°C lower than that of the rectum, at 36.5°C.

Following birth, the temperature is checked half-hourly until there have been two consecutive readings of 36.5°C. After this, it is recorded 4-hourly for the first 24 hours and then, unless there are indications to do it more frequently, twice daily.

The temperature is always measured *before* a baby is fully undressed for a bath or wash, and in some hospitals, *after* the bath as well.

The dangers of hypothermia are discussed on page 198. *Hyper*thermia is also significant, and any elevation of temperature in a baby who is not overwrapped must be reported.

HYGIENE AND SKIN CARE

The buttocks and groins are washed with plain water and dried thoroughly after each wet or soiled napkin is removed. A protective waterproofing substance such as Vaseline or one of the commercial baby-change creams or lotions may be applied. It is important to check that the baby's legs and feet are clean as they can easily become soiled during the napkin changing process.

The baby is fully washed every day in many hospitals and, in most places, this is now done using a bath (rather than as a cot wash or sponge). After observing her baby being bathed once, the mother is encouraged to do the bath herself, with assistance as necessary, so that she gains confidence before going home with the baby. If possible the baby's father is involved and does at least one bath with help himself. If the parents are unfamiliar with baby bathing they may be slow at first, so the importance of setting up and having everything ready before undressing the baby is emphasised so that the baby does not become chilled.

Bathing procedure

The bath should be done before rather than after a feed, if possible, as the movement and handling could unsettle a full stomach. The room should be warm and free from draughts. Clean towels, baby clothes and napkins are laid out and water is added to the bath tub, starting with cold water and adding hot water until the water temperature is comfortably warm when tested with the inside of the wrist or elbow. A bathing solution may be added to the water or pure soap used, depending upon the hospital's policy and the mother's preference.

The baby is fully undressed, and wrapped in a clean towel. His face is washed first, using plain water and cotton-wool swabs or a face washer, then dried carefully. If there is any stickiness of the eyes, they are cleaned with sterile normal saline, using sterile cotton wool, one swab for each wipe, from the nose outwards. A specimen is taken for culture if the stickiness persists. His hair and ears are then washed; if antibacterial solution or soap is used, it is rinsed off carefully over a bath or tub of warm water. Running water is *never* used as it could be dangerous. After the head has been dried with an extra towel, the baby is unwrapped and the front of his body and his limbs are washed. Special attention is given to the skin folds of the neck, axillae and groins. The baby is then turned onto his stomach, and his back and genitals are washed.

The mother or midwife then dries her hands and grips the baby firmly to lift him into the water. The water is then scooped over the baby and special attention is paid to the creases and skin folds. The baby is allowed to stretch and enjoy the water for a few minutes before being lifted out and placed onto a clean dry towel. After being dried he will be dressed without too much delay in clean, warmed clothes. At this stage in the day his cot linen will be renewed.

'Relaxation bath'
An alternative, 'relaxation', bath is now being taught in many hospitals. This method involves turning the baby over onto his stomach in the bath, so that he can float with his limbs down in the water. An ordinary baby bath can be used, with the water deeper than usual. The technique is easily learned, with the important points being—careful support of the baby's head above water by holding up his chin, turning his face to one side, and keeping his arms down in the water. The water must be scooped over the baby's back continuously to keep him warm, but babies do seem to find this floating type of bath very comforting and relaxing. It is not unknown for them to go to sleep in the water.

WEIGHT RECORDING

The baby is bare-weighed every second day while undressed for his wash and check. More frequent weighing is necessary only when there is concern about excessive loss or when the baby's birth weight was below the satisfactory limits for a normal mature baby.

A loss of up to 10% of the birth weight is normal and expected. It is due to the passage of meconium, the use of energy, and the relatively low calorie intake (in a solely breast-fed infant) for the first 3–4 days. The normal baby has the reserves to cope with this weight loss, but his mother may be worried about it and so should be reassured on this point. She should understand the causes and be told the weight is expected to be back to what it was at birth by the time the baby is 10 days old.

A clean sheet of paper is placed upon the scales before each baby is weighed. In some hospitals there is a rule that each weighing must be observed by two members of staff, one a midwife. The scales are checked at regular intervals by maintenance staff to ensure that they are accurate.

NUTRITION AND ELIMINATION

The baby is fed when he is hungry after delivery unless there is any reason to suspect hypoglycaemia. Most newborns are offered a feeding within 5 hours of birth. The practice of the mother putting the baby to the breast soon after delivery is becoming more widespread. This is good, because it is a very natural instinct for the mother, and the baby's sucking instinct is also very strong at this time—it often diminishes after an hour or so and may not be strong again for another 12–24 hours.

Either a 'by the clock' or an 'on-demand' regime is then established. The relative merits of both regimes are discussed on page 183. Whichever the mother chooses, it is important that she be confident in the use of that regime by the time she leaves hospital. For example, if she chooses 'demand' feeding she should be willing to feed at shorter intervals occasionally as well as at longer ones at times. She needs also to be able to defend, if necessary, demand feeding to relatives and acquaintances who 'don't believe in it'.

Hospital policies vary in how long a baby may sleep between feeds but they are now far more flexible than they used to be, while keeping in mind the needs of very small babies. As long as the weight pattern is satisfactory a baby is usually not disturbed to be fed.

Breast feeding is discussed on page 179, and artificial feeding and the types of milks used, on page 188.

Urine

The baby may void only once or twice during the first 24 hours. Urine is often passed at birth and may not be observed. If there is no evidence of voiding within the first 24 hours, the baby's doctor is notified.

After the first day, urine is passed frequently—about 10–12 times per day. It is observed for amount and concentration. It may have a pinkish tinge, which is probably due to the presence of urates; any unusual coloration of the urine should be reported.

Stools

The baby's first bowel action consists of meconium, the dark green tarry substance formed in the intestinal tract during intrauterine life. It should have occurred within the first 24 hours. Meconium must be carefully washed off the buttocks and genitalia straight away, as it can be irritating to the skin and can be difficult to remove if it has been exposed to the air for any length of time.

Following the entry of food into the intestines there is a gradual transition from meconium to the normal yellow stools of the newborn. The transitional stools are dark green-yellow thick curds.

Once the transitional stage has been passed, the stools are observed for colour and consistency as well as frequency. The stools of the breast-fed baby are soft and unformed, yellow to pale brown and have no odour. The artificially-fed baby tends to have firmer, sometimes almost formed, yellow to pale green stools with a distinctive odour. Familiarity with the normal stools will enable recognition of abnormalities such as watery, frothy or abnormally green stools. It is better to ask advice and be reassured that all is normal than to miss the early signs of infection or evidence of underfeeding—or overfeeding. One disadvantage of disposable napkins is that they absorb a lot of the fluid of a fluid stool and so may give a false impression that all is normal.

CORD CARE

The cord is observed at every napkin change until it has separated and the umbilicus has healed. It is kept clean and dry by the use of a spirit solution at least twice daily every 4 hours and more frequently if the cord is moist or sticky. To clean the cord effectively, it must be held away from the skin with one hand while cleaning its base with a swabstick dipped in spirit, with the other hand (Fig. 16.11). Nervous mothers can be reluctant to touch the unattractive cord stump so the importance of correctly cleaning the base of the cord must be emphasised, and the technique demonstrated.

The cord is observed for bleeding at all times. If there is no evidence of bleeding and if the cord stump is dry, the clamp is removed on the 3rd day. The cord separates by a process of dry necrosis on the 6th–8th day. The umbilicus is observed and spirit is applied until it is fully healed. If umbilical care is still necessary by the time the baby goes home, the mother should be advised to continue the spirit applications with a small twist of cotton wool. Swab sticks can sometimes be damaging to an imperfectly-healed umbilicus.

Any redness of the umbilicus should be reported immediately, because the umbilical vein goes straight to the liver. Severe umbilical infection (omphalitis) is potentially fatal; the earliest signs should never be ignored. A swab is taken for culture and sensitivity testing, and local applications of an antibiotic (e.g. Neotracin spray) are started as soon as possible, quite often with systemic antibiotics as well.

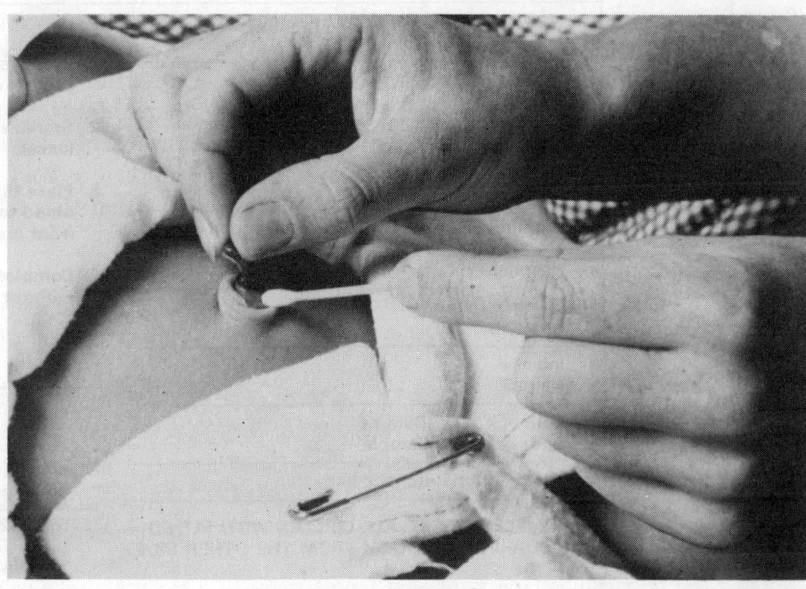

Figure 16.11 The correct method of cleaning the umbilicus, with the cord stump held and lifted away from its base.

PHENYLKETONURIA SCREENING

The Guthrie test is done on the 5th day to test for the presence of high blood levels of phenylalanine. It is a routine screening test for phenylketonuria (PKU), a disorder of protein metabolism. If PKU is not diagnosed in the neonatal period, it can lead to mental retardation. PKU is discovered in 1 in 10 000 babies.

The Guthrie test consists of obtaining sufficient blood from a heel prick (Fig. 16.12) to fill the three circles printed upon the specially impregnated paper (Fig. 16.13). As it is quite a lot of blood to obtain from a heel prick, the procedure needs to be done carefully, warming and massaging the foot before pricking sharply. The heel should not be squeezed to hasten blood flow, because squeezing spreads bleeding into the tissues. The test may need to be delayed if the baby was late to start on milk feedings or if he has had antibiotics.

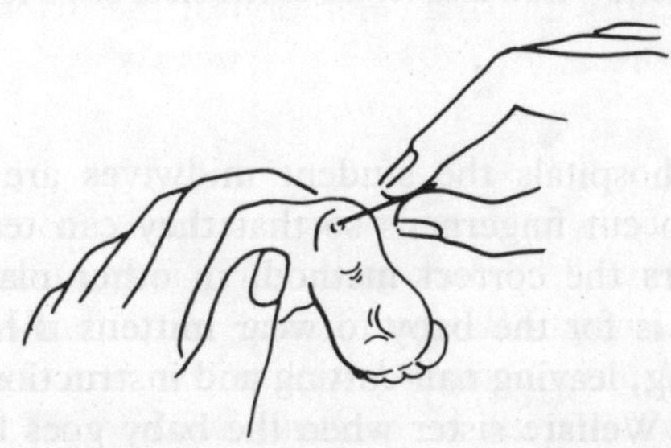

Figure 16.12 Pricking the baby's heel to obtain blood for testing.

Other screening tests

The blood sample taken for PKU screening may also be used to screen for thyroid deficiency, galactosaemia and cystic fibrosis, all rare disorders in which early detection and treatment is vital.

FINGERNAILS

Care of the baby's fingernails can be a problem because teachings and practices vary widely. In

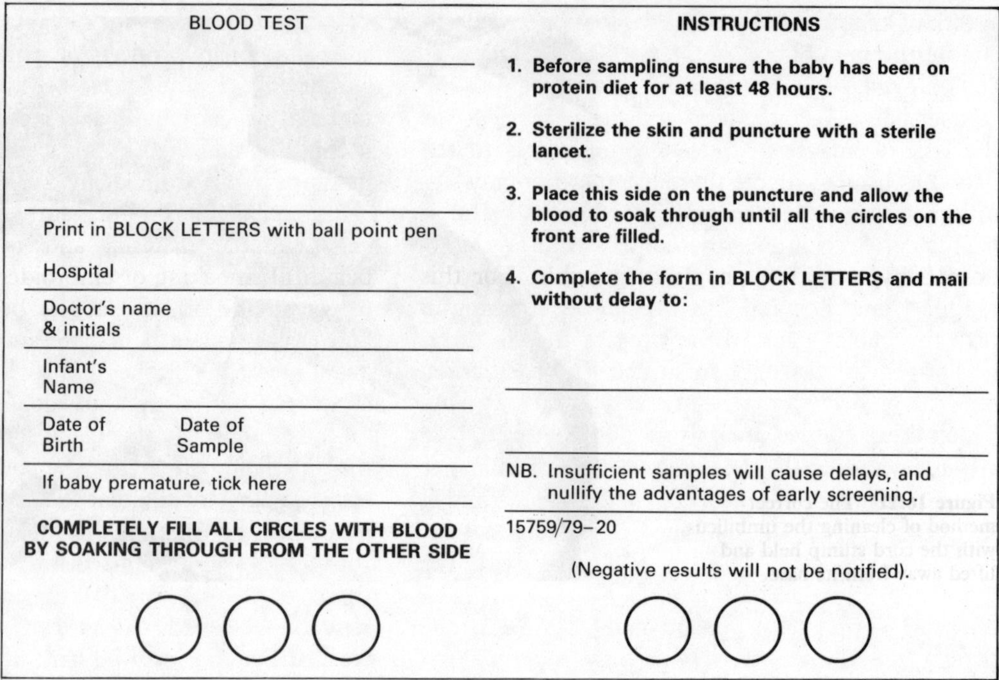

BLOOD TEST

Print in BLOCK LETTERS with ball point pen

Hospital

Doctor's name & initials

Infant's Name

Date of Birth | Date of Sample

If baby premature, tick here

COMPLETELY FILL ALL CIRCLES WITH BLOOD BY SOAKING THROUGH FROM THE OTHER SIDE

INSTRUCTIONS

1. **Before sampling ensure the baby has been on protein diet for at least 48 hours.**
2. **Sterilize the skin and puncture with a sterile lancet.**
3. **Place this side on the puncture and allow the blood to soak through until all the circles on the front are filled.**
4. **Complete the form in BLOCK LETTERS and mail without delay to:**

NB. Insufficient samples will cause delays, and nullify the advantages of early screening.

15759/79–20

(Negative results will not be notified).

Figure 16.13 Card used for the collection of blood for phenylketonuria (PKU) screening.

some hospitals the student midwives are taught how to cut fingernails so that they can teach the mothers the correct method; in other places the policy is for the baby to wear mittens if his nails are long, leaving nail-cutting and instruction to the Infant Welfare sister when the baby goes home.

Fingernails are often long in a newborn baby, especially if the baby is post-mature. They can cause nasty scratches on the baby's face and these scratches can become infected. They can also tear, because although they are long, they are very soft. If they tear they can expose the sensitive underlying tissue to infection.

If mittens are the only solution to the problem, they will need to be worn until the baby goes home. The mittens are likely to become wet through being sucked so they should be changed frequently or they could encourage the growth of microorganisms such as those responsible for paronychia.

Careful nail-cutting is probably the best management of long fingernails in the new baby. The procedure should be demonstrated to the mother, holding the baby's hand firmly, using suitable scissors and working in a good light. If the mother does not know the correct method of cutting a baby's nails she could injure his fingers.

VISITORS

Family and friends of the new parents are usually very eager to meet the baby. The attitudes to visitors in maternity hospitals have changed dramatically over the last 10 years; not so many years ago the father saw his child only through a glass window and did not have an opportunity to hold him until the day they went home. Now the father has free contact with the baby during the hospital period; he is, in fact, able to hold him very soon after birth. In many hospitals a special time is set aside every evening when other visitors are discouraged. Grandparents and brothers and sisters of the new baby are also now often able to cuddle the new baby.

The primary reason for formerly restricting the contact between 'outsiders' and the new baby was the risk of infection. Since greater access to the baby has been available there has not been any significant rise in the neonatal infection rate. But it is still better to limit close contact with any newborn baby to as few people as possible. For this reason some hospitals that practise rooming-in take the babies back to the nursery for the duration of general visiting hours. The visitors can then see the baby, propped-up and with the top bedclothing folded part-way down, through a viewing window. If the mother requests that her visitors all go to the nursery at the same time it saves the baby being disturbed repeatedly.

Where the baby stays in the room with the mother during visiting hours the visitors might be tempted to pick him up and hand him from one person to another. Rarely is any handwashing remembered. The mother often feels quite defenceless and unable to stop this once it starts, and so it is a small but important task for the nursing staff to do rounds at this time—to 'pop in' and ask the mother some innocent question and thus perhaps prevent or stop unnecessary disturbing and handling of the baby. Most visitors would be appalled to think that they could endanger the baby in any way and most respond to a polite request to allow the baby to stay asleep or to let him settle.

CLOTHES

In some hospitals the baby's clothing and napkins are provided and laundered by the hospital linen service; the garments are suitably designed and their cleanliness can be assured because of the rigid rulings that apply to hospital laundry services.

Where the mother provides and launders the baby's garments herself there may be a few problems of which both she and the staff should be aware.

Baby clothing is not always purchased for its suitability or its property of withstanding vigorous laundering. It can often be made of unsuitable material which may be uncomfortable to the baby, it could be damaged by high temperatures or have its appearance ruined by soaking in sterilising solutions. On the other hand, it can be made of very suitable material and be decorated with beautiful smocking or embroidery, yet be difficult to get on and off the baby or be tight at the neck and wrists and so be dangerous.

All new baby clothes and rugs should have been laundered before they are put on the baby. The mother should have been advised about this during the antenatal period, but she could easily forget or else be reluctant to spoil the 'new' look of a baby garment by washing it. Baby clothes probably pass through a lot of hands during manufacture, and there may be no way of knowing what organisms may be on them. As well, the dressing in unwashed material may be hard and irritating to the baby's skin. While admiring and handling the baby's clothing, it is important to look for and tactfully point out any potential problems, such as sleeve elastic that is too tight, a singlet that has not been washed.

If the mother is responsible for her baby's laundry she is best advised to send it home with somebody who can launder it correctly or to use one of the personal linen services that are available (usually only in private hospitals). It is generally unsatisfactory to hand-launder soiled baby clothes in a hospital washbasin. Inability to tolerate water hot enough to kill faecal organisms and the probability of inefficient rinsing of the garments are only two of the associated problems.

Napkins and cot-sheets are taken care of by the hospital. Where disposable napkins are used, the mother may be asked to supply a certain number of these herself. While they have the advantage of reducing the laundry load, and being new and therefore unhandled by people until they are used, the mother should be introduced to cloth napkins and helped to fold and secure them before she goes home. Disposable napkins are very convenient but they are rather expensive, and they are usually plastic backed or secured which some people may not like, including some babies.

MINOR PROBLEMS

Apart from the minor infections already discussed, a newborn baby is prone to minor problems which need special attention.

THRUSH (MONILIASIS)

Thrush is a condition caused by the overgrowth of the fungal organism *Candida albicans*, which is commonly present in the mother's vagina and which may especially flourish during pregnancy. The newborn can encounter *Candida albicans* during his passage through the birth canal or he can be infected through contact with contaminated articles such as teats and 'dummies'.

Thrush causes a sore mouth with white patches on the tongue which cannot be removed by gentle wiping (Fig. 16.14), and, sometimes, sore buttocks. The baby may be disinclined to suck because of the soreness. If the baby is bottle fed, a softer teat should be chosen and kept for his sole use. It should be soaked between feeds in a special individual teat container and the words 'own teat and dummy' be placed in a prominent place at the head of the baby's cot.

Thrush is treated by giving oral nystatin suspension 100 000 units (1 ml) four times daily for 10 days. It is given after a feed so that it can work locally as well as in the gut. Gentian violet solution 0.25% clears the condition in 3 days if used three times daily, three drops each time. It is instilled into the mouth with great care as it can be very messy.

The sore buttocks associated with thrush display typical raised red patches around the perianal area. It can occur without evidence of oral thrush. Nystatin ointment used for 1 week or one application of gentian violet, 1% in spirit, should clear the condition. Exposure of the buttocks (see below) is a good aid in hastening healing. If an electric lamp is used to help heal the buttocks, the ointment or paint is not applied until after exposure to the light.

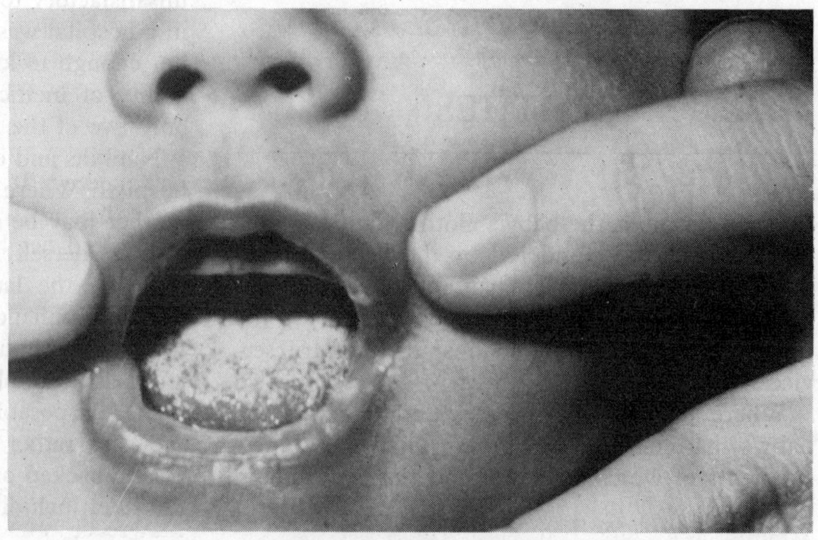

Figure 16.14 Oral thrush.

SORE BUTTOCKS

Sore buttocks are most often caused by:

- inadequate cleansing following the removal of wet or soiled napkins
- not changing napkins frequently enough; they should be changed before and after each feed and should be checked at any other time that the baby wakes
- unsatisfactory methods of laundering; using strong washing powders or not rinsing thoroughly, rarely a problem in hospitals
- irritation from feedings containing too much sugar, or from over-feeding.
- sensitivity to a particular brand of disposable napkin, or to the plastic covering of disposable napkins.

Management

The buttocks are examined closely to distinguish the type of soreness or rash. The cause (e.g. thrush) is ascertained before treatment is begun. General care of sore buttocks includes:

- frequent napkin changing
- thorough cleansing at each change
- using correctly laundered toweling or flannelette napkins in preference to plastic-coated disposable ones
- avoiding the use of plastic pants
- adjustment of feedings if necessary
- application of waterproofing agents to protect the skin e.g. silicone cream or Vaseline
- exposure of buttocks to light and air (see below)
- application of healing creams or lotions, e.g zinc and castor oil, Ungvita, prescribed lotions
- treatment of thrush by oral and local nystatin or gentian violet.

Exposure of the buttocks

The baby's buttocks will heal more quickly if they are not continuously covered by clothing. Exposure to indirect sunlight is ideal if it is possible; care must be taken to prevent the baby from becoming either chilled or sunburnt.

Electric lamps are commonly used in hospitals. The baby is placed on his side or prone, with his hips elevated by a supporting towel placed underneath. The bedclothing is arranged to expose the buttocks while maintaining the baby's temperature. The genitalia and anus are covered.

The electric light is then positioned carefully so that it has no chance of falling down into the cot. If an angle-poise lamp is used, some form of locking device should be fitted to the angles. It is worthwhile having another staff member check the security and placement of the light.

The lamp is positioned at the side of the cot, no closer than 135 cm from the buttocks, with the light shining directly onto the affected area. Total exposure time should not exceed 5 minutes.

NEONATAL BREAST ENGORGEMENT

The breasts of both male and female infants are target tissues for the placental hormones and may respond to withdrawal of those hormones in a manner similar to that of the mother (see p. 180).

The breasts may swell on about the 3rd day and may, occasionally, secrete a milk-like fluid called 'witch's milk' (Fig. 16.6). The swollen breasts are usually quite tender, and care should be taken to wash the chest area carefully so that it does not hurt the baby. Any secretion should be washed away very gently and dried carefully. The breasts should *never* be squeezed.

The mother is reassured that the breast swelling will disappear in a few days time unless handled or squeezed. It is important that she understands what has caused the breast engorgement, particularly if her baby is a boy.

SKIN RASHES

The skin of the newborn baby is very sensitive and may react to its recently changed environment and to articles with which it comes into contact, by erupting into a variety of rashes.

- *Heat rash*, in which overheating can cause generalised fine spotting, particularly in large babies, is managed by temperature control and usually fades within 24 hours.
- *Allergic rash* is due to sensitivity to chemicals present in laundry products, medications or skin applications. Many babies cannot tolerate wool next to their skin. Identification and withdrawal of the cause of the allergy is important. Simpler causes are eliminated first.
- *Cheek burn*, a red sore-looking area on one or both cheeks, may result if the baby has regurgitated mucus or milk from his stomach while lying in his cot. Babies should always be checked between feedings to make sure that regurgitation has not occurred. The checks may be smeared with a soothing ointment to aid healing and lessen the discomfort.

COMMON BIRTH MARKS

Small multiple naevi (red birth marks) occur frequently, particularly on the upper eyelids and on the nape of the neck. Often referred to as 'stork marks', they are not raised above the level of the skin, and they begin to fade after the first few weeks. They have usually disappeared by the time the baby is 12 months old.

Strawberry naevi

These may not appear prominently until a week or more after birth. They are usually bright red and elevated. They eventually regress and disappear completely but this may take 3 or 4 years. Depending upon the size and situation of the mark, problems may arise in the response of the parents to this obvious imperfection in their baby.

Port-wine naevi

These birth marks are purple or dark red, and occur mainly on the face and neck. There is no treatment available, and once again there may be psychological problems for the parents, and later for the child. The relatively recent discovery of an excellent make-up has already helped several people with port-wine birth marks to live normal lives.

Mongolian spots

These areas of dark pigmentation are sometimes found in babies of southern European or olive-skinned people. They are not raised, and are seen mainly on the lower back, buttocks and genitals. No treatment is given. Mongolian spots have no connection with the condition of mongolism (Down syndrome).

THE 'UNSETTLED' BABY

Occasionally a normal, healthy, adequately-fed baby, with no obvious skin or other problems, refuses to settle properly or sleep well between feeds. The mother of such a baby usually becomes very worried and upset, her anxiety is sensed by the baby who responds by further crying and so the cycle continues.

The baby can become unsettled by being handled too frequently, too roughly or too nervously. Overfeeding in response to frequent crying usually only makes matters worse. He will often not settle if his napkin is wet or soiled, if he is too hot or too cold, or if he feels insecure. If his stomach is distended with wind he will feel uncomfortable, and if gas is present in the intestines he may have several hours of misery until it has passed through. Some babies appear to have none of these problems yet continue to cry until they tire themselves out.

Management
The following are suggestions for managing the unsettled baby.

- Every effort is made to ensure that the baby is comfortable: napkin clean and dry, temperature correct, clothing suitable and without tight bands, wrapped securely but not tightly in a light rug (which is not touching his cheek), clean dry cot linen.
- Time must be allowed after each feeding for any swallowed wind to be regurgitated before the baby is lain in his cot. He should be supported upright, with the back, chest and head well supported, and the air allowed to rise naturally. Rubbing the back vigorously as some do, probably turns the milk in the stomach into a 'milk shake', with many small bubbles being retained even though the baby may 'burp'. The mother may not have been shown the correct method of bringing-up wind. Medication may be ordered.
- The handling and feeding of the baby may need investigation. The nervous mother should be assisted if necessary while still allowing her to build up her confidence. She may feel slow and incompetent beside midwives who seen to manage her baby much better than she does. Breast feeding should be observed, but not as though the she is 'on trial'. The baby *may* benefit from being test-weighed (p. 185) over 24 hours. If he is getting the milk too quickly, the mother may need to posture-feed. The bottle-fed baby may benefit by the use of a different type of teat or by adjustment to the strength or type of milk used.
- The baby may simply be lonely or unhappy. Extra cuddling or patting his back as he lies in his cot may help him to relax and so go to sleep. There may be a fine line between extra cuddling and overhandling.
- Quietness, and lowering of the lights may prove useful.
- If the mother does not mind, a dummy or pacifier may comfort the baby sufficiently to allow him to settle. It should probably be a last resort.

CIRCUMCISION

Circumcision is the removal of the prepuce or foreskin of the penis. It is becoming a less frequent practice these days except for religious reasons. They policy of most public hospitals, and of the majority of paediatricians, is *not* to perform the procedure unless there are clear medical indications. These are unlikely to be identified in the neonatal period.

The prepuce of the penis is tightly adherent to the glans, and it cannot be retracted until the child is 3–4 years of age without causing pain and bleeding which leads to scarring.

When a newborn baby is circumcised, it is not usually done before the 8th day, and then only if the baby is healthy, mature, and not jaundiced. The dangers of haemorrhage and infection are kept in mind when caring for the baby after the procedure.

A dressing of ribbon gauze is wound around the circumcision wound, and Friar's Balsam (tinc benz co) is applied to make the dressing adherent and antiseptic. A card may be placed at the head of the cot for the first day, to remind the staff to check frequently for oozing of blood.

The dressing is not usually removed until 3 or 4 days after the procedure; most likely the mother and baby will have been discharged from hospital by then. She is given special instructions for caring for the circumcised penis, and advised how to soak the dressing at the baby's bath time before gently removing it.

MILD (PHYSIOLOGICAL) JAUNDICE

Jaundice is defined as yellow discoloration of the skin due to the staining of the tissues by bilirubin. Approximately 25% of normal babies become mildly jaundiced.

Physiological jaundice is caused by the breakdown of excess haemoglobin which is no longer necessary after birth. The fetus in utero has a high haemoglobin concentration—16 g/100 ml—to compensate for the mingling of oxygenated and deoxygenated blood within the fetal circulation. In addition, the new baby has a red blood cell life of only 80 days as compared with 120 days in the adult so there is further red cell breakdown. The baby's liver is slow to function at first, and its enzyme *glucoronyl transferase*, is not produced until 3–4 days after birth. This enzyme converts unconjugated bilirubin into the conjugated form which is water-soluble and therefore excretable. Unconjugated bilirubin from the haemoglobin breakdown tends to accumulate, and any that cannot attach to albumin in the bloodstream will leak into the tissues (Fig. 16.15).

Satisfactory liver function depends upon satisfactory supplies of oxygen, glucose and many cell substances. Where there have been any problems or deprivations (as is likely in the pre-term baby) jaundice will be more severe.

The normal newborn baby is unlikely to be any more than mildly jaundiced, but even this should be closely observed for its deepening. The baby's activity is watched, if he is sleepy or disinclined to suck he may need extra fluids and more frequent feedings.

Treatment is usually not given for mild physiological jaundice where there is no anaemia. If it progresses and the serum bilirubin levels rise, phototherapy would be commenced.

Other causes of jaundice

Jaundice due to Rhesus factor and ABO incompatibility is discussed on page 100. Breast milk jaundice occasionally occurs, and is believed to be due to impaired liver function. Its incidence is higher in women who have been taking oral contraceptives before conception occurred.

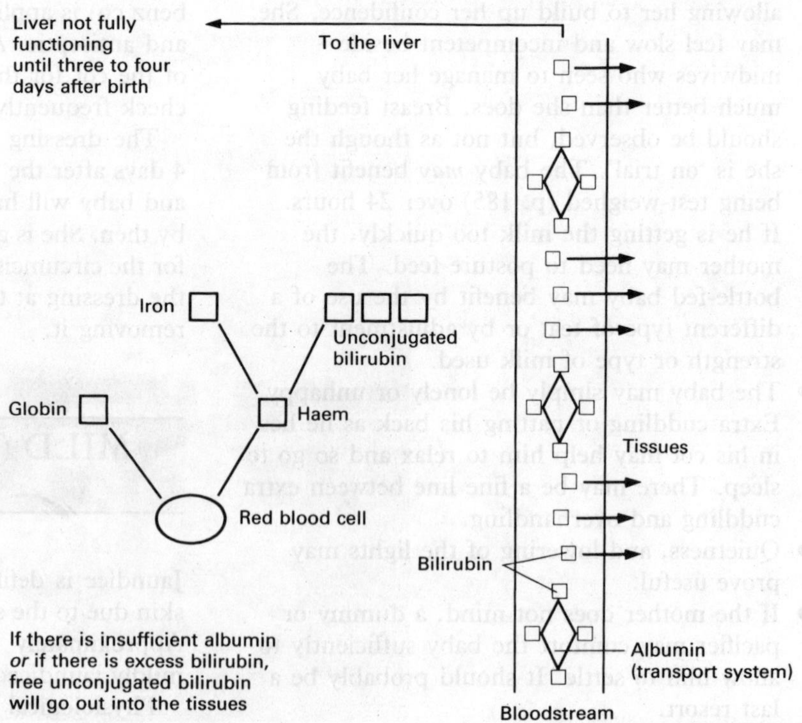

Figure 16.15 **Diagrammatic representation of the cause of physiological jaundice in the newborn.**

PHOTOTHERAPY

Excess unconjugated bilirubin can be converted to water-soluble forms through the process of photo-oxidation if the skin is exposed to white and ultraviolet light. Fluorescent tubes are usually used, and the baby is ideally nursed in an isolette (Fig. 16.16).

Phototherapy is a non-invasive method of treatment and is usually successful in most cases of non-haemolytic jaundice. It has limited results in Rh- and ABO-incompatibility, but it can sometimes bring the serum bilirubin levels low enough to avoid the necessity for an exchange transfusion.

Careful observation and extra care are necessary during the course of phototherapy. The nursing responsibilities involved are as follows (details may vary from one hospital to another).

- Total exposure must not exceed 48 hours.
- Lights are fixed securely 50 cm above the baby.
- The baby's eyes must be protected from the lights at all times. A suitable close-fitting blindfold is secured with Velcro fastening or with light tape.
- Napkins are not worn; a folded napkin is placed under the baby's buttocks.
- The baby is taken out of the isolette to be breast fed if at all possible. The time out should be noted on the chart.
- Feeds should be given approximately 3 hourly, and extra fluids might be offered.
- The baby's skin is washed with water every 6 hours and after the passage of any urine or bowel action.
- Urine and bowel actions are observed and accurately reported. Green loose stools are a typical consequence of phototherapy.
- Every hour the following procedures are carried out:

  security of the blindfold is checked
  the baby is turned a quarter-turn:
  prone—left side—supine—right
  the baby's temperature is recorded
  the cot temperature is recorded (and adjusted if necessary)
  the baby's skin is examined.

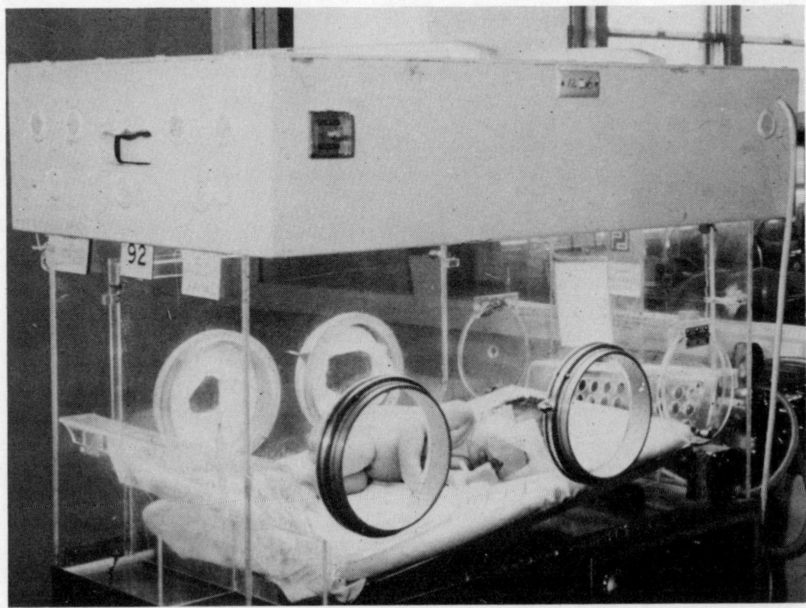

Figure 16.16 Phototherapy.

17

FEEDING THE NORMAL NEWBORN BABY

Chapter outline

Key words

demand-feeding
hind-milk
let-down reflex

Feeding a newborn baby involves far more than giving him food. His needs are for warmth, comfort and security as well as for nutrition. Breast feeding meets these needs most easily and effectively. That is not to say that the artificially-fed baby is necessarily deprived in any way; skilled and loving mothering can be given no matter how the baby is fed. Nor does it mean that breast feeding is without restrictions or problems. But, as it is natural, and as the mother's body has been specifically designed and prepared for it, it is without doubt the best way to feed the normal newborn infant.

In less technologically complex societies mothers instinctively, and without fuss, lift their babies to the breast as soon as they are born. The umbilical cord is exactly the right length for this to be done easily. The stimulation of suckling causes the uterus to contract, and so the placenta separates and is delivered. Such is the design of nature. Those in such societies are fortunate in this respect because they can continue their breast feeding as nature tells them; the babies are fed when they cry, there are no clocks, no critics, no nipple problems, no breast engorgement difficulties.

We, however, live in a complicated society, with a very different lifestyle. which is unnatural in many ways, and artificial things are taken for granted. Our lifestyle does, of course, have its advantages and those from other societies who would aspire to the ways of the wealthy westerners with all their material goods, have begun to imitate them in the practice of bottle feeding. In Papua, for example, the problems of infant sickness and mortality became so great that a law was passed to the effect that teats for feeding bottles were to be issued upon doctors's prescription only.

BREAST FEEDING

Breast feeding has many advantages, both to the mother and to the baby. The milk is suited to the baby's digestive capacity, he absorbs it well, is never constipated and is content. It is free from germs; in fact it contains antibodies and the breasts-fed baby generally has fewer illnesses and allergies than does the artificially-fed baby. And he has to be cuddled to be fed.

To the mother, as well as the physical benefit of aiding involution of the uterus (p. 201) it has many extra benefits. It is emotionally satisfying, giving her a feeling of accomplishment. It is relaxing, convenient, involving very little effort once it has been established, and is both time-saving and money-saving. As well, the incidence of breast cancer is lower in women who have breastfed.

ADVICE TO THE MOTHER

The mother-to-be would have been given many opportunities during the antenatal period in which to discuss her feelings about breast feeding. As stated on page 86, the woman may have feelings of distaste about feeding the baby herself, or she may have to cope with opposition to the idea from people who are close to her. The antenatal clinic midwife or breast consultant can help her to find ways to overcome these feedings or objections as well as giving her advice on breast and nipple care in preparation for breast feeding.

Some women are unwilling to consider breast feeding and have no intention of trying. In such a case, breast feeding is encouraged and the advantages pointed out, but the woman is never pressured. Making a woman attempt to breast feed against her will could cause her to become antagonistic towards the staff and possibly towards her baby.

PHYSIOLOGY OF LACTATION

Breast feeding depends upon four processes:

- the development of milk-producing tissues in the breasts
- the initiation of milk production after delivery
- the maintenance of milk production
- milk ejection (the 'let-down' or draught reflex).

These processes are controlled by the interaction of hormones, as described below.

Development of milk-producing tissues
This is achieved in pregnancy with the stimulation of the glandular tissues and ducts by the hormones produced by the placenta—oestrogen, progesterone and placental lactogenic hormone. Figure 17.1 shows the structure of the breast in cross-section.

Initiation of milk production after delivery
Following the delivery of the placenta, there is a rapid drop in that organ's hormones. The anterior pituitary hormone, *prolactin*, which has been in-

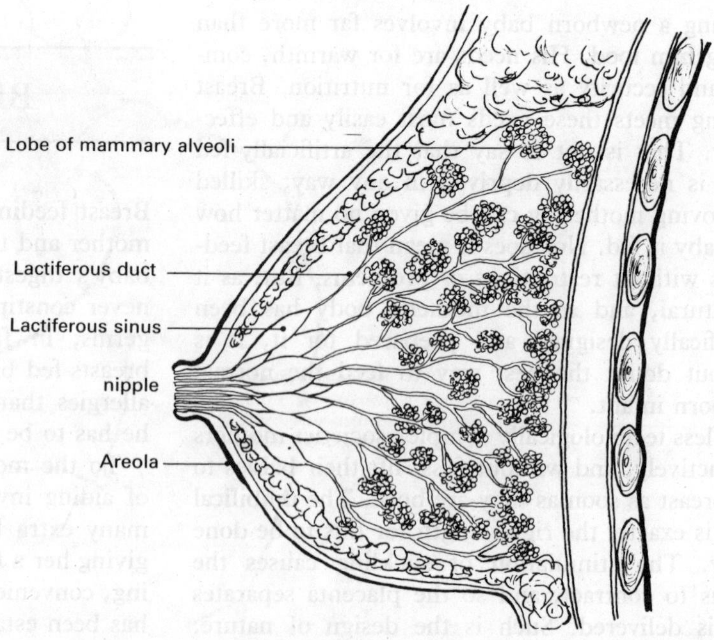

Figure 17.1 The structure of the breast — cross-section.

hibited by the high circulating levels of oestrogen and progesterone, is now released. Prolactin activates the mammary cells to produce milk. Within 3–4 days of the baby's birth, milk production has begun, and mature milk is secreted by the end of the first week.

Maintenance of milk production and the 'let-down' reflex of milk ejection

These processes depend upon another hormone, *oxytocin*, released from the posterior pituitary gland in response to suckling (Fig. 17.2). Oxytocin influences the myo-epithelial cells surrounding the alveoli to contract, forcing out milk which has already been secreted. The let-down reflex is not caused by the negative pressure from sucking, nor by over-full breasts, but by a neurogenic reflex which stimulates oxytocin release.

A nursing mother experiences the let-down reflex about 30–60 seconds after the baby starts to feed. The let-down reflex can also be caused by purely mental factors, such as hearing the baby cry, thinking about the baby, or even just thinking about feeding. Conversely, the reflex can be inhibited by anxiety, fear, insecurity or tension. These factors are thought to increase levels of epinephrine and norepinephrine which, in turn, block the transport of oxytocin to the breast. Once milk production is established, its maintenance is dependent upon the alveolar sacs being emptied regularly.

ESTABLISHMENT OF BREAST FEEDING

The best way to establish breast feeding is for there to be as little fuss and as few problems as

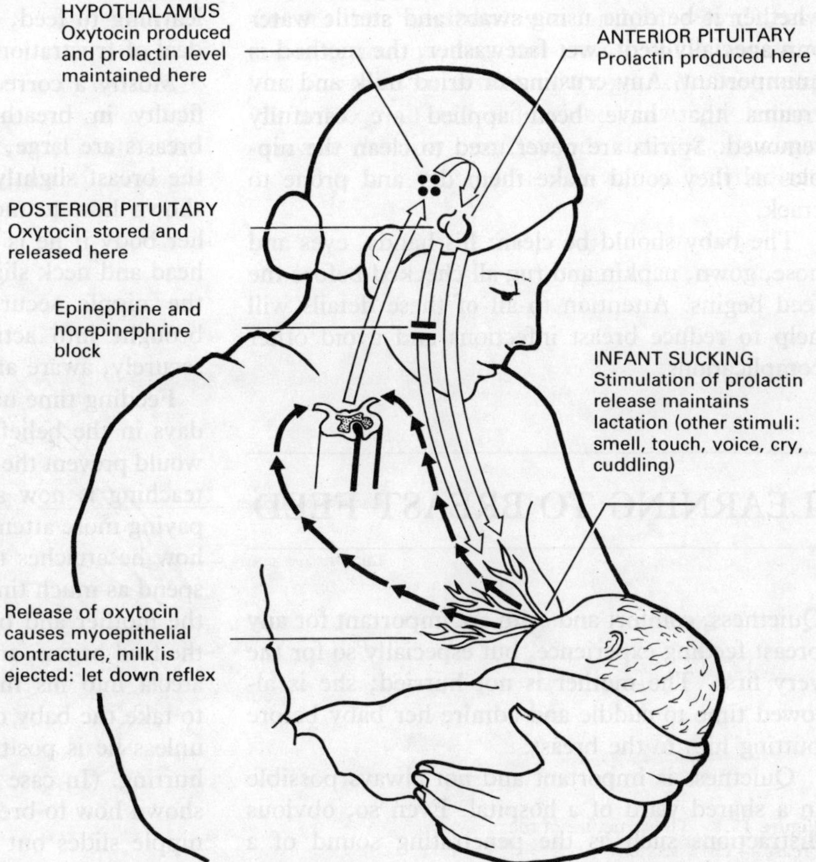

Figure 17.2 Physiology of lactation.

possible. Normal personal hygiene and comfort are important; cleanliness of the hands and fingernails of the mother and of anyone who attends her must be emphasised. Nipples should not be touched with unwashed hands and handkerchiefs should not be warn inside the bras to stop leaking; disposable pads are available for this and can be worn for the relatively short time that leaking is a problem. The mother should wear nightgowns that do not hinder easy feeding; if they have to be pulled up from below they can be uncomfortable—there may also be lochia on the hem. A clean, supporting maternity bra should be worn day and night for comfort and prevention of stasis of milk in the dependent areas of the breast. If the woman does not have a suitable bra, a binder can be fashioned to serve the purpose. The bra is undone in front and the straps let down before each feed. The straps are readjusted after the feed has been completed.

Nipple cleansing procedures differ from one place to another, but as long as the nipple is clean, whether it be done using swabs and sterile water or a specially-kept, wet facewasher, the method is unimportant. Any crusting or dried milk and any creams that have been applied are carefully removed. Spirits are never used to clean the nipples as they could make them dry and prone to crack.

The baby should be clean; his hands, eyes and nose, gown, napkin and rug all checked before the feed begins. Attention to all of these details will help to reduce breast infections and avoid other complications.

LEARNING TO BREAST FEED

Quietness, comfort and calm are important for any breast feeding experience, but especially so for the very first. The mother is not hurried; she is allowed time to cuddle and admire her baby before putting him to the breast.

Quietness is important and not always possible in a shared ward of a hospital. Even so, obvious distractions such as the penetrating sound of a television set or a radio can be eliminated. The woman should sit or lie in whatever position is most comfortable to her. An episiotomy suture line or the would following a caesarean may make sitting up very difficult. As well, the mother who is not used to exposure of her body may feel uncomfortable unless her privacy is assured.

The baby is handed to the mother when she is comfortable, and after she has had time to get used to holding him, she will put him to the breast. The midwife may help her to express a few drops of colostrum before this; it will clear the nipple duct and give the baby something to taste. At this stage it is very important to make sure that the baby is positioned correctly. He should be facing the breast and held so that he has neither to stretch upwards nor tuck in his chin in order to reach the nipple. With the baby's face directly in front of the nipple, and his mouth well open and the tongue down, his face is gently brought forward to the nipple and he will attach easily and correctly. In the early days of mother and baby learning to feed, correct positioning saves a great deal of frustration and discomfort.

Mostly a correctly positioned baby has no difficulty in breathing while feeding. Where the breasts are large, the mother may have to elevate the breast slightly so that his nose is free: she is shown how to move him a little lower (or across her body if he is lying horizontally) to extend his head and neck slightly. Once the baby has hold of the nipple securely his sucking reflex will be brought into action; if he is comfortable, held securely, aware and ready, he will feed.

Feeding time used to be limited for the first few days in the belief that restriction of sucking time would prevent the nipples from becoming sore. This teaching is now superceded (in most centres) by paying more attention to the *way* a baby sucks and how he attaches to the nipples. The midwife will spend as much time as necessary to make sure that the mother and baby are both comfortable before the feed begins, and that the baby takes most of the areola into his mouth. There should be no need to take the baby off the breast while he is sucking unless he is positioned wrongly and the nipple is hurting. (In case this does happen, the mother is shown how to break the vacuum gently so that the nipple slides out of the baby's mouth easily and causes it no damage.) Not only is feeding time no longer limited, but the baby is now allowed to feed on one breast until he stops by himself so that he will obtain the maximum amount of nutrient-rich *hind-milk* (see p. 11). He is then offered the second breast until he requires no more, and the second breast is offered first when he next feeds.

Bringing up the baby's 'wind'

There are several schools of thought about the ways, and even the necessity, of bringing up wind or burping the baby. It is still the practice in most maternity units to encourage the mothers to de-wind their babies between feeding on one breast and the other, and again at the end of the feed.

Working on the theory that air rises, it would seem most logical to assume that if any air has been swallowed, the best way to help to bring that air up is to support the baby in a fairly upright position so that it *can* rise. He can be supported with both hands, one spread over his chest with the index finger and thumb supporting his chin, and the other spread over his back with the index finger and thumb supporting the back of his head.

If he is warm and sleepy, as he could be after a satisfying feed, he could perhaps be unwrapped from his rugs and allowed to stretch his limbs. Some midwives and some mothers like to rub the baby's back; this is useful at times, but often not necessary. If it is done it should be done gently. If done vigorously, any air bubble in the stomach is likely to be broken into hundreds of little bubbles. Even if the baby does bring up some wind, it is likely that a lot of the bubbles will remain.

Sitting the baby upright, without rubbing his back, is usually effective in bringing up wind. It may seem to take longer, but this is probably because nothing is being done to fill in the time. It is a lovely time in which to just look at the baby; his little face seems to 'work' as his body organises itself to bring up the wind. If sitting the baby upright still does not seem to produce results, he can be gently tilted backwards for about 5 seconds and then sat up again. This may help to move the bubble of air if there is one. Some babies, especially if they have not had to cry for long before being fed, simply do not swallow any wind.

When a baby does bring up wind, it seems to happen in two stages. First air comes up, often accompanied by an audible 'burp'. The second part of the process is a visible relaxation of the baby; he simply 'flops'. A little milk may spill from his mouth with the wind.

After the baby has finished his feed and the wind has been brought up, he is checked to make sure that he is clean and dry so that he will settle comfortably to sleep. Any milk that has spilt from his mouth is washed off. If this is not done he could get sore areas on his cheek and chin. When he is returned to his cot he should be laid on his right side to ensure that he is not in any danger of inhaling regurgitated milk. In some centres the head of the cot is elevated for a short time after each feed.

FEEDING REGIMES

Demand feeding

The baby who is fed 'on demand', is fed when he is hungry. Because he does not have to wait to be fed, he is less likely to cry for long periods. Therefore, he is likely to suck well because he is not tired out. Nor is the baby expected to feed when he is not ready or not hungry. The baby usually settles into his own routine after a week or two, and the mother's milk supply adjusts well. In a hospital situation, demand feeding is of advantage to both mothers and midwives because the midwives are more freely available to assist and advise during the feeds when all the mothers are not feeding at the same time. Also, demand feeding mothers appear to have fewer problems with breast engorgement.

Demand feeding is suitable for most, but not all, new mothers. The anxious or unconfident mother may need the security of greater routine for her baby's feeding times. It may also be unsuitable for those babies who are smaller than average, or where there are any medical indications for special care and observation.

Feeding 'by the clock'

Regular 'by the clock' feeding schedules are rarely followed in maternity hospitals now, for normal full-term babies. Under this regime, the babies are usually fed every 4th hour, with the feeds during the day coinciding with that period just after the mother's meal times. This regime is certainly most convenient where the baby is receiving nursery-based care, and it does allow the mother to plan her day. This, however, should not be the major factor in a maternity hospital, where the mother has few urgent responsibilities.

The disadvantage of regular feeding times is that a baby tends to feed differently at different times of the day. He may not always need a feed four hours after the last one, or he may need to be fed earlier than his due time. He may, therefore, have to be woken to feed before he is ready, or have to wait until the right time, when he would probably be tired from crying.

EXPRESSING BREAST MILK

The breasts are expressed for comfort when they are overfull, to rest sore nipples and, when necessary, to stimulate milk production.

Manual breast expression

Manual breast expression can be performed by either the mother or the midwife. It can be tiring and awkward for the mother to have to completely empty her breast by hand expression on her own. She will appreciate assistance if she has to express by hand over an extended period.

The woman should be sitting in a comfortable position. Her hands and those of anyone attending her should be washed before expressing starts. After cleaning her nipples, she begins by massaging her breasts, working right around them, pressing with the flats of her fingers firmly but gently towards the nipple. The areola is then grasped between the thumb and forefinger, squeezing it to compress the underlying lactiferous (milk) sinuses. The expressed milk is collected in a sterile bowl which is held just below the nipple.

Expressing with a breast pump

A hand or an electric breast pump can be used to make expressing a lot easier and quicker. The pump must be positioned absolutely correctly, i.e. centrally. Breast pumps are never used when the nipples are sore or cracked, because they can exert quite considerable suction. The woman using an electric pump should be alert while it is in use; if the pump should slip and she is distracted (e.g. by reading a book) she could suffer from areolar blistering in a very short time.

The type of hand-operated breast pump which converts into a feeding bottle is now in common use. Because the milk does not have to be transferred from an expression bowl into a bottle, there is less risk of contamination. As its suction can be

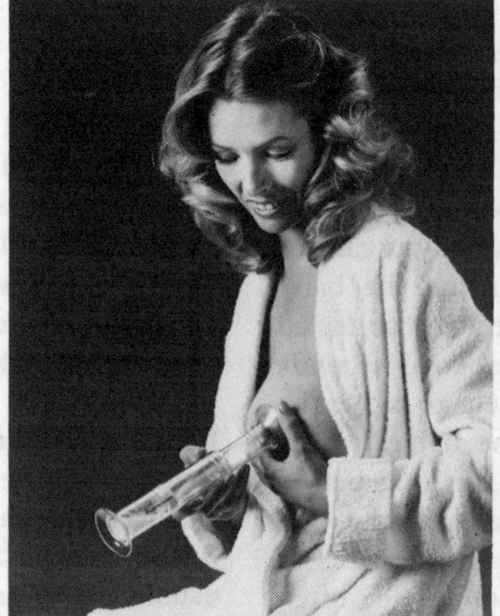

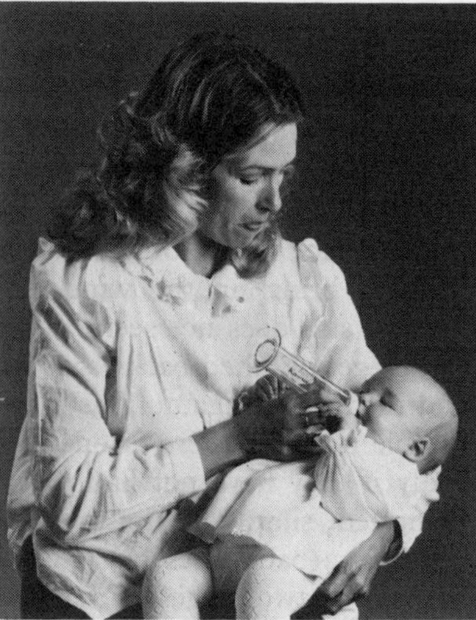

Figure 17.3 Using the Kaneson expressing and feeding bottle (Source: Stylesetter International, 9 Rangers Road, Neutral Bay, NSW).

easily controlled, it is more acceptable to mothers who have sensitive nipples. It is particularly useful after the mother and baby go home from hospital for expressing surplus milk to freeze for later use.

COMPLEMENTARY FEEDS

A complementary feed is a bottle feed given after a presumedly inadequate breast feeding. The practice of giving a bottle of artificial formula to the baby routinely in the first few days because there 'won't be enough milk yet' is now, fortunately, uncommon. In most maternity hospitals water only (or occasionally glucose 5%) is given between breast feedings, and then only to allow the mother to sleep.

Complementary feedings can undermine a mother's confidence in her ability to breast feed. They can also diminish the baby's natural appetite, and cause him to feed less well the next time. As milk is produced on a supply and demand basis, these feedings can seriously affect the establishment and maintenance of lactation.

TEST-WEIGHING

Test-weighing is a procedure carried out in some maternity hospitals as a guide to the amount of milk being taken by the baby from his breast feeds. It is used to be done in many centres on a routine basis but is now uncommon unless there is a specific indication. The procedure is usually carried out as described below.

The baby is prepared for a feed—his napkin is changed and he is wrapped in a clean rug. He is then placed on the scales and his weight is recorded. He is then taken to his mother and is breast fed. After the feed, he is weighed again on the same scales, before having his napkin changed or his rug removed. The weight difference in grams between the recordings represents the amount in ml taken at that feed.

The total intake over 24 hours is significant, rather than the amount taken at individual feedings. Precise electronic scales must be used, and even then the caloric content of the milk will not be known.

Test-weighing can make the mother anxious about her milk supply if the subject is not handled carefully. The important thing for her to realise is that she is *not* 'on trial', that there are likely to be considerable variations in the amount of milk that the baby obtains at different times of the day, and that it is the 24 hour *total* that is important. The entire midwifery staff (*and* student nurses) should adhere to the hospital policy in relation to telling the mother the results of each test-weigh. The most reasonable policy would seem to be that of informing mothers of the results only at the end of the 24 hour period. If *some* mothers are told the results of individual feedings, others will also want to know how they 'did'. Then there is likely to arise a situation in which amounts are compared with neighbours, some getting upset because they do not compare well, others in dismay because this feeding was 10 ml less than the last time. This can mean that the woman starts to worry that her milk supply is failing.

Test-weighing is really only indicated when a baby is continually unsettled or when there is a failure to gain weight according to the usual pattern.

DIFFICULTIES IN BREAST FEEDING

Difficulties and problems may arise during the establishment of breast feeding. Many of these can be prevented by good antenatal care and education, with specific attention to breast and nipple preparation in positive anticipation of breast feeding the baby when he is born, and by consistent, accurate and non-conflicting advice given in the early days of feeding.

Attitude

Breast feeding is rarely likely to succeed if the

woman is antagonistic to the idea. Some women are defensive in their attitude because they have been preached at rather than encouraged and allowed to explore their feelings about feeding their babies. Others are so anxious to succeed that they worry constantly that they will fail; they cannot relax while feeding and the baby senses this immediately. The milk ejection reflex is inhibited and the baby, already unsure and insecure, becomes frustrated. These mothers are likely to need calm and reassuring help while they are feeding.

General health

Difficulties may arise if the mother is unwell or in pain. Breast feeding does make demands on the mother's body, and those who are already physically compromised may find that they are not able to cope with it. Breast feeding may be contraindicated in women who have active tuberculosis, unstable insulin-dependent diabetes, severe or terminal illness, known drug dependence, and certain psychiatric disorders.

Cracked nipples

Nipples can become sore and cracked, making breast feeding very painful for the mother. Nipples become cracked because:

- the baby does not attach properly but 'chews' on the end of the nipple
- sucking is too vigorous—the baby is too hungry—when he has had to wait too long to be fed
- breast pumps may have been applied carelessly or too much suction has been used.

The nipples are inspected every day under a good light to ensure that they are sound. At the first sign of a crack, or if the woman complains of nipple pain when the baby is sucking, and if repositioning the baby does not bring relief, her nipples maybe rested for 24 hours. Milk can be expressed by hand and fed to the baby in a bottle. The nipples are exposed to a healing lamp, or to sunlight if possible.

Inverted nipples

If inverted or flat nipples have not been recognized during pregnancy, the establishment of breast feeding could be very difficult, especially during the 3rd and 4th days when the distended breasts pull the nipples back and make them even flatter. A breast pump may help to pull the nipple forward before feeds, and a soft rubber or latex nipple shield which fits over the areola can be worn during feeds to help the baby attach. Plastic breast shields (see p. 86) can be worn between feeds.

Breast engorgement

The breasts become full and hard on the 3rd–5th day after delivery. This is due to venous engorgement, as the blood supply to the breasts increases in preparation for lactation to commence. The fullness of the breasts stretches and flattens the nipples, occasionally making attachment difficult for the baby. The mother is reassured that this phase is temporary, lasting only about 24–36 hours and symptomatic relief is given. Warm showers, with gentle stroking, and analgesics when the distended breasts are at their sorest are helpful, as is the application of cold compresses, particularly cabbage leaves. These have been shown to contain an as-yet unidentified substance which acts to reduce engorgement. Cold cabbage leaf compresses should, however, be used for a limited period as their continued application can result in a lowered milk production. They are usually effective quite quickly—within a few hours. If a small amount of milk is expressed before attempting to put the baby to the breast, he may be able to attach more easily and the milk will flow more readily through the cleared nipple ducts.

Infective mastitis

Infective mastitis is now fairly uncommon, affecting about 1% of maternity patients. It rarely arises during the first 2 weeks of lactation. The usual causative organism is *Staphylococcus aureus* which gains entry through cracks in the nipple. The woman becomes sick and feverish, with tenderness and induration over the affected part of the breast. There may be a distinct area of redness.

A sample of milk from the affected side is expressed and sent for culture and sensitivity testing. Antibiotic treatment, usually with methacillin or cloxacillin, is begun while awaiting the results.

The breast are supported with a firm binder or bra. Pain relief is important.

Lactation need not necessarily be suppressed for mastitis. Many doctors allow the baby to feed from the unaffected breast and the mother expresses the milk manually from the affected side. Some doctors recommend continuing to feed from the affected side, reasoning that maintaining the flow of milk reduces the number of organisms.

Inadequate lactation
An inadequate supply of breast milk is frustrating for both the mother and the baby, especially if the mother is very keen to breast feed. Sometimes the milk is slow to come in but this does not mean that breast feeding cannot be established. An established milk supply can, in fact, take up to 2 weeks–sometimes even longer—to achieve.

Failure of the breast alveoli to produce milk is rare. The most common cause for an inadequate milk supply is the failure of the 'let-down' reflex. This reflex can be inhibited by many psychological factors (p. 181), by pain associated with suckling, such as nipple pain and strong uterine contractions, and by insufficient stimulation.

As the supply of breast milk depends upon the demand, the answer to the problem of an inadequate milk supply is for the baby to feed more frequently. This should be accompanied by a lot of reassurance, plenty of real rest and sleep, and a calm and positive approach to prevent the mother from becoming upset and exhausted. Manual expression to stimulate the supply may be advised. This can be effective, but should not take too long or be too tiring. Oxytocin nasal spray is sometimes prescribed to induce the let-down of milk.

Overabundance
The problem of too much milk is less common than that of too little, but it can be very distressing for the mother, who can have painfully full breasts, and for the baby, who might get his feed so quickly that he splutters at the breast, vomits or gets indigestion. The pain of indigestion can make him cry, and unless the fact that he has been overfed is recognised, he may be given even more. He will develop loose stools of a greenish colour.

The overabundant milk supply is managed by lessening the demand. The baby is fed less frequently, for shorter times at each feed—perhaps feeding on only one breast, with minimal expression (for comfort only) of the other. To prevent him from becoming distressed by the speed of the flow, he may be 'posture-fed', with the mother lying down and the baby lying on top of her, sucking uphill. The baby should finish one breast before feeding on the other side.

These measures are usually sufficient for the overabundant milk supply to reduce. Rarely are fluid restriction or diuretics necessary. The mother is reassured that it is usually a temporary problem, and that the associated leaking will not continue for long.

Problems due to the baby
The baby who cannot suck well enough at the breast is another difficulty in the establishment of successful lactation. Sometimes the problems are temporary, such as the baby who has the 'snuffles' and cannot breathe properly unless he lets go of the nipple, the baby with oral thrush, whose mouth is very sore, or the sleepy jaundiced baby. Premature babies usually do not have the strength that is necessary to suck effectively at the breast. Mentally subnormal babies often cannot use their tongues properly, and the baby with a cleft palate cannot form proper suction.

Each baby is assessed individually and support and encouragement is given to the mother. It is important that the baby's fluid needs in particular are satisfied.

THE SUPPRESSION OF LACTATION

Although the establishment of lactation depends mainly upon the stimulation of the breasts by the sucking of the baby, the unstimulated breasts will still undergo the process of physiological engorgement to a certain degree with its associated discomfort, and possibly the secretion of milk, unless measures to prevent these occurring are taken.

When it is known in advance that the mother is going to suppress lactation, her doctor may order the administration of a single dose of methyl testosterone and ethinyl oestradiol (Mixogen SL), which is given intramuscularly immediately after the second stage of labour. This drug is given to suppress the action of the hormone prolactin. Bromocriptine is another medication which inhibits prolactin. It is given in tablet form, twice daily, for 14 days. It is given with meals as it can cause nausea.

In most cases, lactation can be suppressed simply by the avoidance of stimulation of the breast, the wearing of a proper, firmly-supporting bra or breast binder, and the administration of suitable analgesics when required. A normal diet and normal fluid intake in moderation is allowed.

For many women, suppressing lactation is rather a sad thing. Therefore, it should be done without fuss, so that it causes as little discomfort as possible.

DRUGS EXCRETED IN BREAST MILK

The following relatively common drugs are known to be excreted in breast milk and are therefore best avoided or at least used minimally by the mother:

- alcohol
- nicotine
- caffeine
- quinine
- laxatives
- diazepam
- salicylates
- barbiturates
- cytotoxic drugs

The mother should be reminded to take only *prescribed* medications and to tell her doctor or dentist that she is breast feeding. She can also aim to protect her baby from pesticides and other chemicals by scrubbing or peeling all fruits and vegetables which might have been exposed to spraying—this includes most commercially-produced crops. Fatty meats should also be avoided, and saltwater fish are less likely to be contaminated than those from rivers.

ARTIFICIAL FEEDING

Although breast feeding is obviously the best method of feeding a newborn baby, bottle feeding can be managed in such a way that the baby misses out on very little. He can still be cuddled while being fed, so that the important warmth and security are still there. The milk can be warmed to the correct temperature, the teat checked and the bottle held at such an angle that the baby can drink at the right speed, and above all he can be fed gently and without being hurried.

MILK FORMULAS

Most of the milk formulas available are based on cow's milk. Because cow's milk is unsuitable for the newborn human baby, it must be modified in order to be effectively digested. Table 17.1 compares the constituents of human breast milk with unmodified cow's milk.

The modification of cow's milk involves its dilution to reduce the protein content and the addition of sugar to make up the resulting deficiency in caloric content. As well, the cow's milk must be subjected to heat in order to render the protein digestible. Even after modification, the protein in cow's milk cause large curds in the stomach, which is why the baby's stools are firmer and paler. Additional vitamins must be given to the artificially-fed baby as those in cow's milk are inadequate or are destroyed by heating.

Most hospitals offer a choice of commercial formulas for artificially fed babies. Home-modified cow's milk is no longer recommended for babies under 6 months. In consultation with the midwife and, perhaps, the doctor, the mother will decide which formula will be best to use at home, and the baby's feedings will be changed to that preparation.

Commercial formulas are available in dried or

Table 17.1 Comparison of human breast milk with cow's milk

Composition	Human milk	Cow's milk
Carbohydrate	7%	5%
Protein	1.5%	3.5%
lactalbumin	(0.8)	(0.5)
casein	(0.7) fine curd	(3.0) tough curd
Fat	3.5%	3.5% large molecules
Minerals	0.2% low in iron	0.8% very low in iron
Vitamins	contains:	A depends on cow's diet
	A	B1 unstable to heat
	B	B2 unstable to exposure
	C group	B6 deficient
	D	C most perishable
		D inadequate
Water	88%	88%
Kilocalories	70 per 100 ml	70 per 100 ml

liquid form, and now contain iron, vitamins and minerals. All formulas, regardless of their content must be freshly made up and sterile. In hospital, milk mixtures may be pre-packed or made up once a day by an experienced midwife or mothercraft nurse. The made-up mixtures are carefully labelled and kept in the refrigerator until just before they are used, when they are warmed to room temperature (or to blood heat).

Before the mother goes home with her artificially-fed baby she will be shown how to make up the formula that she will be using. She will be shown how to reduce the margin of error by making up individual feeds, and told the importance of correct storage of formula, both before and after making it up, especially in hot weather. Student nurses should try to be present at least one of these demonstrations, in order to learn the many points involved. Whichever formula is chosen, it is always important to use the *exact* quantity, the correct equipment (e.g. the spoon or scoop designed specifically for that particular formula), to follow precisely the directions for the formula, which may be either to *pack* or to *level off* the mixture when using a scoop, to pay the greatest attention to hygiene and to realise the importance of sterility for the protection of the baby.

METHOD OF BOTTLE FEEDING

After washing her hands, the nurse selects the correct feeding for the baby from the refrigerator and warms it in a jug of hot water. After it has warmed sufficiently, she removes it from the water and wipes the outside of the bottle dry. A teat is taken from its container or sterilising fluid, and lifted up to the light to see that its holes are patent. It is then attached to the bottle. A little of the milk is then tipped onto the nurse's arm, to ensure it is the correct temperature and that it drops readily from the holes in the teat.

Before the feed, the baby's napkin and rug are changed. A suitable lint-free cloth or paper square is placed under the baby's chin as a bib. If vitamins or medications are prescribed, they are checked and given before the feed. The nurse, or the baby's mother, then sits comfortably to feed the baby, holding him in the crook of the arm. The bottle is held in the palm of the other hand, with the forefinger placed under the baby's chin. The bottle is held so that milk fills the teat and the baby does not swallow air. The tilting of the bottle should be gentle, so that the milk does not flow too quickly. The teat should be placed above the baby's tongue, taking care not to push it too far into the baby's mouth.

The baby should suck steadily for the first 3 or 4 minutes, or for the first half of his feed. When he slows or starts to get sleepy, the teat should be eased out of his mouth and he should be given a rest. He is then sat up and de-winded. If he seems to be sucking hard without result, the teat is checked to make sure that milk is able to flow from it or to ensure that it has not collapsed.

The rest of the feed is then offered. A baby is never forced to finish a feed. The finger under his chin is simply to help the baby's mouth grip the tear well, and should *not* push the chin up and down on the teat. Overfeeding can cause hiccoughs and regurgitation. Most babies will stop sucking and go to sleep when they have had enough. If the feeding is not finished, the remaining milk is discarded. If the baby is obviously still hungry, he should be offered an extra 30 or 40 ml of the same formula.

At the conclusion of the feeding the baby is once again sat up and de-winded. His napkin is then changed if necessary and he is returned to his cot to lie on his right side with the head of the cot elevated. After an hour the cot is laid flat again and the baby may then be turned onto his left side to sleep until the next feeding.

The details of the feed and how it was taken are entered upon the baby's chart.

Care of bottles and teats

The bottles are rinsed under running cold water, washed in warm soapy water, brushed with a bottle brush and rinsed with cold water. They are then sterilised by autoclaving or by boiling for 20 minutes.

Teats are tested for patency by forcing water through the holes. They are then turned inside out and rubbed to remove any milk particles that may be clinging to the inside. They are rinsed several times in cold water and placed into a special soaking solution. A sodium hypochlorite solution, such as Milton solution, is used in many maternity hospitals for this purpose.

18

THE BABY WHO NEEDS SPECIAL CARE

Chapter outline

Key words

Dextrostix
intrauterine growth retardation –IUGR
lanugo
lecithin/sphingelomyelin –L/S– ratio
pre-term
retrolental fibroplasia
Shirodkar suture
surfactant

THE LOW-BIRTH-WEIGHT BABY

The low-birth-weight baby is one who weighs less than 2500 g at birth. Low birth weight can be due to either pre-term birth or intrauterine growth retardation (IUGR)

Pre-term birth is defined as that which occurs before the 37th week of gestation is completed.

Intrauterine growth retardation (sometimes called 'small-for-dates') is diagnosed when the baby's birth weight is below the 10th percentile for gestational age.

The pre-term baby need not necessarily be below 2500 g at birth; in fact, in cases like diabetes the baby could be of the size and weight of a full-term baby, but his organs will be immature and will make him prone to the complications of pre-term birth. These are watched for, and preventive management given.

It is also possible for a baby to be born both pre-term *and* growth-retarded. Figure 18.1 shows the average intrauterine growth pattern, with the upper (90th percentile) and lower (10th percentile) limits of normal. Table 18.1 shows the differentiating characteristics of prematurity and intrauterine growth retardation.

Table 18.1 Differentiating characteristics: prematurity and intrauterine growth retardation

Premature baby	Growth-retarded baby
Small (usually), thin, sleepy	Long, thin and wasted, but vigorous
Poor muscle tone; no resistance to head rotation or passive movement of limbs (e.g. Fig. 18.2)	Good muscle tone
Skin transparent and shiny, no creases in palms and soles, covered with fine downy hair (Fig. 18.3)	Skin dry and cracked: nails firm; ear cartilage, breast tissue, palm and sole creases all present
Reflexes absent or poor; sucking nil or poor; cough absent, grasp absent, Moro poor	All reflexes present, sucks strongly and hungrily (often 'starving')

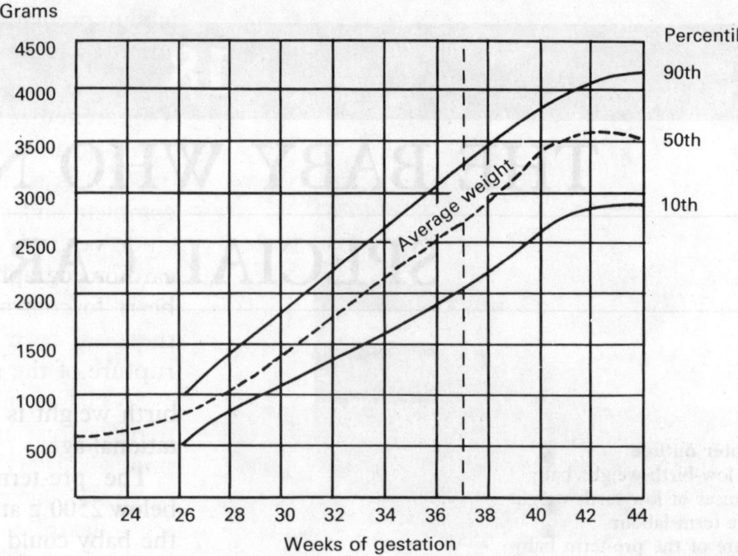

Figure 18.1 Intrauterine growth chart.

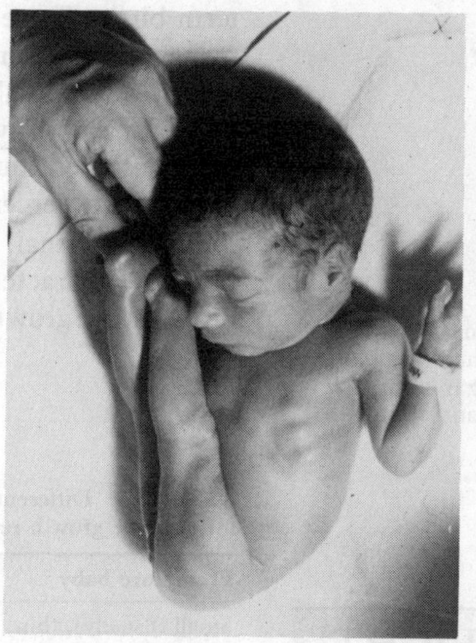

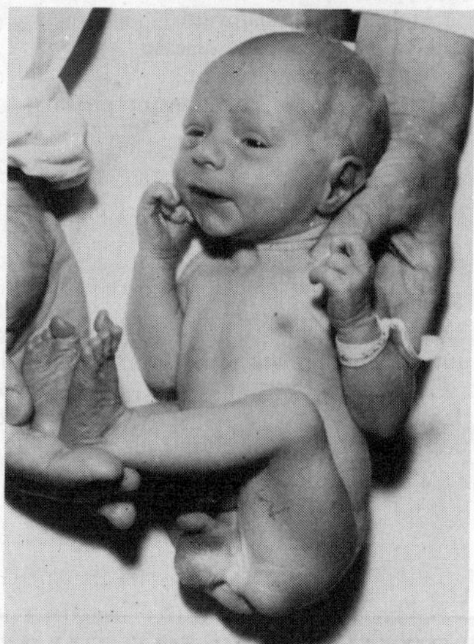

Figure 18.2 The heel of the pre-term baby (left) can be taken up to his neck without the resistance shown by the growth-retarded baby (right).

CAUSE OF LOW BIRTH WEIGHT

In 50% of cases of low birth weight the exact cause is not known, but there is a significant association with poor socio-economic conditions and also with smoking.

Pre-term birth

The known causes of pre-term birth include:

- early induction of labour, e.g. for pre-eclampsia, hypertension, Rh incompatibility, diabetes, low oestriol count
- multiple pregnancy, e.g. twins
- polyhydramnios (excessive amniotic fluid) as occurs with fetal malformations.
- infection

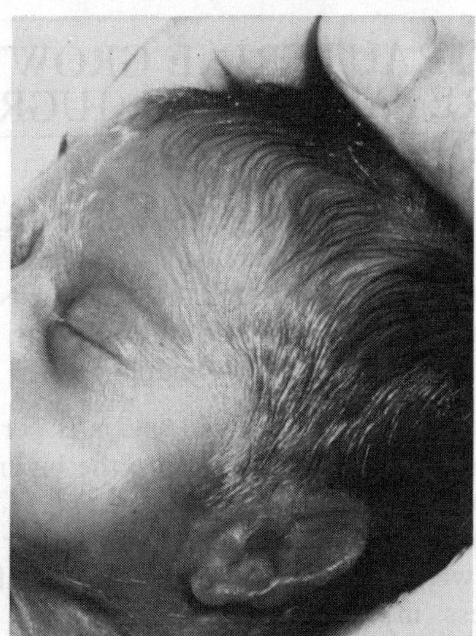

Figure 18.3 Lanugo: the fine downy fetal hair which is often found on the face, shoulders back and arms, especially in pre-term babies.

Intrauterine growth retardation
The known causes of intrauterine growth retardation are:

- placental insufficiency—premature aging of the placenta
- multiple pregnancies, sometimes; occasionally only one baby is affected
- maternal conditions, e.g. pre-eclampsia, hypertension, chronic renal disease, malnutrition
- uterine factors, e.g. chronic intrauterine infection, antepartum haemorrhage.

PRE-TERM LABOUR

One of the aims of antenatal care is to maintain the pregnancy until the fetus is mature enough to cope well with extrauterine life, i.e. until term. Those women who are at risk of coming into labour prematurely are seen more frequently and admitted to hospital earlier if necessary.

Threatened pre-term labour
The woman who shows any of the signs of labour (p. 113) is admitted to hospital immediately, for complete and strict rest in bed. Investigations include oestriol studies, fetal monitoring using the cardiotocograph to show the response of the fetal heart to contractions, and vaginal examination if there has been no evidence of placenta praevia or rupture of the membranes.

Special attention is given to the women's nutritional status, and sometimes hyperalimentation is prescribed. Hyperalimentation involves a carefully programmed regime of intravenous fluids, e.g 25% dextrose solution 1 litre, alternated with Aminofuson 500 ml.

Salbutomol may be given intravenously (10 mcg per ml infusion) in suitable cases, to relax contracting uterine muscles. If it is effective intravenously it may be continued orally (4 mg, 6 hourly at first). The dose is reduced over 2 or 3 days to a maintenance dose of 4 mg per day until 37 weeks gestation is reached.

Betamethasone may be ordered if delivery is anticipated within the next 24–48 hours. Betamethasone is effective in stimulating surfactant production in the fetal lungs (see p. 196).

A Shirodkar suture may be inserted for premature dilatation of the cervix.

Hypnosis sometimes works in reversing pre-term labour.

Psychological and social care is important for the woman in threatened pre-term labour.

Inevitable pre-term labour
The labour is often 'actively' managed (p. 145) if there is no response to attempts to stop it from progressing. Fetal response to contractions is monitored throughout.

Epidural analgesia may be given to eliminate the need for 'depressing' analgesia.

An episiotomy is often performed to shorten the second stage of labour and so protect the softer fetal skull from pressure.

The baby is given careful, gentle resuscitation, and transferred to a special care nursery in an isolette.

CARE OF THE PRE-TERM BABY

The basic aim of the management of the pre-term baby is to provide the environment, nutrition and support which enables him to overcome the handicaps of pre-term birth and their associated complications. Table 18.2 summarises the baby's usual pattern of care in relationship to these complications.

Bottle feeding is started when sucking reflexes appear. It is introduced by offering one bottle every 24 hours. When part bottle fed/part gavaged, the baby is bottle fed first. Sucking is tiring, so usually it is limited to 10–15 minutes duration. If the feed is not finished, the remainder is gavaged after a wait of 20 minutes to allow the first part of the feed to settle.

Breast feeding is begun as soon as the baby is sucking properly, providing that he is well enough to leave the insulcot to be fed.

Once the baby's condition is stable, with satisfactory temperature maintenance, weight and respiratory function, he is taken out of the insulcot and placed in a warmed cot using an electric blanket under the mattress. The extra heating is gradually withdrawn and is removed when the baby has adjusted to the changed conditions.

The pre-term baby is usually kept in hospital until he has reached maturity (40 weeks). Normally, his weight must be at least 2500 g before being allowed to go home.

Visitors to the baby under special care

The mother and father of the baby are usually allowed contact with their baby at all times. Nowadays most special care nurseries allow other children of the family and the baby's grandparents to visit as well, provided they are known to be free from infection. All visitors are asked to observe the hygiene protocol of the nursery.

The social worker attached to the special care nursery endeavours to maintain contact with the baby's parents, seeing each mother at least weekly if possible.

INTRAUTERINE GROWTH RETARDATION (IUGR)

The mother whose baby is at risk of IUGR, or who has a significant present history (sluggish or poor fetal movements, low weight gain, uterus small for gestation, reduced amniotic fluid) may be admitted to hospital for investigations:

- a series of urinary oestriol assays is performed
- ultrasound is used to measure the biparietal diameter of the fetal skull
- an amnioscopy may be performed after the 36th week, to look for evidence of fetal distress (meconium-stained liquor)
- fetal monitoring is done, to record the response to Braxton-Hicks contractions
- an amniocentesis may be performed to assess fetal lung maturity.

Antenatal management is directed towards the treatment of any causative factors such as hypertension, the improvement of placental circulation and transfer of oxygen and nutrients, and the assessment of the best time to induce the labour.

Labour and the growth-retarded fetus

The fetus is monitored throughout labour, using electrodes attached to the fetal scalp to transmit the heart beat (internal monitoring).

The second stage is shortened, using forceps (instrumental delivery) and an episiotomy.

The baby is gently and carefully resuscitated. Treatment of acidosis with IV sodium bicarbonate and of hypoglycaemia with IV glucose may be necessary.

Dangers of intrauterine growth retardation

Immediate dangers are:

- birth asphyxia
- respiratory distress
- meconium inhalation
- hypothermia
- hypoglycaemia.

The baby is subsequently prone to:

- hypoglycaemia
- vomiting

Table 18.2 Handicaps of prematurity

System	Handicap	Complications	Management
Respiratory	Poor development of respiratory centre, lung tissue and thoracic muscles; cough reflex poor, decreased surfactant, more likely to be affected by maternal drugs	Birth asphyxia, recurrent apneoa; very prone to respiratory distress, mainly due to hyaline membrane disease; more likely to aspirate; bronchopulmonary dysplasia (complication of oxygen therapy)	Positioned to drain secretions; oxygen therapy for specific indications only, eg respiratory difficulty, sternal retraction, cyanosis; may need positive pressure ventilation, either intermittent (IPPV) or continuous (CPAP)
Cardiac	Immature conductile tissue	Cardiac irregularities	Careful observation and monitoring
Digestive	High requirements and inadequate stores; poor feeding reflexes, poor tolerance of cow's milk; poor muscular development, affecting peristalsis and cardiac sphincter	Prone to nutritional deficiencies, particularly hypoglycaemia and anaemia; digestion slow; prone to abdominal distension, vomiting and aspiration	Intravenous therapy to supply essential nutrients; milk feedings introduced gradually, diluted, in small amounts, frequently (e.g. 1- to 2-hourly); gavaged to prevent baby becoming tired from sucking; multivitamin preparations, iron and folic acid prescribed
Liver	Deficient glycogen stores, deficient clotting factors, decreased enzyme activity	Prone to hypoglycaemia, haemorrhagic disease, jaundice; difficulty in excreting drugs	As above, plus phototherapy if serum bilirubin levels high, vitamin K, observation; minimum of drugs prescribed
Brain	Skull bones soft, increased permeability of blood-brain barrier, increased capillary fragility	Very prone to intracranial haemorrhage, hypoxia, kernicterus	Gengle handling, maintenance of oxygen, care with jaundice
Eyes	Immature retina	Prone to damage from high levels of oxygen, leading to retrolental fibroplasia	Minimum necessary oxygen administered according to blood gas estimations (arterial oxygen); routine examination by eye specialist
Body temperature	Temperature regulation centre immature, heat production poor, heat loss excessive, deficient brown fat (special fat that babies have which is easily burnt up)	Hypothermia	Nursed in heated cot; temperature recorded hourly, brought up slowly; heat tunnel, plastic film or bubble plastic may be used; baby wrapped in cotton wool or foil for transporting
Kidneys	Poor mineral clearance, poor acid-base balance; poor excretion of drugs	Prone to electrolyte imbalance, disturbances of acid-base balance	Observation
Blood	Immature cells, excessive breakdown and over-formation of red blood cells; increased fetal haemoglobin	Very prone to anaemia; jaundice of prematurity common	Observation, fluids maintained; phototherapy
Antibody formatioon	Inadequate transfer of maternal antibodies; poor manufacture of own antibodies	Prone to infection, particularly thrush, skin infection, pneumonia, septicemia	High standard of preventive care; septic 'work-up' if infection suspected; prophylactic antibiotic therapy

- infection
- jaundice
- bleeding tendency, in the first week of extrauterine life.

Care after birth
Neonatal care is aimed at preventing or treating the above problems. It consists of:

- special attention to provision of warmth
- administration of oxygen if necessary
- early and frequent feeding to prevent hypoglycaemia; Dextrostix readings are done hourly for the first 4–6 hours, then before each feed for at least 24 hours.
- jaundice is treated early.

Paediatricians attempt to follow up IUGR babies for the first 5 years if possible in order to evaluate the results of their antenatal and neonatal care.

OTHER NEONATAL CONDITIONS

A number of serious conditions often complicate a low birth weight and pre-term birth and can possibly arise in the normal full-term baby. The conditions outlined here are:

- hypoxia
- atelectasis neonatorum
- hyaline membrane disease
- necrotising enterocolitis (NEC)
- umbilical cord infection (omphalitis)
- hypoglycaemia
- hypothermia
- kernicterus
- neonatal heroin additcion
- persistent vomiting.

HYPOXIA

Hypoxia is diagnosed when there is a lowered arterial oxygen, i.e. PaO_2 less than 50 mmHg (normal is 80–100 mmHg). Clinical signs such as cyanosis are unreliable in the newborn, so babies at risk of hypoxia are constantly monitored by frequent, hourly at first, blood gas sampling. Oxygen is administered to the baby in relation to the blood gas results. The minimum effective oxygen concentration is used because of the danger of causing retrolental fibroplasia and subsequent blindness.

Hypothermia worsens the effects of hypoxia.

ATELECTASIS NEONATORUM

Atelectasis neonatorum is an imperfect expansion of the lungs of the newborn baby. The respirations are rapid and shallow, with associated abdominal retraction on inspiration. Occasionally an audible grunt is present.

The lungs may not be able expand fully because of hyaline membrane disease (see below) or because there is an obstruction such as mucus or inhaled meconium in the upper bronchial tree.

Whenever there are signs suggesting respiratory distress a chest X-ray is performed to diagnose and reveal the extent of the inexpansion and its possible cause. Positive pressure ventilation using a respirator is usually necessary (Fig. 18.4).

HYALINE MEMBRANE DISEASE

Hyaline membrane disease occurs in approximately 50% of pre-term babies. Their underdeveloped lungs lack a secretion called surfactant, a detergent-like substance consisting of the phospholipids lecithin and sphingomyelin. When these are in a certain proportion, a ratio of two parts lecithin to one part sphingomyelin, the surfactant produced is adequate in its function of preventing the collapse and adherence of the alveoli walls. Surfactant does not have an L/S ratio of 2:1 until at least 35 weeks gestation.

The L/S ratio can be measured by amniocentesis

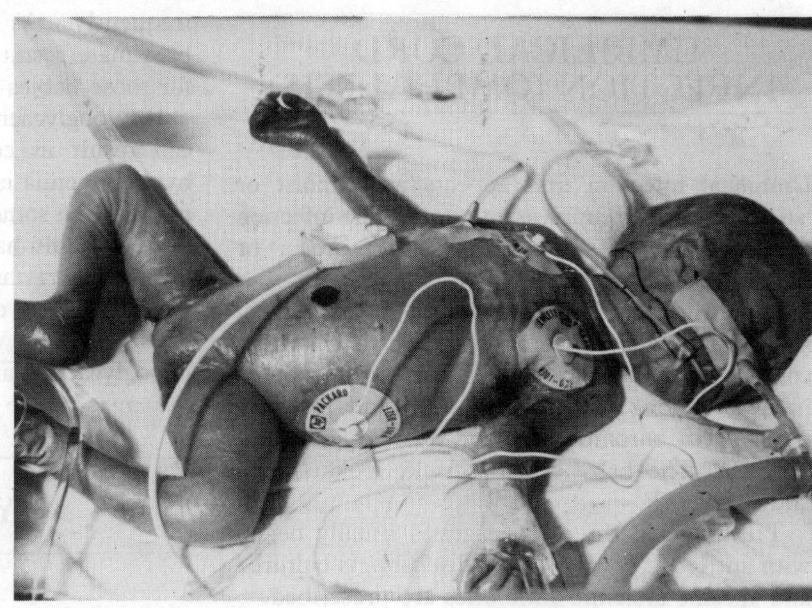

Figure 18.4 Pre-term baby attached to a respirator.

to indicate fetal lung maturity because surfactant works its way through the bronchial tree to the mouth and is thus present in the liquor.

The baby lacking sufficient or effective surfactant will have respiratory distress because the alveoli are tight, do not inflate easily, and collapse after each breath. Lung cell damage occurs, and eventually the damaged cells combine with white blood cells and serum to form a fibrous material, 'hyaline membrane'. This material fills the air sacs and prevents sufficient oxygen from reaching the infant's bloodstream.

At about 3–5 days after birth, the baby will have responded to the changed conditions and the lungs will produce sufficient surfactant to allow better alveolar inflation. Until this occurs assisted ventilation is often necessary using continuous positive airways pressure (CPAP).

NECROTISING ENTEROCOLITIS

Commonly referred to as 'NEC', necrotising enterocolitis is a condition in which part of the baby's gastro-intestinal tract undergoes necrotising changes. Prematurity, with its many complications, predisposes to the condition. It is a serious condition which can be fatal without urgent treatment.

Necrotising enterocolitis is usually associated with hypoxia, leading to ischaemia of the gut which leads in turn to tissue death. As well, the baby may have had intravenous therapy or a history of infected liquor, perhaps following early rupture of eh membranes.

Early signs are vomiting, abdominal distension and gastro-intestinal bleeding. The temperature is usually elevated.

X-rays of the affected baby's abdomen will show gas within the bowel and also in the peritoneal cavity. If the condition progresses, there may be bowel perforation, peritonitis and septicaemia. Bowel obstruction and stenosis may also result.

Necrotising enterocolitis is managed by intravenous therapy (not via the umbilical route), broad-spectrum antibiotics and, if there is no response to these, by surgical removal of the affected part of the gut.

UMBILICAL CORD INFECTION (OMPHALITIS)

Umbilical infection first appears as a moist or 'sticky' cord, with unpleasant odour. The infection may be due to staphylococci, streptococci or Gram-negative bacilli.

If the infection is not treated at the first signs, it spreads to the area around the cord which becomes red and swollen. It may also spread internally along the umbilical vein and result in portal vein thrombosis, liver abscess and septicaemia. The baby becomes sick, looks 'grey', and is feverish.

Treatment in the early stages is usually begun with antibiotic powders. Any discharge is cultured and specific systemic antibiotics are prescribed.

The importance of careful routine cord care and the early reporting and treatment of any redness or discharge from the cord stump is once again emphasised.

HYPOGLYCAEMIA

Hypoglycaemia is diagnosed when the plasma glucose level is below 1.75 mmol per litre (30 mg%) in a term baby, or below 1.15 mmol per litre (20 mg%) in a premature baby. Normal blood glucose level is 3.5–5.5 mmol per litre (60–100 mg%).

Newborn babies need glucose for energy production and for cell metabolism, and therefore for cardiac, respiratory and cerebral functioning. Low blood glucose levels will jeopardise these vital functions.

Babies most at risk of hypoglycaemia are those born pre-term, those with growth retardation or respiratory distress, or babies of diabetic mothers.

Signs of hypoglycaemia (lethargy, poor sucking, hypertonicity, jittery movements) may not be evident *until brain damage has occurred*. All babies at risk are screened frequently using Dextrostix to assess blood glucose levels, and are fed early and frequently. As Dextrostix give only an approximate result, biochemical testing is necessary for those babies most at risk.

If hypoglycaemia is not discovered very early it can result in cerebral impairment. Even when hypoglycaemia is treated *before* signs appear there may still be some central nervous system dysfunction. If signs have appeared before treatment is given, there is high (30–60%) incidence of central nervous system dysfunction.

All babies who have been diagnosed as hypoglycaemic are carefully followed up.

HYPOTHERMIA

A baby's rectal temperature of below 35°C is defined as hypothermia, but in practice any temperature below 36°C is cause for concern and the institution of heat-preserving procedures.

As his heat-regulating mechanism is still immature at birth, even the full term normal baby is unable to withstand heat loss without serious complications. Therefore, the environment of the new baby must be maintained at a temperature which will not demand a great increase in his metabolic rate to maintain his temperature. The sick or preterm infant can ill-afford to waste any precious oxygen and calories on this function.

Those most at risk of hypothermia are the preterm, hypoxic and hypoglycaemic babies, and those whose delivery has been difficult or prolonged. Babies can get very cold through excessive handling by staff or parents while still in the labour ward.

The hypothermic baby is weak and lethargic, disinterested in sucking and feels cold to touch. If not treated, hypothermia can lead to neonatal cold injury in which there may be solid oedema (sclerema), a 'marble baby'; a serious and often fatal state.

Prevention of hypothermia is of the greatest importance. The usual measures taken are described on pages 45 and 165.

Any episode of hypothermia is treated by the gradual rewarming of the baby in an insulcot until his temperature is at least 36.5°C. He will need to stay in a controlled temperature environment for several hours until he has proved that he can maintain a normal temperature. He is closely observed for any signs of respiratory difficulty and for maintenance of satisfactory blood glucose levels.

KERNICTERUS

Kernicterus (bilirubin encephalopathy) is a serious complication of jaundice, in which there is bile staining and necrosis of the fatty cells of the brain. It is caused by the deposition of unconjugated and unbound bilirubin in the brain cells.

Kernicterus is an irreversible condition which may result in mental subnormality, deafness, spastic paralysis or death. Early recognition of jaundice and its prompt treatment are therefore vital.

NEONATAL DRUG ADDICTION

The baby of the drug-addicted mother is himself physically addicted at birth, when his source of the drug is withdrawn and he may undergo withdrawal symptoms usually after 18–24 hours. The symptoms, particularly in heroin-addicted babies, are:

- a high pitched cry
- irritability, with convulsive movements (jittery)
- strong sucking at first, but often unable to finish feeds
- loose stools.

The baby is kept in a nursery rather than rooming in with his mother, as he will need close observation.

Sedation such as phenobarbitone is often necessary. The dose is reduced as the tremors become less frequent.

In many cases there has been little or no antenatal care and the mother's background and lifestyle is unstable. Pre-term birth, growth retardation and fetal distress add to the problems of these babies.

The question of breast feeding is difficult, but it may not be encouraged because if the mother continues to take the drug it would be present in the milk and the baby could need alternative 'carers' at any time.

PERSISTENT VOMITING

Small 'spills' or possets are common and usually insignificant. They should always be recorded on the baby's chart to assess their frequency and to took for a pattern in relation to feeds.

All episodes of vomiting are observed for:

- time, in relation to the feed
- frequency
- type, e.g. whether forceful (projectile) or 'dribble'
- amount
- constituents, e.g. undigested milk, curds and mucus.

It should also be noted whether or not the baby sucks well, and whether there is any associated diarrhoea.

From these observations the cause is usually able to be determined and treated. Until then the baby may be limited to glucose feeds or he may be fed intravenously if necessary. Milk feedings are resumed with caution, using half-strength and half-quantity feedings, gradually resuming full strength and quantity as each increase is tolerated.

The baby may need to be gavaged for a period, and perhaps postured after feeds. Some hospitals use a plastic bucket with the front removed or a car-seat type of baby support to assist gravity to retain the feeding. Milk may be thickened with an additive such as Gaviscon.

Vomiting can be indication of serious disorders including increased intracranial pressure, intestinal obstruction and establishing infection. It should never be ignored.

19

PHYSIOLOGY OF THE PUERPERIUM

Chapter outline
Involution
Findings at the postnatal examination

Key words
involution
lochia
puerperium
puerperal psychosis

The puerperium is the period of time during which the reproductive organs return to the non-pregnant state. This takes about 6 weeks. The progression of changes in the organs is called involution.

INVOLUTION

Uterus

At the end of the third stage of labour the fundus of the uterus is at the level of the umbilicus, and the uterus weighs 1000 g. It involutes rapidly for the first 7–10 days, then more gradually (Fig. 19.1).

By 12 days postnatal it is not usually able to be felt abdominally, and by 6 weeks it has returned to the non-pregnant size, 8 cm high and 50 g in weight.

Involution is caused by:

- the continued contraction and retraction of the uterine muscle fibres, causing compression of the blood vessels, resulting in localised anaemia—ischaemia
- autolysis—self-digestion of excess cell cytoplasm, leaving traces of fibro-elastic tissue as evidence of the pregnancy
- atrophy—the tissues, which proliferated in the presence of high levels of oestrogen, atrophy in response to its withdrawal with the removal of the placenta.

As well as the atrophic changes in the muscle of the uterus, its lining (decidua) undergoes atrophy and is shed, leaving the basal layer to regenerate a new endometrium. The site of placental attach-

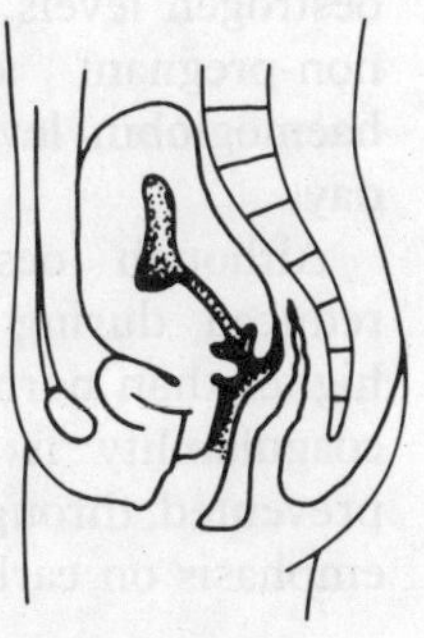
Following labour

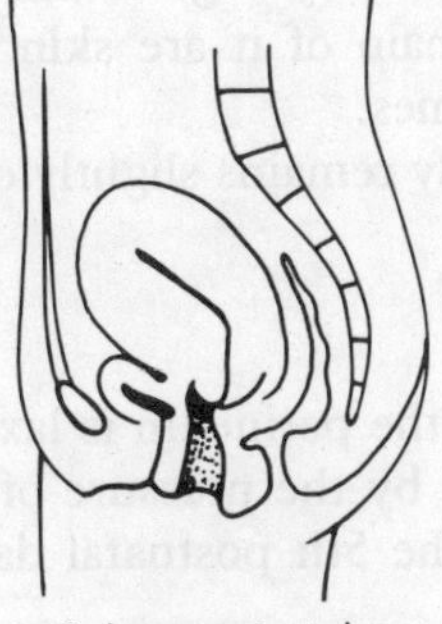
3 days postnatal

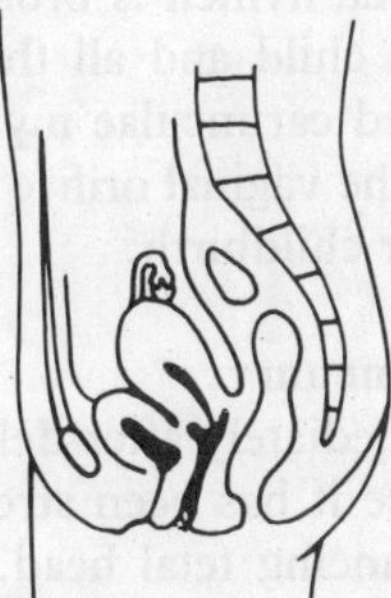
10 days postnatal

Figure 19.1 Involution of the uterus.

ment takes 8 weeks to heal completely. Return of menstruation varies; in the non-lactating woman it is usually at 6–8 weeks, but where the baby is fully breast fed it may not return for some months.

Lochia

Lochia is the name given to the passage of blood and necrotic decidua from the uterus during the puerperium. It progressively decreases in amount and colour:

- *lochia rubra* (days 1–4)—moderate in amount, red, and mainly blood
- *lochia serosa* (days 4–8)—reduced amount, and pink (haemoserous)
- *lochia alba* (days 8–14)—scant in amount, white or almost colourless.

Cervix

The cervix involutes along with the uterus. After labour, the external os can admit two to three fingers; by 6 weeks postnatal the cervix is closed.

Because of tiny tears occurring during dilatation, the cervix never returns to its pre-pregnant (nulliparous) state of a pinpoint opening, only to the non-pregnant state of a healed, closed, but slit-shaped opening. The parous cervical os is, therefore, one of the signs of a previous vaginal childbirth.

Vulva and vagina

The vulva and vagina undergo considerable pressure and stretching during the delivery of the baby, and for the first few days afterwards they may remain lax. By 3 weeks they are almost back to the pre-pregnant state, with rugae gradually reappearing in the vagina and the labia becoming less prominent.

The hymen is broken down by vaginal delivery of a child and all that remain of it are skin tags called carunculae myrtiformes.

The vaginal orifice usually remains slightly open after childbirth.

Perineum

Immediately after delivery the perineum is lax because it has been stretched by the pressure of the advancing fetal head. By the 5th postnatal day it should have regained most of its tone although it will always be more lax than in the nulliparous state.

Some relaxation of the pelvic floor and the abdominal muscles may also persist.

Breasts

In contrast to the atrophic changes occurring in the pelvic organs, the breasts reach their full maturity during the puerperium unless lactation is suppressed. They become larger, firmer and initially tender, in response to the changed hormonal status and the initiation of lactation.

Urinary tract

Voiding is often difficult for the first 24 hours. There may be spasm of the sphincter and oedema of the bladder neck following its compression between the fetal head and the pubic bone during labour.

Large amounts of urine are produced from 12–36 hours after delivery. When the placenta is expelled there is a marked reduction in levels of oestrogen which has a water-retaining property. This causes the diuresis. The dilated ureters return to normal in 6 weeks.

Gastro-intestinal system

Bowel function often takes 3–4 days to return to normal. Although the progesterone level drops after delivery, there may be a reduced intake of food for a day or two, less bodily exercise and, when a pre-delivery enema was given, often an empty lower bowel. Soreness of the perineum may inhibit early attempts to open the bowels.

The cardiovascular system

Following the marked diuresis due to the fall in oestrogen levels, the blood volume returns to the non-pregnant amount. Red cell count and haemoglobin level returns to normal by the 5th day.

Although oestrogen levels are considerably reduced during the puerperium, they are still higher than normal. The plasma is less fluid, and coagulability is therefore increased. Clotting is prevented through careful management, with the emphasis on early ambulation.

Psychological changes

The sudden and dramatic changes in the woman's hormonal status makes her sensitive to factors with which she would normally otherwise be able to cope. In addition to hormonal changes, her physical reserves are often drained by the demands of pregnancy and labour, loss of sleep, unfamiliar surroundings and anxieties about the baby or her husband and other children. Her body may not respond well to unfamiliar drugs such as narcotic analgesics given in labour.

Mild depression, '4th day blues', is common and many new mothers find themselves in tears, at least once, often about the smallest problem. Some women feel inadequate for a short time, but this generally disappears as their confidence in themselves and their babies grows. Should depression or insomnia persist for more than 1 or 2 days, specialist psychiatric help is sought in order to exclude the development of puerperal psychosis (p. 215).

FINDINGS AT THE POSTNATAL EXAMINATION

The normal time for the postnatal physical examination is 6 weeks after delivery. Findings should be:

- the uterus is not palpable abdominally
- on vaginal examination the uterus is well involuted and has returned to its non-pregnant size
- the cervix has healed
- the vaginal rugae have reappeared and there is no vaginal wall laxity or prolapse
- the vulva is not gaping excessively
- the perineum is firm and any episiotomy or tear wound has healed
- there is no unusual or abnormal physical or mental distress caused by the examination
- the muscle tone of the pelvic floor can be satisfactorily demonstrated by squeezing the levator ani muscles
- the vaginal loss has ceased—unless menstruation has started again.

Table 19.1 shows the permanent changes caused by pregnancy and vaginal delivery.

Table 19.1 Permanent changes in the parous woman

	Nulliparous	Parous
Breasts	Firm, no striae (unless there has been obesity or significant weight loss)	May be flabby (not if lactating), striae may be present
Nipples	Pink	Brown, more prominent
Abdomen	No striae (unless as above), muscles usually firm	Striae may be present, muscles often lax, skin may be loose, linea nigra may be evident
Uterus	Ovoid in shape	Round in shape
Cervix	Round, pinpoint opening, admits a fingertip only	Transverse slit opening, admits one finger
Vagina	Orifice small, hymen present or partly evident	Orifice enlarged, may gape slightly, tags only of hymen (carunculae myrtiformes)
Perineum	Firm, and without scarring	May show evidence of repair of episiotomy or tear, may be lax

20

POSTNATAL CARE

Chapter outline

Key words

'after pains'
lochia
postpartum haemorrhage (PPH)
puerperal
stress incontinence

To many women the labour experience is rather a hazy memory; there was a lot going on, it was exciting and fairly exhausting, and it was of comparatively short duration. So it is the time spent in the *postnatal* area that is usually remembered most by the maternity patient. It is also the one that she is likely to talk about to her friends and family, so her happiness and satisfaction with the hospital and its staff is important. For many young women, this will be their first-ever stay in hospital. They are often shy, uncertain, on their best behaviour, and may not like to be dependent, even for a short time, upon others. The newly-delivered mother often has to be convinced that small tasks are no trouble for us, and that we *want* to do things like escort her to the toilet for the first few times after she is allowed up, as well as it being for her own safety.

Most new mothers settle in well to the particular daily pattern of a postnatal floor or ward. They usually want, first, to rest, then to learn as much as they can before they go home. With good care and friendly help they find that the time they spend in the postnatal department is an enjoyable experience.

The nursing student will find that the postnatal area is one in which she can practise quite a lot of her learned skills. She may find that the new mothers often want to engage her in conversation, seeing the nurse as one who has more time to talk about things not 'important' enough to bother the midwife or doctor about. The nurse should make the most of such conversations and encourage the woman to voice these matters. Any item of information that may be significant will be welcomed by those in charge, and discussion will enhance the nurse's basic maternity and general knowledge.

AIMS OF POSTNATAL CARE

All aspects of postnatal care are aimed towards discharging from hospital a healthy mother with a healthy baby that she knows how to care for. This is achieved if the mother:

- has sufficient rest, so that her body and mind are able to recover from the physical and emotional tasks of pregnancy and labour
- avoids infection, which may inhibit satisfactory healing of injured tissues
- establishes satisfactory lactation, or becomes confident with an artificial feeding method

- learns to handle, change, feed and comfort her baby so that he is settled and contented.

Nearly every contact with the new mother is an opportunity for learning, often for the mother and the nursing staff to learn from each other.

Length of stay in hospital

The postnatal hospital stay is ideally about 5–7 days following normal delivery; perhaps a day or two longer following complications or interventions. Social or economic factors may make this impractical; mothers who have very little in the way of rest and recovery are still able to manage.

The ideal is encouraged when possible, especially with mothers who already have small children at home. Most of them are understandably keen to be back with their families, yet once they are back they may find that they cannot get the rest that they need. The little toddler who comes to visit his mother in hospital in clean clothes and well fed by his grandmother, can be a lot more of a handful than she remembered him to be.

Some mothers find it valuable to go to an aftercare hospital for a few days before going home. These centres (e.g. Torrens House in Adelaide, Queen Elizabeth Hospital or the Grey Sisters in Melbourne) allow the transition from hospital care to be made gently. They either give the woman going home to a very full life extra rest, or help the unsure mother gain extra confidence and skills in handling her baby.

POSTNATAL OBSERVATIONS

The immediate care and observation of the newly-delivered woman is described at the end of Chapter 14 because many centres regard that time as the 'fourth stage' of labour.

When the mother has rested after delivery, when her vital signs are stable and satisfactory, her fundus firm and central, vaginal loss minimal and when she has voided, she is transferred to the postnatal department. For the next 6 hours the pulse, fundus, loss and bladder are observed hourly, after which, if everything is normal, they are made 4 hourly for the first 24 hours.

After the first postnatal day, the woman is checked twice daily unless there is any indication to observe her more frequently.

Temperature

The temperature is recorded morning and evening. In midwifery, a temperature of over 37.2°C is always reported to the midwife in charge of the ward, who will contact the doctor should it rise above 37.5°C.

Minor rises in temperature are common on about the 4th day and may be associated with breast activity. On the other hand, any elevated temperature could be due to puerperal sepsis, a potentially serious disorder which must be treated immediately with antibiotics.

Pulse

The pulse rate is recorded twice daily. It is normally comparatively slow for the first week after delivery. A fast pulse may be due to infection, especially if it is accompanied by any elevation in temperature. A high vaginal swab, mid-stream specimen of urine and throat swab may be ordered for laboratory investigation.

Postpartum haemorrhage may also cause a rise in the pulse rate and a weakening of pulse volume. The nurse, if unsure, should always ask someone more experienced to check her findings.

Blood pressure

After the first 24 hours, the blood pressure is recorded twice daily until day 4 then daily. It is recorded more frequently when indicated, such as for a previously pre-eclamptic patient, or when the vaginal loss is excessive or the pulse rapid. A low blood pressure may indicate postpartum haemorrhage. A high blood pressure may warn of the development of pre-eclampsia which can arise at any time during the puerperium, although it does so rarely.

The uterine fundus

Fundal height is measured and recorded daily, and the fundus is palpated twice daily to ensure that it is firmly contracted and centrally situated.

The woman should empty her bladder just before the fundus is checked. A full bladder will displace the uterus upwards and may prevent firm uterine contraction.

The fundal height decreases by approximately 1 cm daily until it can no longer be felt abdominally, usually by the 11th or 12th day (Fig. 19.1).

Lochia

The lochia, which include blood, decidua and any retained products of conception, are observed twice daily.

Lochia should progressively decrease in amount and colour until by the 14th day there remains only a scant white or almost colourless discharge from the vagina.

For the first day or two the woman may worry that she is losing too much because when she gets up from lying down there may be a 'rush' of blood. This can be explained by the fact that the blood drains to the vaginal vault and collects there while she is lying down.

The lochia should not contain blood clots. If they, or any other solid matter, are evident in the lochia, the pad or pan should be saved for inspection by the midwife.

The smell of the lochia is normally no different from that of menstrual blood. If it is offensive, it should be reported immediately as it could indicate puerperal sepsis.

The pad onto which the lochia drain is handled by its tapes or ends only and is disposed of into a clean bag without contaminating the hands or the outside of the bag. Blood is an ideal medium for the growth of infective organisms.

The breasts

The breasts are inspected and palpated twice daily, and the mother is asked whether they are comfortable, sore or painful.

Using a good light, the midwife looks for any red areas on the breasts and inspects the nipples for oedema, cracking or bleeding. She feels right around the breasts, including the axillary area, for any unusual hardness or for lumps which might indicate blocked milk ducts. She then works inwards, palpating carefully and noticing any areas of tenderness.

The perineum

The perineum is examined twice daily in a good light. The midwife observes for redness, oedema, bruising, discharge and tightness or 'cutting-in' of sutures. The mother is asked whether she feels that her perineum is comfortable, tight or painful.

Lower extremities

There is a small but definite risk of venous thrombosis and pulmonary embolism following childbirth. The calves are checked for tenderness and heat each day and the mother asked to report any leg discomfort.

REST

Satisfactory rest for the new mother is extremely important yet sometimes not very easy to achieve. There is no doubt that she ought to rest; pregnancy with its heavy weight and many discomforts, plus the work of labour, is not good preparation for the busy time that follows. Yet the postnatal days can be full: there is so much to learn, milk is coming in to the breasts, there is the excitement of cards, flowers, presents and visitors, and there may be worries and concerns unconnected with the present situation. So, with a tired body and probably a very active mind, she will often need to be reminded and helped to get sufficient rest.

Night rest

For the first night or two the new mother may benefit from some form of mild sedation. This is usually ordered to be given if needed. Often her body takes over and she sleeps, barely disturbed by the checks of vital signs and fundus. Some find the strange surroundings distracting and others may find the discomfort of an episiotomy, when the local anaesthetic has worn off, prevents sleep. Pain or discomfort are always investigated and an analgesic given before sedation is administered.

After the second postnatal night sedation is usually unnecessary, and is inadvisable if the woman is to feed her baby during the night. She is helped to settle early, and not disturbed without reason. Small distractions such as squeaking doors or dripping taps ought to be reported during the day so that they can be dealt with before they disturb sleep.

The new mother who is unable to sleep is observed closely and the fact reported to her doctor. Insomnia is one of the warning signs of puerperal psychosis (p. 215).

Daytime rest

The new mother's day in hospital need not be frantic, but many say that it is. 'I had to come home to have a rest!' is a commonly-heard statement and one to which those involved in maternity care must listen and find out why.

In almost every maternity hospital, a definite rest period is set aside at a regular time, often for the hour preceding the patients' lunch. The curtains are drawn, radios are turned off, the staff work quietly, visitors are discouraged and telephone calls not put through to patients' extensions unless they are urgent. The woman is helped to organise herself for this rest time; going to the toilet, putting away knitting, lying down prone (perhaps with a pillow under her hips) to aid uterine drainage if that position is comfortable. This rest period is generally of great physical and psychological benefit. Some hospitals repeat a definite rest-time again in the afternoon.

When asked to say what it was that made the day in the postnatal ward so busy, the answers of some mothers are revealing. The routine and regular events like the doctors' visits, exercise sessions, demonstration baths or even feeding the baby do not seem to be the problem. It is the activities that demand some emotional output, like coping with visitors, especially outside visiting hours, and incoming telephone calls, or writing thank-you notes for cards and gifts which tire them. Perhaps nurses who sense that a mother is becoming overwhelmed by such things could help by discussing priorities, 'Does everybody who sent you a card really want a reply? Won't you be seeing some of them soon?', and by being careful at visiting time to see that the mother is coping with her visitors.

VISITORS

The subject of visitors deserves its own heading because it *can* be a real postnatal problem.

People do want to visit their relations and friends who have just had a baby. It is 'nice' hospital visiting—nobody is sick or sad, and there is the long-awaited baby to see. The mother and father are happy and excited and the grandparents proud.

Visiting hours can be very tiring for the mother. Because people come from far and wide, she often ends up entertaining people who do not know each other and may not be interested in anything about each other but sit there hoping that the other will go away first. Or else they visit *each other* and almost ignore the patient. Then there are those who feel that their claims upon the attention of the mother are more important than those of other visitors and let it be known, and those who expound their own ideas about baby care and how that compares to the what the mother is being taught at this hospital.

The problem is perhaps, that while visitors know that the mother is not sick, some of them do not understand or have forgotten how soreness or tiredness can make one feel. The postpartum 'blues' are usually at their worst after evening visiting hours.

Many midwives do a round before and during visiting hours, to check how well their patients feel able to cope or are coping with company. Some hospitals have signs announcing that there be only two or three visitors per patient at a time. It may be up to the nurse to ensure (politely) that the mother has no more than this number of visitors. Few new mothers protest at this; most are rather grateful. Those visitors who are visiting each other usually do not mind at all.

Husbands must be allowed an opportunity to visit alone. Most hospitals now have a special time set aside in the evening for husbands to visit. The other children in the family also need to spend time with their mother without the noise and interruption of other people.

Midwives and nurses who have worked in postnatal departments tend to be very considerate visitors themselves after their experiences.

GENERAL CARE

General care of the postnatal patient is based around the maintenance of hygiene and comfort, the prevention of infection and the relief of minor disorders as they arise. Sample nursing care plans for normal delivery and caesarean section are shown in Tables 20.1 and 20.2.

HYGIENE

The patient who is confined to bed (e.g. because of hypertension, intravenous therapy, caesarean section) is given a full daily sponge, another wash to freshen up later in the day, and perineal wash-downs twice daily and after using bedpans. Even though the mother is usually young and healthy, her pressure areas still need attention and protective care.

Once the mother is able to shower (ideally at least twice daily) she can usually perform her own perineal washdowns using a jug set aside for her use alone. Pad changing should be done frequently, at least after each wash and after every bedpan or visit to the toilet.

Table 20.1 Example of nursing care plan (Vaginal delivery)

Problem/need	Goal	Nursing action
Potential for postpartum haemorrhage related to vaginal delivery and uterine atony	Mother able to recognise normal lochia and report if abnormal Normal involution of the uterus	Education re normal colour, consistency, amount, odour and duration of flow and reportable abnormalities. Education re pelvic floor exercises. Assessment of fundal height, position and tone 4-hourly for 24 hours then twice daily until discharged. Uterus massaged as necessary.
Potential for infection related to labour, vaginal delivery and possible blood loss	Mother able to recognise early symptoms of the onset of infection and able to demonstrate	Education re abnormalities of lochia, particularly odour, general malaise, differentiation Instruction in perineal hygiene, use of salt baths, ray lamps etc. Preventative education regarding the use of tampons, vaginal deodorants, swimming during the puerperium. Assessment of temperature twice daily or 4-hourly if febrile until 24 hours of afebrile readings is reached. Report to doctor if T>38°. Administer antipyretic and or analgesia prn.
Potential for anxiety because of inexperience and lack of knowledge of baby care and feeling	Mother able to demonstrate a secure ability in both care and feeding of her baby	Facilitation of bonding experiences as soon as possible after delivery. Encouragement and supervision of baby handling and feeding, with emotional support and positive reinforcement. Where appropriate, referral to literature and community support groups.
Potential for constipation related to reduced intestinal muscle tone, changes in diet and normal activity, and perineal soreness.	Return of normal, comfortable bowel action	Encouragement and assistance with ambulation and activity. Advice on suitable foods, fluids and fibre. If necessary, gentle aperients given.

Table 20.2 Example of Nursing Care Plan — caesarean section (specific points)

Problem/Need	Goal	Nursing action
Potential for haemorrhage — related to caesarean delivery and possible complications	Early detection/prevention	One return to ward ½-hourly pulse, BP, wound and perineal pad check (observe for colour, amount and odour) for 4 hours then once hourly for 2 hours; then if satisfactory, 4-hourly for 48 hours. Therefore BD until discharged. Teach patient to recognise normal lochia, colour, amount, odour and duration of flow, and when to report to midwife.
Potential for paralytic ileus — due to operative procedure	Prevention/early detection	IV therapy until bowel sounds heard — peristalsis returned. Restrict fluids and food until the return of bowel sounds. After flatus passed return patient to normal food and fluid intake as desired.
Discomfort or pain due to operative procedure	Minimise pain/provide relief	Give analgesia as ordered. As soon as sensation begins to return after epidural and thereafter as ordered or needed. Position patient for comfort, assist with position change.
Potential for emboli/thrombi due to rest in bed	Prevent formation/early detection	Observe legs BD; promote circulation with special leg exercises hourly whilst non-ambulant. Encourage early ambulation.
Potential for infection: wound — related to impaired skin integrity respiratory — related to impaired mobility; operative procedure	Prevention/early detection; mother able to report abnormalities	Temperature to be taken on return to ward then 4-hourly for 48 hours. If satisfactory to be taken BD until discharge. If febrile, temperature to be taken 4/24 until afebrile. Report temperature of 38° and above to doctor. Observe abdominal wound for inflammation, tenderness, discharge. Apply dressing PRN. Notify doctor if abnormality detected. Advise patient re chest physiotherapy — deep breathing and coughing. Encourage early ambulation. Alert patient to report offensive lochia, abdominal pain, general feeling of being unwell. Advise patient re hygiene — perineal care, frequent changing of perineal pads.

The breasts are given special attention at the twice daily sponges or showers. They are washed first, keeping a face-washer reserved for them alone. They are gently massaged and the nipples are carefully pulled out. Soap is not used on the nipples.

PERINEAL CARE

A perineal wound from an episiotomy, tear or laceration is in an area which is not easy to keep clean and dry. Special observation and care are necessary to ensure that it heals quickly and easily. The perineal toilet gives an opportunity for inspecting the perineum closely and it makes the area much more comfortable.

Infrared ray lamp

An infrared ray lamp may be ordered to be used twice daily to assist in the drying and healing of the perineal wound.

The mother usually lies in an exaggerated left lateral (Sims') position, with her hand elevating her right buttock to expose the wound properly.

A ray lamp is set up no closer than 50 cm away and is positioned securely so that it cannot slip. The rays are directed towards the perineum.

The mother's privacy is ensured, she is handed a buzzer and asked to ring it when 10 minutes have elapsed. The midwife notes the time, and returns within 10 minutes. She should, in fact, return every few minutes, to make sure that the mother is still elevating her buttock properly and that she has not fallen asleep. The lamp is warm and soothing and often makes people feel drowsy.

In some centres a hand-held hair dryer is used on a low setting instead of the ray lamp.

Perineal soreness

The perineum may feel especially sore on about the 6th postnatal day, when the blood supply to the area is properly restored.

Local treatment

The hygiene measures of showers and perineal toilets, and the use of the ray lamp, help to relieve some of the soreness. Sitz baths (a tub bath with salt added) are sometimes used to give comfort and aid healing. A small soft towel is placed on the bottom of the tub before use, and the bath is disinfected afterwards.

An analgesic spray (e.g. Dermoplast) may be prescribed. These sprays are often rather expensive, but are usually very effective.

Oral analgesia

The woman should be assured that it will not harm her or her baby if she takes simple oral analgesics for the few days during which perineal soreness is at its worst. 4-hourly paracetamol or codeine combination-type analgesics may be prescribed at this time.

Air cushions

Foam rubber rings provide great relief for the mother with a sore perineum. They enable her to sit up to eat or feed the baby much more easily. If foam rings are not available, an inflatable ring is used, but care must be taken not to over-inflate it; it needs just enough air in it to lift the perineum off the bed. The air cushion that is blown up too hard can feel like a beach ball to sit upon and the woman will be reluctant to move for fear of falling off. The woman should be told that air cushions are available so that she can ask for one when she needs to sit up.

Perineal wound infection

The discomfort of a perineal wound is made worse and healing is delayed in the presence of infection. Perineal infection may be due to a haematoma, or to failure in aseptic technique.

A swab is taken of any discharge from the wound, and is sent for culture and sensitivity testing. Antibiotics are prescribed and the patient is reminded that she must complete the full course. The ray lamp is used three times a day following careful perineal toilets, unless there is oedema or bruising. Sitz baths may be ordered. An antiseptic drying paint may be applied *after* the ray lamp is used. Extra analgesia is usually prescribed.

The swollen perineum

When the perineum is swollen or oedematous, the stitches cut into the tissues and the area is extremely sore.

Small ice-packs placed inside the perineal pad are useful in reducing swelling and relieving discomfort. They need to be replaced frequently—1 to 2-hourly.

Perineal and vulval haematomata

Bleeding from a relatively small vessel can quickly distend the loose tissues of the vulva or the superficial perineum. If swelling becomes severe, it may be necessary for the wound to be re-opened, to allow drainage of the blood and to identify and tie the bleeding vessel. Figure 20.1 shows a severe vulval haematoma.

Analgesics, air cushions and ice-packs are also usually given and, of course no heat is applied.

'AFTER PAINS'

'After pains' are lower abdominal cramping (contraction) pains which commonly arise in the first 7–10 postnatal days.

They are more usual in the multipara because her uterus, having been fully stretched twice, tends to be slacker than the uterus of a primipara and so has to contract harder to involute. After pains usually occur when the mother is breast

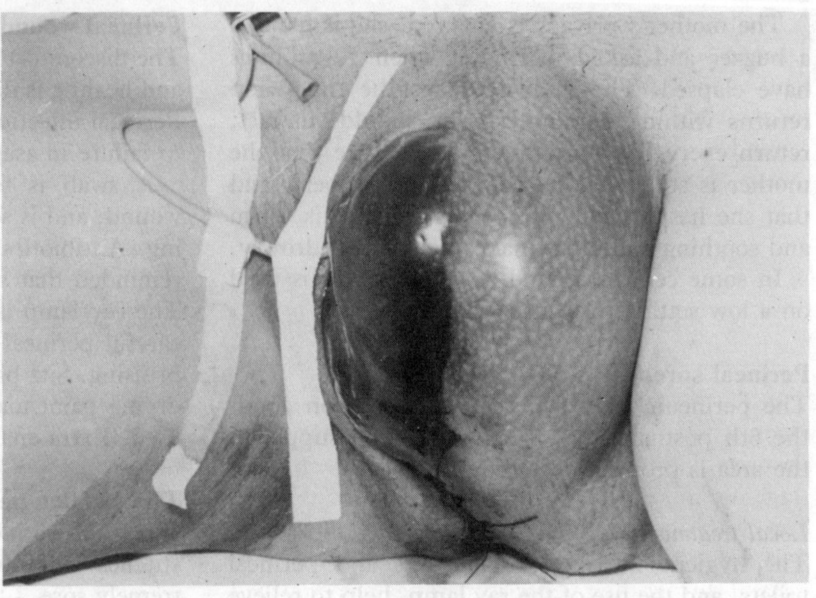

Figure 20.1 Vulval haematoma.

feeding her baby, because suckling leads to the release of oxytocin which makes the uterus contract. These postnatal contractions when breast feeding are a natural way of preventing postpartum haemorrhage.

The pains can be quite severe, enough to make the mother cry and, in fact, sometimes dread feeding the baby. Some mothers are frightened of the pain because it did not happen after the first baby.

Explaining the cause will help to reassure the woman. Giving analgesics such as codeine or paracetamol, about an hour before the baby is due to be fed, will take away the worst of the discomfort of after pains.

BLADDER CARE

There is a marked diuresis for the first day or two following delivery, and the mother sometimes has difficulty in emptying her bladder because of soreness, bruising and loss of muscle tone. She is helped up to sit out of bed on a commode if she is not yet ambulant and is having difficulty voiding on a pan in bed.

Catheterisation, although avoided whenever possible, is preferable to urinary tract infection from static urine.

Stress incontinence may occur, but is generally transitory, clearing when the pelvic floor muscle tone has improved. Postnatal exercises (Fig. 20.2) will help; occasionally specialist physiotherapy will be necessary.

BOWEL MANAGEMENT

Because the bowels tend to be sluggish and the woman is prone to constipation (p. 59) bowel medication is often useful. A typical pattern of management if the bowels have not opened by the second postnatal day is:

- 2nd night—Agarol or Milk of Magnesia 15 ml
- 3rd night—coloxyl tablets (ii)
- 4th day—glycerine suppositories (ii) or a small enema.

Caesarean section patients undergo the same regime 1 or 2 days later than this.

Dietary factors are important in the re-establishment of satisfactory bowel function. The mother may need assistance in selecting suitable foods from a menu. She may also need to be reminded of the benefits of early ambulation in of taking extra fluids and avoiding constipation.

HAEMORRHOIDS

Haemorrhoids may appear for the first time postnatally (recall the 'pouting' anus in the second stage of labour), or they may have been a problem during the pregnancy.

Haemorrhoids can become swollen, itchy and painful during the puerperium. They are managed in the following ways:

- the use of ice-packs held to the area by a firm perineal pad
- the avoidance or treatment of constipation
- the provision of air cushions
- the application of soothing ointments—proprietary haemorrhoid ointments usually have both anaesthetic and vasoconstricting properties
- the administration of satisfactory analgesia either oral or local (e.g. Dermoplast spray).

The ray lamp is never used for the perineal wound in the presence of haemorrhoids because heat will increase the blood supply to the area causing irritation and further discomfort.

NUTRITION

The new mother will require a full nourishing diet in order to help her body recover from the demands of pregnancy and labour, resist infection, prevent constipation and begin the process of full lactation. The diet should be high in protein, iron and calcium, vitamins and fibre, and must include 3000 ml of fluid of which 1000 ml should be milk. Caloric intake should be increased to 2700 calories (11500 kilojoules).

The food supplied in most hospitals is adequate for the needs of the postnatal woman. She may, however, need help or advice in selecting the best foods offered on the menu. She may also need to be reminded that the sweets and chocolates visitors bring to her may spoil her appetite for the proper meals that her body needs.

Meal service is important. When the mother is feeling tired she may need to be tempted to eat. The tray should not be overloaded with food; in some hospitals the main courses only are served on the tray and a dessert trolley brought around afterwards so that the more valuable food is offered first.

It is hard to eat properly if the food cannot be seen. The mother may need help to sit well up, perhaps with a foam ring, so that she can manage her meals more easily.

When the mother goes home, she is reminded to buy 'as much from the butcher, greengrocer and dairy, and as little from the grocer, as possible'. Ideally, she is given printed nutrition advice and meal suggestions.

An iron supplement may be prescribed to be continued for the first 4 postnatal weeks.

EXERCISES AND AMBULATION

The newly-delivered mother may be reluctant to move around very much, because she is weary and sore.

Early ambulation is of great importance in the prevention of venous thrombosis. Following a normal delivery, if not restricted by intravenous or other tubings, and if her vital signs are satisfactory, the mother is usually able to go to the shower and toilet with assistance an hour or two after normal delivery. Before this she should be asked to do deep breathing and simple leg exercises, and should sit up and swing her legs from the side of the bed. Caesarean section patients usually begin to ambulate 24–36 hours after delivery. If she has had epidural analgesia, full return of sensation

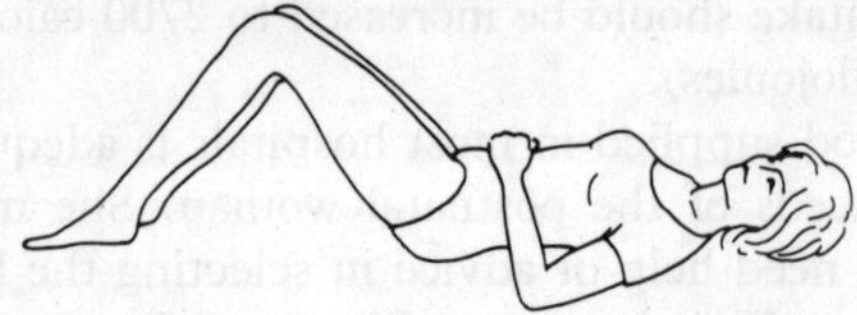

1 Lie on back, knees bent. Place hands on abdominal area below ribs. Breathe in slowly and deeply through the nose and then exhale through the mouth, tightening the abdominal wall to help empty the lungs.

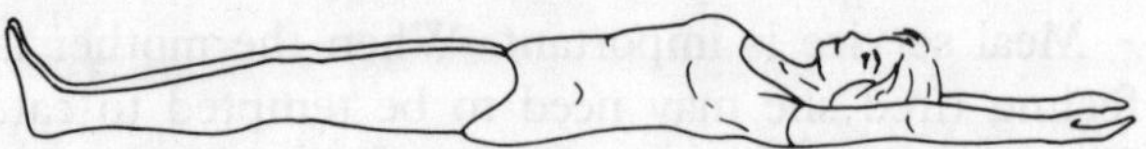

2 Lie on back, arms extended above head, palms up. Release left arm slightly and stretch right arm. At the same time relax left leg and stretch right leg so there is full stretch of the entire right side of the body. Repeat on the opposite side.

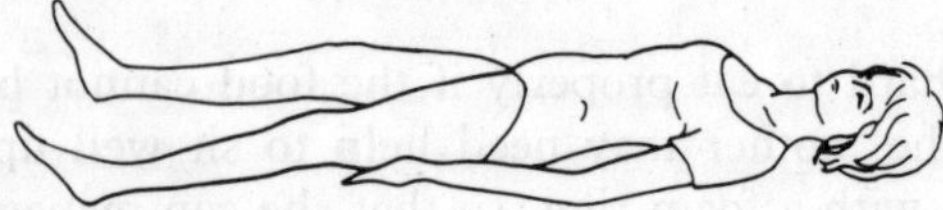

3 *Vaginal contraction*
Lie on back, or front if you have stitches—it is more comfortable. Legs slightly apart. Draw up the pelvic floor, hold three seconds and then relax. Progress to standing and sitting.

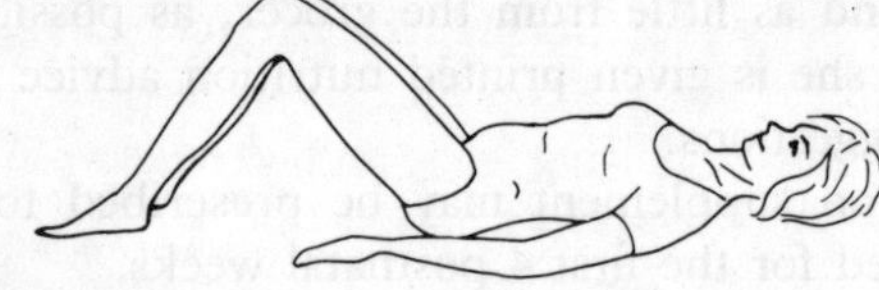

4 *Pelvic tilt.*
Lie on back, knees bent. Contract abdominal muscles to flatten spine and tighten buttock muscles—hold 3 seconds then relax.

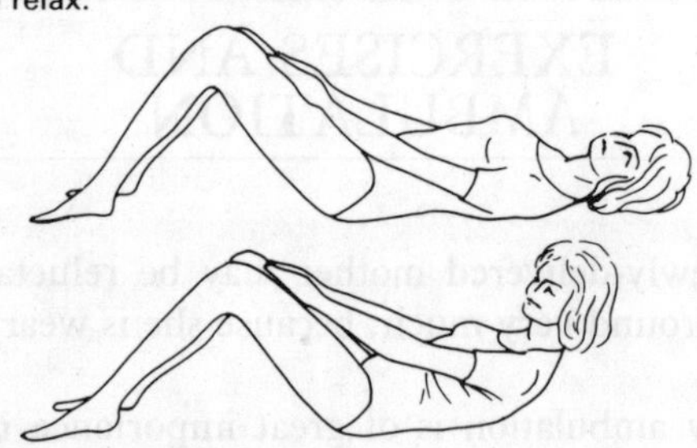

5 *After the third day*
Lie on back, knees bent, arms outstretched. Raise head and shoulders to about 45 degrees, hold three seconds and slowly relax.

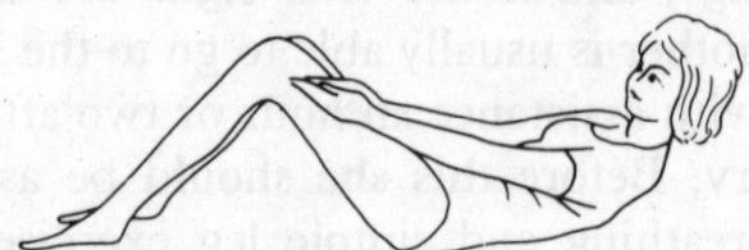

6 Same position as above. Take arms to outside of left knee. Repeat to outside right knee.

Figure 20.2 Typical instruction sheet for postnatal exercises following normal delivery.

must be demonstrated before ambulation is commenced.

Good posture is encouraged from the start to help to prevent backache.

Postnatal exercises are performed as described in Figure 20.2. They usually begin on the first day and are performed once daily under the supervision of a midwife. In some hospitals a physiotherapist conducts postnatal exercise classes on certain days each week.

The purpose of these exercises is explained to the mother so that she will realise the importance of setting aside time for them while she is in hospital, and will continue them when she goes home. They help to strengthen the abdominal muscles and so help to regain good physical shape, they tone up the pelvic floor, thus preventing or improving any stress incontinence, and they assist with proper circulation of the blood throughout the body.

A printed sheet, such as the one illustrated in Figure 20.2, is given to each patient in most hospitals.

POSTPARTUM HAEMORRHAGE (PPH)

Primary postpartum hemorrhage is excessive bleeding (600 ml or more) from the genital tract occurring within 12–24 hours of delivery.

It can happen after any labour but is more common where there has been a large baby, hydramnios, multiparity, prolonged labour or difficult delivery. The main cause of primary postpartum haemorrhage is failure of the uterus to achieve or maintain a state of contraction. This occurs with incomplete placental separation or retention of placental fragments. Laceration of the cervix or vagina can also cause significant blood loss.

Primary PPH is treated by first ensuring that the uterus is contracted, by fundal massage or by the administration of an oxytocic drug (e.g. IV ergometrine). Manual removal of the placenta is often necessary. A careful assessment of blood loss is made. For non-uterine causes, the bleeding points must be stopped by direct pressure (vaginal packing if necessary) until they can be isolated and secured.

Secondary postpartum haemorrhage, occurring from 24 hours after delivery, is almost always the result of infection caused by retained products in the uterus. The uterus is slow to involute and the lochia become brighter in colour and heavier. Treatment involves oxytocics and antibiotics and, in some cases, dilatation and curettage to empty the uterus.

PSYCHOLOGICAL CARE

The psychological impact of the events of the first few postnatal days is discussed on page 203. As the responses to the many emotions during this time are so varied and influenced by so many factors, the main emphasis of the nursing approach is one of help, sympathy and encouragement.

Many of the fears and worries of new mothers are simple and can be easily allayed, or in fact prevented, by alert staff. By attending to the comments of the woman, her attitude to staff, visitors, her husband and her baby, the midwife can often anticipate the sort of things that may cause psychological stress. By meeting and getting to know the woman's husband or other people close to her, the midwife will have greater insight into any underlying problem.

It is especially important to encourage the nervous or insecure mother, especially the primipara, in the business of handling her baby. It is easy for her to be discouraged by the apparent competence of professionals who take over the baby and manage to settle him when she has been unable to. Midwives are usually aware of this and are able to remind the mother that they have had time to learn various skills that she will gradually learn, and that they have not just been through the draining process of pregnancy and labour.

If a new mother's behaviour is unusual or irrational, the staff should be alert for the development of puerperal psychosis, a relatively rare but often serious psychiatric condition.

PUERPERAL PSYCHOSIS

Mental illness (as distinct from the common, transient, mild depression) arising for the first time during the puerperium is termed puerperal psychosis. It usually occurs before the 14th postnatal day but can occur later. The mother may have appeared to be completely normal until the time of its onset or she may have had persisting mild depression. The first warning sign is (almost always) insomnia over two or more days; inability to sleep should always be reported in the apparently normal postnatal patient. Another early sign is that of the mother becoming unusually talkative, bright and lively. It is often the husband or other person close to the mother who first recognises this change of behaviour and comments upon it to the staff.

Puerperal psychosis may manifest itself in aggressive behaviour, hallucinations, suspicions and accusations about the staff or husband. The woman may reject her baby or, alternatively, become very possessive of him.

Very careful observation and *constant* supervision are vital when puerperal psychosis is suspected. If the condition is diagnosed, the woman is usually transferred, with her baby if possible (depending upon her condition), to a psychiatric hospital for specialist care. Lactation is normally not suppressed unless violence is feared, or the mother needs medications which are known to be secreted in breast milk and which might harm the baby.

GOING HOME FROM HOSPITAL

Before the woman is due to go home with her baby, the midwife in charge of the postnatal area will spend time talking with her on a one-to-one basis. It is important that the mother feels confident in her ability to cope and that her worries about herself and the baby are aired. Once she gets home she is likely to be given advice from a variety of sources and this may well unsettle her. Most hospitals issue printed handouts to reinforce their advice.

She should understand how to manage her baby's feeding, whether it be by breast or bottle. If bottle feeding she may be given enough made-up formula to last for the first 24 hours, so that she does not have the bother of buying and preparing milk mixtures that day. She will also be given written instructions on the making-up and storage of feedings and the care of bottles and other equipment.

She will be given appointments for herself and the baby for the postnatal checkup, usually 6 weeks after the date of delivery.

A referral to the nearest infant welfare centre (Baby Clinic) would have been made at the time of birth, so the infant welfare sister will be expecting her to visit. In some areas the sister calls upon the mother and baby a few days after they arrive home to introduce herself and explain the facilities and services offered by the centre. Even if this does not happen, the mother should go to the centre within 10 days of leaving hospital. The hospital midwife will supply the address and show the mother its location in a street directory.

Some hospitals have their own domiciliary service which visits all primiparae and any multiparae who are referred to it with special needs, particularly if their stay in hospital has been short.

The midwife will introduce the subject of the resumption of intercourse and make sure that the woman understands that conditions will be changed, at least for a while.

When to resume intercourse depends upon a number of factors. Once the drainage of lochia has finished, and the perineal wound (if any) has healed (usually by 3–4 weeks following delivery), there is no reason why the couple should not have a normal satisfactory sexual relationship. It will probably be several weeks before full pelvic floor muscle tone returns and vaginal lubrication may be diminished for up to 6 months. Where there is still vaginal loss (blood or haemoserous) the placental site may not be fully healed and intercourse is probably unwise. A sutured perineum may feel tight at the first attempts at intercourse, and if the wound is not well healed it could be painful or even damaging. In such cases it is wise to wait until after the postnatal check-up at 6 weeks, or to contact the doctor earlier.

The woman is warned that her sexual feelings and interest may have changed after the birth of her child. She may have more, or less, interest in intercourse than before, and these feelings may continue for some months. If she or her husband is worried about this change, they should be told that it is a known problem and that they should not be nervous of discussing the matter with their doctor.

The return of menstruation following childbirth varies according to whether the woman is fully, partially, or not, lactating. If lactation is suppressed at the time of delivery, the first period usually occurs about 6 weeks afterwards. When fully breast feeding, a woman can have amenorrhoea until she starts to wean the baby. Most women will ovulate *prior* to the first menstruation following childbirth.

21

THE MOTHER WITHOUT A BABY

The nurse may have under her care a mother without a baby. The baby may have been stillborn, may have died after birth, may have been given for adoption or may be very sick or premature. In each case the woman is going to have special and extra psychological needs. These must not be ignored. This chapter relates mainly to the situations that may arise in cases of stillbirth or neonatal death.

In some hospitals the mother without a baby is transferred to a general ward because it is felt that being with mothers who do have babies might be distressing for her. This is a debatable point; some mothers seem to cope better if they are able to face the situation by seeing and hearing babies from the start.

It is often easy to do less for the mother without a baby because the usual reasons for spending time with a postnatal woman are centred around the baby management and feeding. Yet she still has the same needs for physical care and observations as the mother with a baby has, and she may very well need the opportunity to talk about her feelings when she is ready.

Extra awareness of the mother's response to her visitors is necessary. In the case of a stillbirth or neonatal death her visitors may themselves be finding the situation difficult to cope with and may bring little comfort to the mother. She should be asked who she wants to see most and who she might find difficult to be with at this stage. The set visiting hours should be relaxed to suit her needs. The husband should be allowed to visit his wife whenever he is able, both for her sake and his own.

While the mother is protected to some degree from the outside world, her husband is not. It is usually he who has to 'let people know'; who has to go home, often to an empty house, and pack away the bits and pieces that the couple had gathered for the baby. Often he has to do his daily work as well, having to concentrate and take care at his job and drive safely.

No amount of good nursing can ease the hurt and disappointment of the death of a longed-for baby. But it helps to allow the couple time and privacy to be together.

The policies of different hospitals vary in regard to the parents' contact with their baby after it has died. In most places they are offered the opportunity to not only see and hold, but to bath and dress, the baby. Their time together is very precious and very short, but this contact can help the couple to accept the fact of the baby's death and so start them in the process of working through their grief. Tangible reminders of the baby—a lock of hair, a name band, a cot card, a photograph—are often all that the parents can take with them. They are usually greatly appreciated. Where there is a quite unsightly abnormality, the baby can be wrapped carefully to obscure the worst-looking features. It is best if the parents are able to see and hold their baby as soon after death as possible, because a post-mortem is usually performed, and even if it is done very carefully, its evidence could be a further hurt for the parents.

Funeral arrangements may be made by the parents or by the hospital; most hospitals have an agreement with one or more funeral directors to provide a simple burial in an unmarked grave at minimal cost. An experienced midwife will spend time with the parents discussing this. If the parents wish, she will arrange for a priest or minister to visit them.

There are a few extra points that any nurse looking after a mother without a baby should consider:

- The parents may not like the term 'lost'. They have not lost her baby; it has died. Some people feel that 'lost' minimises the value or personhood of their baby who, to them, is very real.
- Where a birth announcement has been put into the papers it may not have been fully read by those who work for the companies that send mail (samples, free offers, etc) to new mothers. If they have not noticed the word 'stillborn' or 'lived only for a few hours', they may send their insurance offers or pink or blue money boxes. The arrival of these items can be very upsetting. The woman's mail should therefore, be scanned for any of these or similar items and they should be put aside to check with the husband when he next visits.
- Lactation will need to be suppressed (p. 187) without fuss, and as quickly as possible. The staff can offer to wash out any bras or nightgowns that milk has leaked on to; such laundry could be a hard task for the husband or woman's mother to cope with emotionally.
- The mother should be encouraged to stay in hospital long enough to recover and allow wounds to heal and lactation to be suppressed. That is, if she wants to. Sometimes she will want to go home early to be with her husband. Often mothers feel that they do need the time in hospital to recover and prepare to face the world, yet they get the impression (by small, usually well-meant comments) that they should not stay. After the subject has been discussed by the parents with the midwife in charge and the doctor, the other staff should not make suggestions about early discharge from hospital.
- Going home can be hard. The process of getting dressed to go home, perhaps packing up unused baby clothing, saying farewell to the staff to who have helped her through this crisis can be difficult. When she gets home the mother will have to face the disappointment of other people, and other people react in different ways; either coming to visit when she is unable to manage, or avoiding her through embarrassment (e.g. turning their backs when they see her, joining the queue farthest away at the bank or the supermarket). If she has some warning that these things may happen, she may be less upset when they do.

It may help the couple to know about two groups of people who can share their experience. The Compassionate Friends is an international organisation of bereaved parents who offer friendship and understanding to others; and their telephone number can be found in the directories listed under 'C'. Sands (The Stillbirth and Neonatal Death Support group) works with the same basic aims, perhaps more specifically for parents of *babies* who have died. Their telephone number is also listed in the directories.

22

FAMILY PLANNING

Chapter outline

Suppression of ovulation—the 'pill'
Preventing the ovum and sperm from meeting
- Sterilisation operations
- Alteration of cervical mucus
- Mechanical barriers
- Chemical contraceptive agents
- Limiting intercourse to infertile periods

Preventing implantation of a fertilised ovum
Family planning during the puerpeium

Key words

amenorrhoea	'peak' mucus
gonads	proliferative phase
luteal phase	spermicidal
'mini-pill'	vas deferens

A basic knowledge of family planning is important for the nurse. She will be expected in her professional capacity (and quite often privately as well) to be able to interpret and explain the various ways of both achieving and avoiding pregnancy. Family planning discussion and advice can be centred around revising the ways in which pregnancy is achieved, i.e. the factors necessary for the establishment of pregnancy, as shown in Figure 22.1. The ways of avoiding pregnancy can then be looked at in detail by showing how the absence of one or more of these factors prevents pregnancy. In essence, contraception can be achieved by:

1. the suppression of ovulation
2. allowing ovulation to occur, but preventing the ovum and sperm from meeting.
3. allowing the ovum and sperm to meet, and fertilisation to occur, but preventing successful implantation in the uterus.

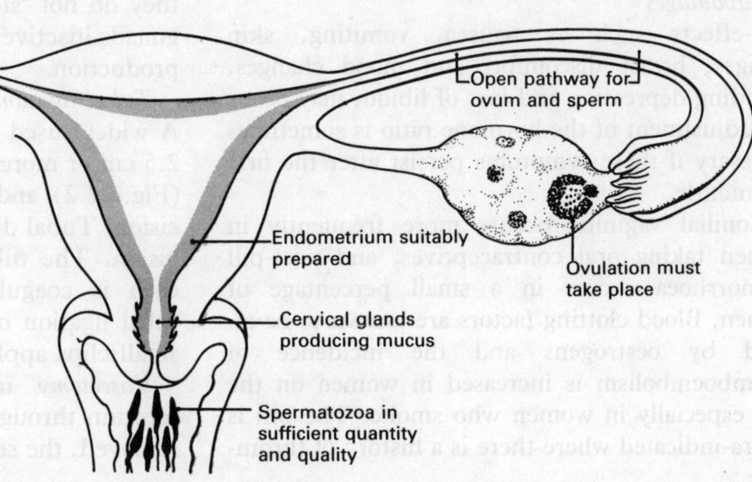

Figure 22.1 Factors necessary for the establishment of pregnancy.

SUPPRESSION OF OVULATION—THE 'PILL'

Oral contraceptives—the 'pill'—are tablets containing the hormones oestrogen and progesterone in various combinations. Low levels of oestrogens cause the release of follicle stimulating hormone (FSH), so when oestrogen levels are maintained artificially, FSH is not released. Without FSH, ovarian follicles are not ripened and ovulation does not occur. Progestogen is included to balance the oestrogen and prevent undesirable side-effects. The endometrium proliferates to a lesser degree than during a normal cycle, and the menstruation (withdrawal bleeding) is slight. Oral contraceptives are issued on prescription only, and therefore the woman must return regularly for renewal of the prescription, enabling assessment of her response to the hormones and any side-effects to be discovered.

Advantages
Oral contraceptives are almost 100% effective if taken according to the instructions, which are clearly stated and illustrated on the literature included in the packs. The woman will have regular 'periods' with reduced blood loss, with little pain or discomfort and with fewer premenstrual problems. The habit of taking the pill each day is soon acquired, and there is no interruption to the spontaneity of intercourse.

Disadvantages
Side-effects such as nausea, vomiting, skin changes, breast discomfort and mood changes, including depression and loss of libido, may occur and adjustment of the hormone ratio is sometimes necessary if these symptoms persist after the first few months.

Monilial vaginitis occurs more frequently in women taking oral contraceptives, and post-pill amenorrhoea occurs in a small percentage of women. Blood clotting factors are known to be altered by oestrogens and the incidence of thromboembolism is increased in women on the pill, especially in women who smoke. The pill is contra-indicated where there is a history of thrombophlebitis or pulmonary embolism, and may doctors require that it be discontinued 4–6 weeks before elective operations, especially those involving the pelvic or abdominal regions.

PREVENTING THE OVUM AND SPERM FROM MEETING

Interruption of the pathway of either the ovum or the sperm can be achieved by:

1. 'Sterilisation' operations—to block the fallopian tubes in the woman or the vasa deferentia in the man
2. Altering the cervical mucus so that it is impenetrable to sperm
3. Blocking the ascent of the sperm by mechanical barriers
4. Destroying the sperm by chemical agents
5. Limiting intercourse to the woman's infertile periods

STERILISATION OPERATIONS

Tubal ligation or diathermy in the female, and vasectomy in the male involve the severing or blocking of the tubes which carry the germ cells: they do not 'sterilise' in the sense of making the gonads inactive, and so they do not affect hormone production.

Tubal ligation may be done by several methods. A widely used procedure involves the removal of 2.5 cm or more of the central portion of each tube (Fig. 22.2) and involves a small abdominal incision. Tubal diathermy is done under laproscopic vision. The tubes are elevated and a portion of each is coagulated by diathermy. 'Temporary' tubal ligation methods are now being tried using small clips applied under laproscopic vision.

Vasectomy involves small incision into the scrotum through which about 6 cm of each vas is removed, the severed ends turned back and sealed

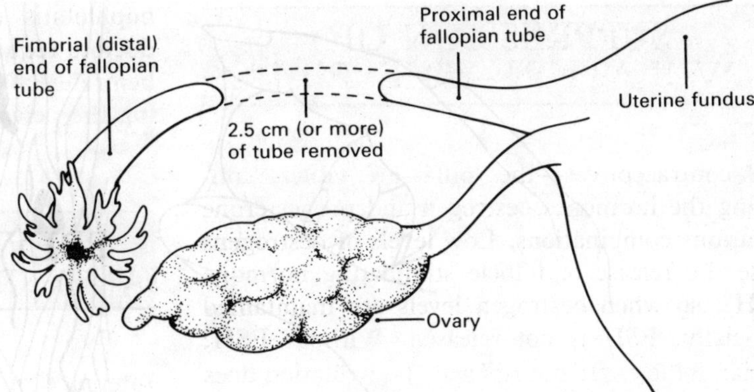

Figure 22.2 Tubal ligation.

by diathermy. Temporary vasectomy procedures are also being researched. The contraceptive effect of vasectomy is not achieved until all remaining sperm above the excised portion of the vas have been expelled from the body. This may take 20–30 ejaculations.

Sterilisation operations provide a permanent and almost 100% effective means of contraception, acting immediately in the woman and usually by 4 months in the man. Hormone production and general body functioning are not affected.

The permanency of the sterilisation procedure, however, is not always an advantage as life situations can change. Reconstruction operations have some success but are rarely guaranteed. In some, the effect of loss of fertility can show itself in disorders such as depression, difficulty with intercourse, frigidity or impotence. Most doctors now feel that the early days following childbirth are a time of stress in themselves and few will offer permanent sterilisation operations to the mother at that time.

ALTERATION OF CERVICAL MUCUS

Cervical mucus is of great importance in assisting the spermatozoa to ascend thrugh the cervix and uterus. At the time of ovulation the mucus has been prepared by high levels of oestrogen to a state in which it is thin, clear, stretchy and easily penetrable. After ovulation and the formation of corpus luteum, progesterone is produced, and it acts upon the cervical glands to produce thick mucus which is impenetrable by sperm (Fig. 22.3). Studies of cervical mucus changes have led to the development of the Billings method (see p. 223), and also to the administration of low doses of progestogens (the 'mini-pill') to achieve this state.

The mini-pill is particularly suitable for women who are breast feeding as it does not affect the hormonal balance necessary for the maintenance of lactation. It is available only by doctor's prescription.

MECHANICAL BARRIERS

Male barriers—*condoms*—are fine rubber coverings rolled on to the erect penis and worn during intercourse to prevent sperm from being deposited in the vagina. They are widely available and can be bought from dispensers or over the counter.

If used correctly (especially in combination with a spermicidal agent) condoms are an efficient form of contraception. They form a physical barrier against infective organisms as well as against pregnancy. Condoms do, however, necessitate interruption to the spontanaeity of intercourse, as they cannot be put on until the penis is erect. Some find that they reduce sensation. If the penis

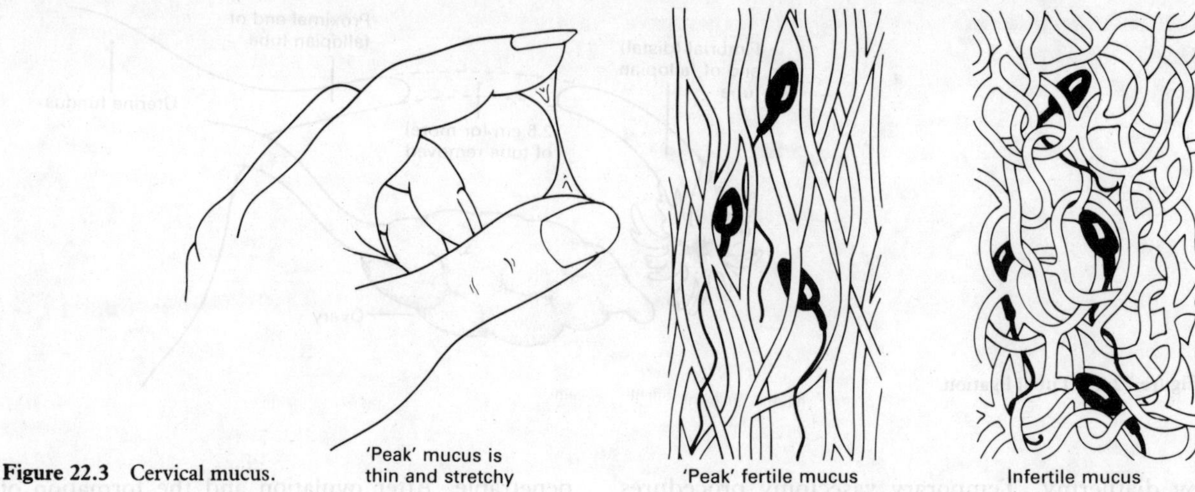

Figure 22.3 Cervical mucus.

is not withdrawn soon after ejaculation, the condom could slip off, and sperm be allowed to enter the vagina. Cost factors may also need to be considered.

Female barriers—*the diaphragm and the cervical cap* (Figs. 22.4 and 22.5)—are the two most commonly used female barrier methods of contraception. The diaphragm is a saucer-shaped rubber cap with a spring inside the circular rim.

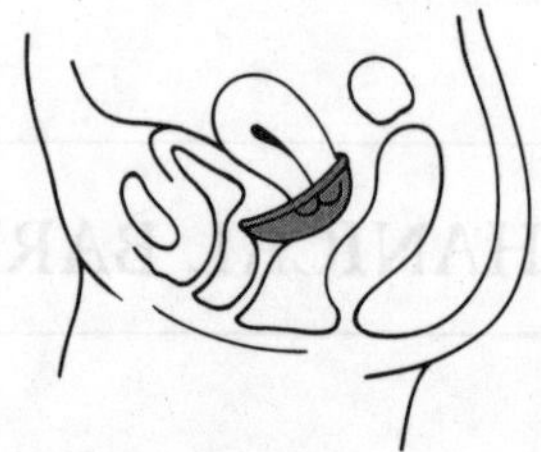

Figure 22.4 Correctly placed diaphragm.

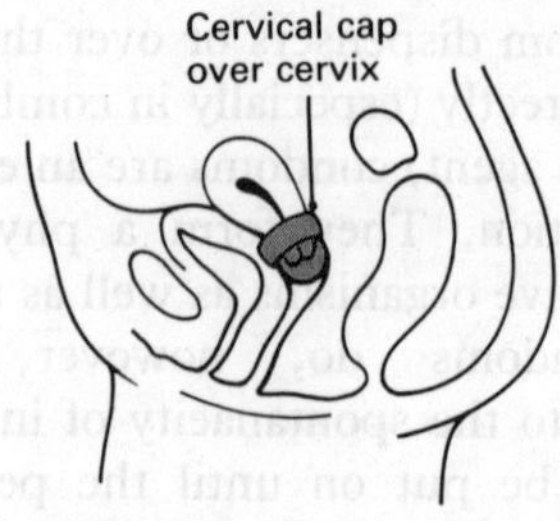

Figure 22.5 Cervical cap in place.

When inserted it lies in the formices of the vagina and so occludes the cervix. The cervical cap, less commonly used, is thimble-shaped and fits directly onto the cervix. A spermicidal agent is normally recommended for use in conjunction with these barriers.

The diaphragm or cap has no effect upon the body and may even afford protection to the cervix. They can be inserted up to 2 hours before intercourse and so need not interfere with spontanaeity. Women who use them are usually instructed to retain them in place for at least 6 hours after intercourse to allow the spermicidal agent to be effective.

The disadvantages of female barrier methods are that they are not suitable for everybody, especially where there is displacement of the uterus or laxity of the vaginal walls. Also, following childbirth or significant weight loss or gain they must be refitted, and an annual check is necessary. The diaphragm or cap needs to be checked frequently for damage.

CHEMICAL CONTRACEPTIVE AGENTS

Chemicals which destroy or inactivate spermatozoa are combined with a base agent that serves to form a blocking flim across the vagina. They are available as creams, pastes, dissolving pessaries and foam (the most effective) or jellies. Most health professionals would recommend that they be used in conjunction with a physical barrier such as a diaphragm or condom rather than on their own. They may be purchased without prescription, and help to lubricate the vagina. They can, however, be messy to use, in most cases have to be applied just before intercourse, and sometimes cause reactions such as itching and burning.

LIMITING INTERCOURSE TO INFERTILE PERIODS

Abstaining from intercourse during the time around and after ovulation is the basis of natural family planning. There are, basically, three methods of identifying the time of ovulation: the ryhthm method, the temperature method and the ovulation (Billings) method.

The rhythm method

Based upon simple calculation of days since the last menstrual period, the rhythm method relies heavily upon regularity of the cycle and constancy of the luteal phase. It is unsuitable for women with irregular cycles and those nearing the menopause. It cannot be applied during lactation. Unless the period of abstinence is extended it has a fairly high failure rate, and is no longer taught by health professionals.

The temperature method

This temperature method is based upon the knowledge that progesterone has a thermogenic (temperature raising) effect. The woman records her early morning (basal) temperature daily (Fig. 22.6) and with ovulation the progesterone produced by the corpus luteum will cause the temperature to rise by approximately 0.5°C. This elevation remains until the corpus luteum degenerates, a few days before the onset of the period. The woman cannot predict when ovulation will occur by this method, she can only realise it after it has happened. Therefore, strict application of this method will involve abstinence from intercourse from the onset of menstruation until 3 full days after the temperature rise. Confusion can be caused by temperature variations from other sources, e.g. infections.

Basal temperature charting is an improvement upon the rhythm method but as not all cycles are ovulatory, it can involve long periods of abstinence from intercourse.

The Ovulation (Billings) Method

This method has now supereded both the rhythm and temperature methods for those couples who wish to avoid or space pregnancies without using artificial methods of contraception. It is based upon the recognition of ovulation by noting the changes in the amount and consistency of cervical

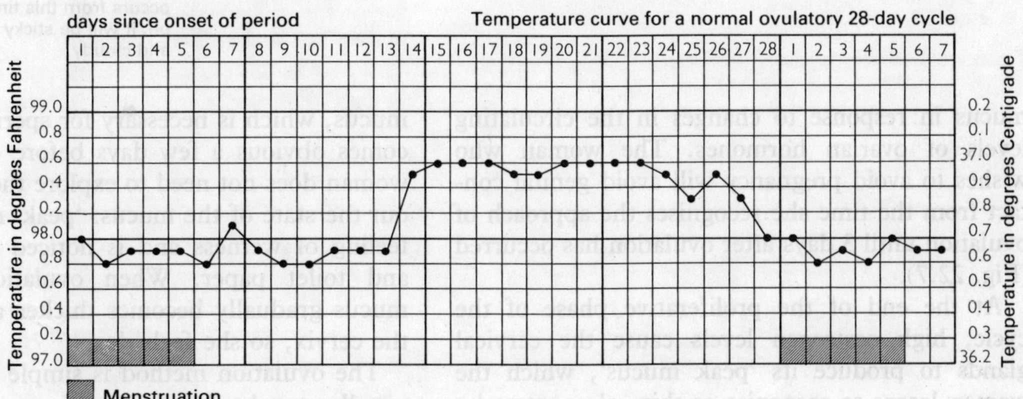

Figure 22.6 Basal temperature charting showing temperature changes around the time of ovulation.

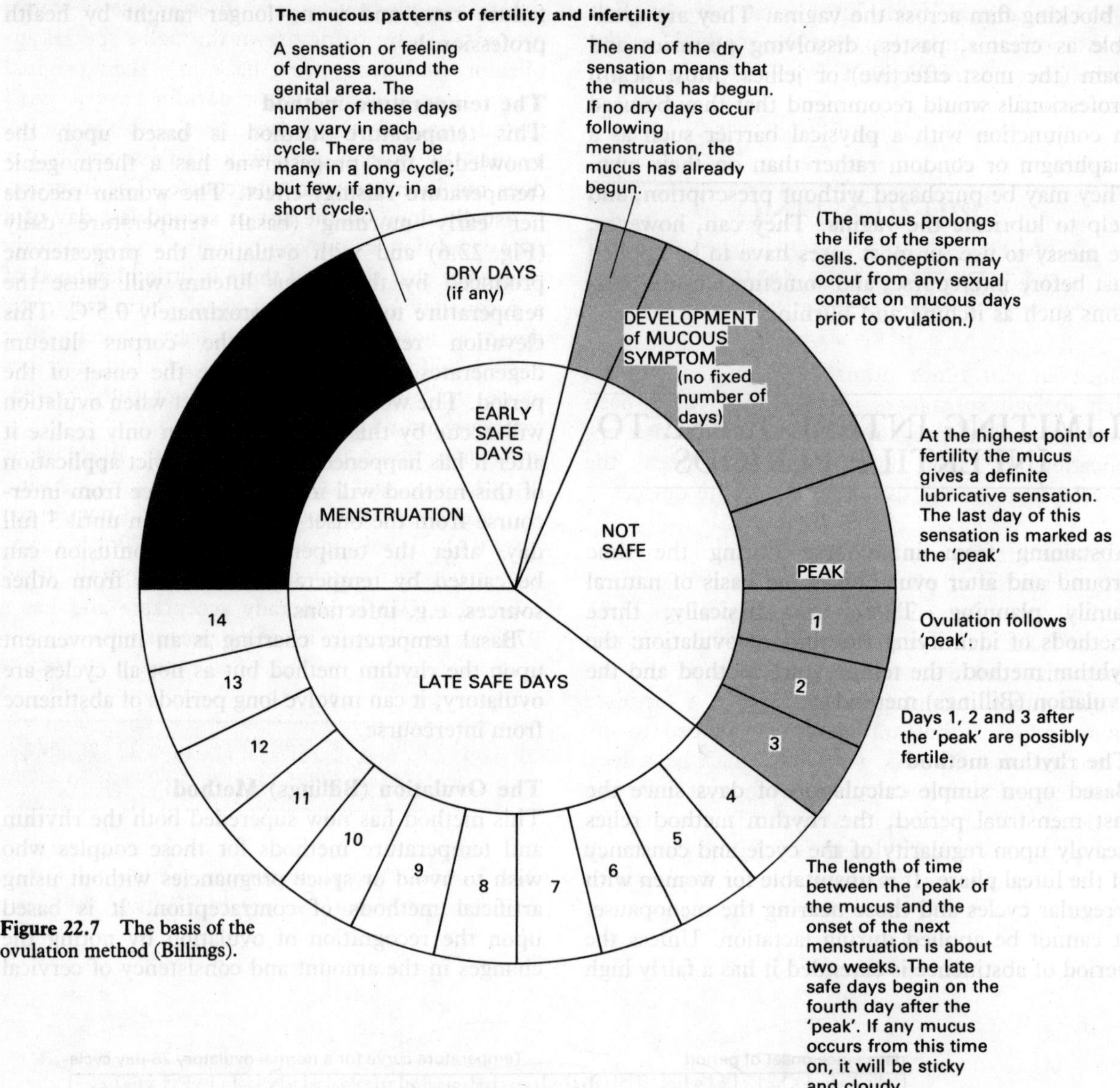

Figure 22.7 The basis of the ovulation method (Billings).

mucus in response to changes in the circulating levels of ovarian hormones. The woman who wishes to avoid pregnancy will avoid genital contact from the time she recognises the approach of ovulation until 3 days after ovulation has occurred (Fig. 22.7).

At the end of the proliferative phase of the cycle, high oestrogen levels cause the cervical glands to produce its 'peak mucus', which the woman learns to recognise as thin, clear, stretchy and slippery (Fig. 22.3). This 'peak' or 'fertile' mucus, which is necessary for sperm survival, becomes obvious a few days before ovulation. The woman does not need to explore the cervix to find out the state of the mucus: 'peak' mucus causes a feeling of wetness and is noticed on underpants and toilet paper. When ovulation occurs the mucus gradually becomes thicker and remains in the cervix, so she feels dry.

The ovulation method is simple to learn and is usually taught by trained instructors who are themselves experienced in its use. The woman is asked to abstain from intercourse for the first month, while she is learning the method, as the presence of seminal fluid from intercourse can cause confusion.

PREVENTING IMPLANTATION OF A FERTILISED OVUM

Since ancient times human beings have known that foreign substances in the uterus have been able to prevent pregnancy. The modern-day application of that knowledge has been the development of the various intrauterine devices

Intrauterine devices (IUDs)
These are small plastic and/or metal objects inserted into the endometrial cavity (Fig. 22.8). Their exact action is unknown. One theory is that they may cause increased peristalsis of the fallopian tubes, bringing to the uterus a fertilised ovum which is not sufficiently developed to implant successfully. As well, they may be a local endometrial reaction to the presence of a foreign body or foreign chemicals and this changed endometrium is unsuitable either for implantation or for the provision of nutrients should implantation occur.

Intrauterine devices are inserted (as a sterile procedure) after being drawn through a special applicator, and they spring back into their original shape after insertion. Most devices have a small thread attached: this hangs down into the vagina so that the woman can check its presence, but it does not interfere with intercourse. The insertion is usually done on the last or second last day of a menstrual flow as the cervix is likely to be slightly relaxed at that time and there is little likelihood of a pregnancy being present then. Postnatally, the device is not inserted until at least 6 weeks have passed: before this it might be expelled and, because the placental site is still not fully healed, infection must be avoided.

Regular check-ups are necessary. Bleeding is often heavier, and pain and cramping worse, during the next one or two periods but should not persist after that. Expulsion occurs in about 20% of cases, and may sometimes go unnoticed. Overall, however, the IUD is generally acceptable and has a 97% success rate in avoiding pregnancy.

FAMILY PLANNING DURING THE PEURPERIUM

The couple's usual or former method of family planning may not be suitable during the early

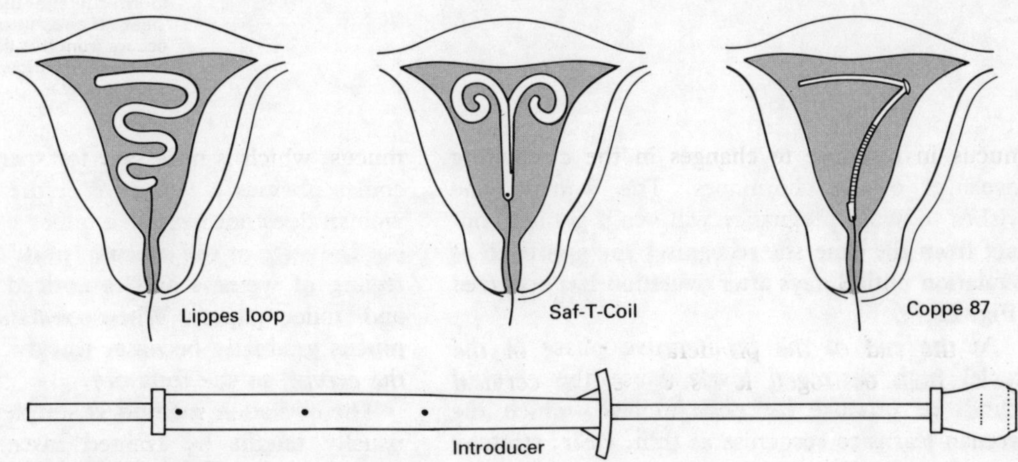

Figure 22.8 Types of intrauterine devices.

weeks following childbirth. Specific points to be noted are given below.

- The ordinary'pill' is unsuitable for breast-feeding mothers. A low dose progestogen-only 'mini-pill' which works by making the cervical mucus impenetrable to sperm is available: it needs a doctor's prescription and accompanying advice. The mother should know this, or she might go home and resume a course of 'left-over' contraceptive pills.
- The intrauterine device is usually not a suitable form of contraception until the placental site is healed. Few doctors will insert these devices before the check-up at 6 weeks after the birth.
- The diaphragm or cervical cap, if used previously, may no longer be the right size and may not sit securely in the upper vagina or on the cervix, both of which will have been stretched by childbirth. These contraceptives will need to be fitted no earlier than 6 weeks postnatally.
- The only easily available and suitable methods that usually provide protection for the lactating mother in the early weeks after childbirth are the condom, the ovulation method and the 'mini-pill'
- Long-term injectible hormones, acting for 3–6 months, are usually offered only in special circumstances during the puerperium.

23

COMMUNITY CARE AND SUPPORT

Chapter outline
Baby Clinic services
Community support groups

Most new mothers are glad to return home from hospital, no matter how much they appreciated their time there. Arriving home brings new excitements and challenges, and sometimes a welcome relief from visitors, who may be reluctant to disturb the new family, for a while at least. The parents realise, though, that now it is they who have full responsibility for the care and safety of their baby. No longer is there advice and help a few steps away. It is important that they understand that they are not entirely alone—that there are people out in the world who are ready and very willing to help them in their transition. Not only family and friends, but professional helpers such as the Baby Clinic (Infant Welfare or Maternal and Child Health) Nurse for their area. As well, they will find community support groups formed for different purposes, but all aimed to support and encourage the new parents to settle and adjust to the days and months ahead.

BABY CLINIC SERVICES

Maternity care is continued in the community by the Maternal and Child Health nurse who has the specialised knowledge and facilities to ensure that both the mother and infant continue to do well. She has the power of referral to several types of extra assistance for special needs and circumstances. Because she can usually establish a close relationship with the parents, the Maternal and Child Health nurse will, in most cases, understand how parenting affects their particular resources of emotion, energy, time, money and freedom. She is often able to identify those who may find the pressures great or their resources limited.

Notification of the birth is sent routinely by the hospital to the local government authority (council) and the Maternal and Child Health nurse usually visits the woman within a week of her arrival home.

The services offered by the Maternal and Child Welfare Department in Victoria and similar bodies in other States are:

- routine assessment of progress of the baby (e.g. weight gain, mental and physical development)
- information and advice to the mother on the baby's feeding, clothing, skin care and behaviour, and on the mother's general well-being
- antenatal clinic and childbirth preparation (in some centres)
- family planning
- immunisation programmes
- playgroups for the pre-kindergarten age group
- new mothers' groups
- dental care—up to 7 years of age
- provision of literature covering all aspects of child care
- authorisation of housekeeping assistance
- referral to other agencies, e.g. social welfare, child-care co-ordinators, behaviour clinics, emergency accommodation.

COMMUNITY SUPPORT GROUPS

There are a number of support groups for parents who have special needs after the birth of a baby. Being able to meet with other parents in a similar situation can be very reassuring and the support and services offered by such groups can be most valuable. The midwives in hospital postnatal wards and nurseries can provide information about support groups and arrange for visits from members when suitable, but not all people are ready to hear or absorb many details in the early days following birth or diagnosis of a problem. Some, in the first shock of distress, do not want to know that others might have suffered as they are suffering now, and might resent suggestions that they are not alone.

After some time has passed, however, many parents are very willing to consider making contact with support groups, many of which offer individual contact with other parents who have successfully adjusted to their particular situation. The following brief descriptions simply give an outline of the work of some of the support groups: there are many more, and their services are more comprehensive than can be shown here. Most groups have branches in all States, sometimes listed under slightly different names. Many groups offer speakers to talk to meetings.

Association for the Welfare of Children in Hospital (AWCH)
Works towards greater involvement of parents in the care of children admitted to hospital. Counselling and support, newsletter, publications, meetings.

Australian Multiple Birth Association—AMBA
Provides a support service for parents who have twins (or other multiple births). Has meetings, outings, library, newsletter, equipment hire.

Congenital Abnormality Support Association—CASA
Parent group concerned with the care of children born with any congenital abnormality—not only those diagnosed at birth. Personal meetings, newsletter, library, research, publications.

Down Syndrome Association
Promotes improvement in quality of life of persons with Down Syndrome. Parent support and encouragement. Literature, newsletter, library, meetings, research.

Nursing Mothers Association of Australia—NMAA
Promotes breast feeding, but membership is open to all. Telephone advice service, using trained counsellors. Meetings, social activities, publications, baby products, library, newsletter, research.

Premature Birth Support Association
Parents share information about the special needs and problems in the continuing care of premature and low-birth-weight babies. Newsletter, library, meetings, research.

Post and Ante Natal Depression Association—PaNDa
Self-help group which assists mothers who have experienced depression associated with pregnancy and birth. Meetings, literature, newsletter, research.

Stillbirth and Neonatal Death Support group—SANDS
Group caring for other parents who have experienced pregnancy loss, whether from miscarriage, stillbirth or death in the early weeks following birth. Meetings, research, publications, newsletter.

Sudden Infant Death Research Foundation—SIDRF
Support group for those who have experienced 'cot death'. Research, meetings, literature, personal contacts and counselling for parents and wider family.

Associations for single parents
The Council for the Single Mother and her Child, the Australian Birthright Movement, Parents without Partners, and the Lone Fathers Association are some of the groups for single parents:

meetings, mutual help, advice and crisis counselling.

Emergency services
In an emergency, parents may telephone the following.

- Lifeline
- Personal Emergency Service
- Parents Anonymous
- Telephone Interpreter Service.

Their numbers are given in the 'Community' section at the front of the telephone directories.

INDEX